Global Health and Security

T0203963

The past decade has witnessed a significant increase in the construction of health as a security issue by national governments and multilateral organizations. This book provides the first critical, feminist analysis of the flesh-and-blood impacts of the securitization of health on different bodies, while broadening the scope of what we understand as global health security.

It looks at how feminist perspectives on health and security can lead to different questions about health and in/security, problematizing some of the 'common sense' assumptions that underlie much of the discourse in this area. It considers the norms, ideologies, and vested interests that frame specific 'threats' to health and policy responses, while exposing how the current governance of the global economy shapes new threats to health. Some chapters focus on conflict, war and complex emergencies, while others move from a 'high political' focus to the domain of subtler and often insidious structural violence, illuminating the impacts of hegemonic masculinities and the neoliberal governance of the global economy on health and life chances.

Highlighting the critical intersections across health, gender and security, this book is an important contribution to scholarship on health and security, global health, public health and gender studies.

Colleen O'Manique teaches at Trent University, Canada. Her research has focused on feminist political economy and rights-based perspectives on health and health policies in the context of neoliberal globalization.

Pieter Fourie teaches at Stellenbosch University, South Africa. His research focuses on HIV/AIDS, global health governance, political epidemiology, and the political economy of global development.

Routledge Studies in Public Health

https://www.routledge.com/Routledge-Studies-in-Public-Health/book-series/RSPH

Global Health and Security

Critical Feminist Perspectives

**Edited by Colleen O'Manique
and Pieter Fourie**

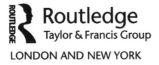

LONDON AND NEW YORK

First published 2018 by Routledge

2 Park Square, Milton Park, Abingdon, Oxfordshire OX14 4RN
52 Vanderbilt Avenue, New York, NY 10017

Routledge is an imprint of the Taylor & Francis Group, an informa business

First issued in paperback 2019

British Library Cataloguing-in-Publication Data
A catalogue record for this book is available from the British Library

Library of Congress Cataloging-in-Publication Data
Names: O'Manique, Colleen, 1962- editor. | Fourie, Pieter, 1972- editor.
Title: Global health and security : critical feminist perspectives / edited by Colleen O'Manique and Pieter Fourie.
Other titles: Routledge studies in public health.
Description: Abingdon, Oxon; New York, NY : Routledge, 2018. |
Series: Routledge studies in public health | Includes bibliographical references and index.
Identifiers: LCCN 2017048589| ISBN 9781138677364 (hbk) |
ISBN 9781315559568 (ebk)
Subjects: | MESH: Global Health | Exposure to Violence | Feminism | Gender Identity | Health Policy | Social Security
Classification: LCC RA441 | NLM WA 530.1 | DDC 362.1—dc23
LC record available at https://lccn.loc.gov/2017048589

ISBN: 978-1-138-67736-4 (hbk)
ISBN: 978-0-367-45750-1 (pbk)

Typeset in Times New Roman
by Keystroke, Neville Lodge, Tettenhall, Wolverhampton

Contents

Contributors

Vanessa Farr is an independent consultant specializing in gender, peace and security, particularly in the Islamic world. She holds a PhD from the School of Women's Studies at York University, Toronto. She has published widely on issues related to gender and armed conflict, including in Afghanistan, Libya, Yemen and Palestine. She is the co-editor of two books: *Back to the Roots: Security Sector Reform and Development* (Münster: LIT, 2012) and *Sexed Pistols: The Gendered Impacts of Small Arms and Light Weapons* (UNU Press, 2009).

Pieter Fourie teaches Political Science at Stellenbosch University (South Africa), and was trained at the universities of Stellenbosch, Paris, London and Johannesburg. He has worked for the United Nations, the Australian Department of Foreign Affairs and Trade, in civil society, and he has taught International Relations at universities in South Africa and Australia. His research focuses on HIV/AIDS, global health governance, political epidemiology and the political economy of global development.

Adrienne Germain is President Emerita of the International Women's Health Coalition (IWHC), and has received the 2012 United Nations Population Award for her lifetime work on women's health and rights. Following 14 years with the Ford Foundation, including four as Bangladesh country representative, she led IWHC's partnerships with women's health and rights organizations in Africa, Asia and Latin America, and, with them, helped create the international movement for women's health and human rights. Serving on US government delegations to the UN's 1994 International Conference on Population and Development (ICPD), and 1995 Fourth World Women's Conference, she shaped US positions and the final conference agreements.

Teresa Healy is an Associate Professor of Community Economic and Social Development at Algoma University. She earned her doctorate in Political Science from Carleton University. Her research focuses on social movements' struggles for equity and community-based sustainability in times of economic crisis. Teresa worked as a senior researcher within the Canadian labour movement and is also a recording singer-songwriter. She is the author of *Gendered Struggles against Globalisation in Mexico* (Ashgate, 2008), the editor of *The*

Harper Record (CCPA, 2008) and the co-editor of *The Harper Record 2008–2015* (CCPA, 2015). She also is Adjunct Research Professor at the Institute for Political Economy, Carleton University, and Research Associate at the Canadian Centre for Policy Alternatives.

Tessa Hochfeld is an Associate Professor at the Centre for Social Development in Africa, University of Johannesburg. Her work includes research on social justice, social welfare, social policy, transformative social protection and gender and development, with a focus on the social impacts of the Child Support Grant in South Africa. Tessa has a BA in Social Work from the University of the Witwatersrand, an MSc in Gender and Development from the University of London, and a PhD in Development Studies from the University of the Witwatersrand.

H. Patricia Hynes is a retired professor of environmental health from Boston University School of Public Health. She has directed community-based environmental justice projects in Boston Public Housing and diverse, low-income neighborhoods in Boston. For her work, she has received many awards, including Lifetime Achievement Awards from the Boston Natural Areas Fund and Environmental Protection Agency New England, as well as Boston University teaching awards and an American Public Health Association Best Practice Award. An environmental engineer, Pat designed her passive solar home, worked for EPA in the Superfund Program and subsequently wrote *The Recurring Silent Spring* on the impact of Rachel Carson's groundbreaking critique of pesticides in agriculture. A longtime feminist, she co-founded Bread and Roses in 1974, a feminist restaurant and cultural center in Cambridge, Massachusetts. Currently, she chairs the board of the Traprock Center for Peace and Justice in Massachusetts and writes on peace and justice issues.

Helen Liebling is a Senior Lecturer-Practitioner in Clinical Psychology and Associate of the African Studies Centre at Coventry University and has an M.Phil. from Edinburgh University, and PhD from the University of Warwick. She has carried out research with survivors of conflict and post-conflict sexual violence and torture including refugees, in Africa and UK since 1998. She has numerous journal publications and two books *Ugandan Women War Survivors* (Liebling-Kalifani, 2009), and *Justice and Health Provision for Survivors of Sexual Violence* (Liebling & Baker, 2010). Helen has provided consultancies, training and interventions to improve support for survivors in conjunction with Isis-WICCE, Uganda and as part of an EU project involving training police to support survivors. Helen was invited as an expert panel member to help plan a five-year international research agenda on sexual and gender-based violence (SGBV) in conflict settings. She is also a member of the Tearfund/SVRI steering group on the role of faith-based organizations in preventing conflict SGBV.

Colleen O'Manique has a PhD in Political Science from York University and has been a faculty member at Trent University for 17 years, teaching in the departments of Political Studies, Gender and Women's Studies, and International Development Studies. Her research has focused on feminist and rights-based perspectives on health and health policies in the context of neoliberal globalization. Among her publications is the book *Neoliberalism and AIDS Crisis in Sub-Saharan Africa: Globalization's Pandemic* (Palgrave 2004).

Sarah Pugh is an independent consultant based in Cape Town, South Africa, with a background in international development, migration, gender and health. She worked for several years in Vancouver, Canada, at a provincial healthcare network, before pursuing a PhD in International Development and Political Science through the University of Guelph, in Ontario, Canada. From 2014 to 2016, Sarah held a Social Sciences and Humanities Research Council postdoctoral fellowship in the Department of Political Science at Stellenbosch University. She is currently a Research Associate with the Centre for International and Comparative Politics in the Department of Political Science at Stellenbosch University, and Managing Editor of the journal *Reproductive Health Matters*.

Simon Rushton is a lecturer in the Department of Politics at the University of Sheffield, UK and an Associate Fellow of the Centre on Global Health Security at Chatham House, UK. He has written widely on international responses to HIV/AIDS and other diseases, the links between health and security, and the changing nature of global health governance. His most recent books have been *The Routledge Handbook of Global Health Security* (Routledge, 2014 – co-edited with Jeremy Youde) and *Disease Diplomacy: International Norms and Global Health Security* (Johns Hopkins University Press 2015, with Sara Davies and Adam Kamradt-Scott).

Jade S. Sasser is an Assistant Professor of Gender and Sexuality Studies at the University of California, Riverside. She holds a PhD in Environmental Science, Policy and Management and an MA in Cultural Anthropology from the University of California, Berkeley, and an MPH from Boston University. Her forthcoming book, *Making Sexual Stewards: Population, Climate Activism, and Social Justice in the New Millennium*, explores activism linking climate change with women's reproductive rights. Her broader research interests are focused at the intersections of gender and environment, international development, and women's health.

Chloe Schwenke is the Director of the Global Program on Violence, Rights and Inclusion at the International Center for Research on Women in Washington, DC. An openly transgender woman, she is a human rights and social inclusion researcher, feminist author, scholar and international development practitioner with over three decades of international practitioner and research experience – nearly half in Africa and Asia. She served as a political appointee during the Obama Administration, as Senior Advisor on Human Rights at USAID. She was also a Fulbright Senior Scholar in Uganda, and has served as an adjunct professor for the past 18 years.

Abbreviations

AIDS	Acquired Immune Deficiency Syndrome
ART	antiretroviral therapy
BPHS	Basic Primary Health Services
CBHC	Community Based Health Care
CDC	Centers for Disease Control and Prevention
CHW	community health worker
CSG	Child Support Grant
DAWN	Development Alternatives with Women for a New Era
DOE	Department of Energy
DoPH	Department of Public Health (Provincial)
DRC	Democratic Republic of Congo
EPA	Environmental Protection Agency
EU	European Union
FAO	Food and Agricultural Organization
FCHW	female community health worker
FfD	Financing for Development
FGM	female genital mutilation
FIGO	International Federation for Obstetricians and Gynaecologists
GBV	gender-based violence
GDP	gross domestic product
GGE	greenhouse gas emission
HAART	highly active antiretroviral therapy
HDC	highly developed country
HERA	health, empowerment, rights, and accountability
HIV	Human Immunodeficiency Virus
HPAI	highly pathogenic avian influenza
HRP	Special Programme of Research on Human Reproduction
ICPD	International Conference on Population and Development
IFI	international financial institution
IHR	international health regulation
IISS	International Institute for Strategic Studies
IMF	International Monetary Fund
IOM	International Organisation for Migration

IPCC	Intergovernmental Panel on Climate Change
IR	International Relations
ITECH	International Training and Education Center for Health
IWHC	International Women's Health Coalition
KAP	knowledge and practices
KII	key informant interview
KIWEPI	Kitgum Women's Peace Initiative
LDC	less developed country
LGBTI	lesbian, gay, bisexual, transgender, and intersexual
LGBTQ	lesbian, gay, bisexual, transgender, and queer
LGBTQI	lesbian, gay, bisexual, transgender, queer, and intersex
LRA	Lord's Resistance Army
MCH	maternal and child health
MCHW	male community health worker
MDG	Millennium Development Goal
MNC	multinational corporation
MoPH	Ministry of Public Health
MSM	men who have sex with men
MSW	men who have sex with women
MVA	manual vacuum aspiration
NASA	National Aeronautics and Space Administration
NATO	North Atlantic Treaty Organisation
NFPB	National Family Planning Board
NGO	Non-Government Organisation
NID	National Immunisation Day
NPO	mon-profit organization
OECD	Organization for Economic Co-operation and Development
OHS	Occupational Health and Safety
OPV	oral polio vaccine
OWFI	Organization for Women's Freedom in Iraq
PEI	Polio Eradication Initiative
PEPFAR	President's Emergency Plan for AIDS Relief
PHC	primary health care
PHEIC	Public Health Emergency of International Concern
PLWHIV	people living with HIV
PTSD	post-traumatic stress disorder
SASSA	South African Social Security Agency
SDG	sustainable development goal
SM	social mobilizer
SRHR	sexual and reproductive health and rights
STD	sexually transmitted disease
STI	sexually transmitted infection
TBA	traditional birth attendant
TOW	Transforming Our World
TPO	Transcultural Psychosocial Organisation

UN	United Nations
UNAIDS	Joint United Nations Programme on HIV/AIDS
UNESCO	United Nations Educational, Scientific and Cultural Organization
UNFPA	United Nations Population Fund
UNICEF	United Nations International Children's Emergency Fund
UNIFEM	United Nations Development Fund for Women
UNSCR	United National Security Council Resolution
US	United States
USA	United States of America
USAID	US Agency for International Development
USTS	US Trans Survey
VA	Veterans Administration
WB	World Bank
WHAM	Women's Health Advocates on Microbicides
WHO	World Health Organization

1   Global health, gender, and the security question

Colleen O'Manique and Pieter Fourie

Insecurity has always been a feature of human societies, as has the impulse to mitigate and control risks, and to protect oneself and one's kin. The new millennium has been marked by increased attention to human health as a security issue by a range of actors, including nation-states, multilateral organizations and private interests. New health "threats" such as novel influenzas, SARS and Ebola, have joined terrorism, refugee "crises" and environmental disasters in contributing to the normalization of a culture of fear and heightened insecurity. The WHO 2007 World Health Report was aptly titled *A Safer Future: Global Public Health Security in the 21st Century*. In it, the Director General of the WHO states that '[s]hocks to health reverberate as shocks to economies and the business community in areas well beyond the affected area. Vulnerability is universal' (2008: vi).

Appeals to the dangers that specific "health security" risks pose for nation-states and the global economy are in tension with ones that point to the impacts of broader health "threats" for all of humanity. The latter include chronic and non-communicable diseases that are endemic to many parts of our planet, the erosion of the social determinants of health, and the deepening of market relations in the provision of basic health services (O'Manique and Fourie, 2010: 248). While disease outbreaks have become more central to the lexicon of globalization and foreign policy, a focus on the foundations of human health insecurities around the world has shifted further away from foreign policy and local and global governance agendas. It is indeed *not* the case that "vulnerability is universal". We are not all equally at risk. In order to understand the state of health security for all people on the planet we need to understand the *embodied* realities of people's lives that result in health security for some people, and in insecurity for others. This means drawing attention to the narrowness of the mainstream discourse of global health security that renders invisible the actual people who are impacted by global health emergencies, and illuminating how current ideologies and structures of governance shape the life chances of individuals the world over.

As we have noted elsewhere (Fourie, 2015; O'Manique, 2015) the utility of securitizing any issue – including health – is manifold. By making appeals to *states'* security a number of effects can be achieved: a sense of imminent peril is evoked and a common enemy can be identified; an instant increase in the political commitment to address the issue, domestically, multilaterally, as well as globally, can be justified, and institutions, budgets and expertise and personnel can be mobilized. The issue can be moved from the domain of "normal" and low politics to "exceptional" and high politics, which allows for easy mythmaking around who the heroes or victors are, so that public health interventions can be activated. As we have seen with the security responses to recent infectious diseases, human rights concerns can take a backseat, while interfering laws, rules, and regulations can be suspended to enable rapid intervention that is crafted as serving the "greater good". We see this reflected, for example, in the above-mentioned WHO 2007 World Health Report. The document navigates the tension between state sovereignty and human security by unequivocally accepting the state as the global unit of analysis in terms of security while drawing special attention to the obligation that states have to protect individuals' rights to health. The two are constructed as mutually compatible. In the words of the conclusion to the 2007 WHO report:

> Although the subject of this report has taken a global approach to public health security, WHO does not neglect the fact that all individuals – women, men and children – are affected by the common threats to health. It is vital not to lose sight of the personal consequences of global health challenges. This was the inspiration that led to the "health for all" commitment to primary health care in 1978. That commitment and the principles supporting it remain untarnished and as essential as ever. On that basis, primary health care and humanitarian action in times of crisis – two means to ensure health security at individual and community levels – will be discussed at length in The World Health Report 2008.
>
> (WHO 2007: 19)

It is worth stating that the "health for all" commitment to primary health care was to be realized by the year 2000. The goal remains as elusive as ever. And the value of people's lives is shaped by the accident of whether one is born into security or insecurity – by one's economic class, nation, skin pigmentation, religion, sex, and sexuality.

A year later, the WHO's 2008 report, *Primary Health Care: Now More Than Ever*, documents some of the shortcomings of contemporary health systems, among them the disproportionate focus on hospital care, fragmentation of health services, and the proliferation of unregulated commercial care. It admits that global health gains have been "unevenly shared", particularly on the African continent where health has stagnated or worsened (WHO, 2008). However, the report is largely silent on the global political and financial context, and on the architecture of health policy reform. Furthermore, "health" has become increasingly synonymous with health care, rendering invisible the foundations of persistent health insecurities that shape life chances: the deepening wealth inequality both within and among countries, declining conditions labour and the increasing precariousness of livelihoods, permanent war and political violence, refugee movements, and the destruction of the ecosystem upon which all life depends. Neoliberal globalism, as Janine Brodie (2003: 47) states, is marked by '. . . a deep and perilous gap between [its] promises, and the insecurities of daily life for the majority of humankind'. Health insecurities arise from this foundation.

This volume endeavours to begin to make this mostly tacit, complicated reality explicit, and to demonstrate how across various levels of analysis and normative frames *critical feminist analyses* expose and challenge the dominant framings of global health security, by casting a light on the many chronic and every-day gendered, classed and racialized violences that shape access to health's social determinants, and by extension, the health of differently situated and gendered bodies. Remarkably, feminist perspectives have remained on the borders of the evolving body of scholarship that has situated global health within a security frame, and in particular, feminist analyses that address the flesh-and-blood impacts worldwide on different bodies. This can be said of both of the competing conceptions of health in/security reflected in contemporary global health governance: first, health as a "human" security issue linked to the study of the ideological and structural forces shaping both the governance of global health and the conditions that shape human health, and, second, the increasingly hegemonic view of health as a national security issue in which intensified globalization produces new pathogens and "health threats" with potential impacts on stability and wealth accumulation. Some contributions to this volume specifically engage in this question of securitization, while others amplify more tacit cognate narratives.

Social and political life is profoundly gendered and feminist scholarship has a critical role to play in illuminating both the foundations of health insecurities and the effects of different policies and practices on different bodies. For example, we need only look to some of today's sites of conflict to see the ubiquity of sexual violence as part of militarized violence, state violence targeted at queer and trans people, the structural violence of the austerity response that has undermined basic health care and which has left impoverished women struggling to fill the care gap, or the absence of the most basic occupational health conditions for women in parts of the global south.

The overarching aim of this volume is to begin to illuminate some of the critical intersections across health, gender, and security, through an approach that focuses on the quotidian violences – those everyday insecurities – emerging from the socio-economic and cultural organization of society that shape the health and life chances of people occupying different spaces and identities around the world. The chapters in this book address how one's experience of "health security" has much to do with gender to the extent that specific "risks" and vulnerabilities are located in culturally constructed gender roles, and one's sex and gender can circumscribe access to health care and the social determinants of health. In/security is constituted through and by sex and gender as key components of the matrix of power that governs the global life economy. Within most scholarship of global health and accounts of health's social determinants, gender tends to be seen as one of a collection of variables, with sex and gender often conflated. The reality is more complicated.

The politics and ideology of global neoliberalism contribute to emerging health "crises" and the frameworks though which they are addressed: the general acceptance of international competitive rules, the hollowing out of the state, and a belief that market arrangements should play a central role in the provision of a minimal social safety net. Neoliberalism is largely consistent with the biomedical construction of disease, which reduces it to its individual and clinical dimensions. What is erased and obscured are the material conditions that allow disease to thrive, the broader factors that condition access to treatment, and the daily realities of affected bodies and households where the tangible impacts are felt. The overwhelming focus on clinical management and education obscures gendered and racialized crises of production and social reproduction at the local level, a key feature of epidemics in many regions of the world. A central concern of the contributions in this book is to document what is missing in global health scholarship that is both gender-blind to the individuals and communities who are subject to both the physical violence of conflict and insecurity, and to the more ordinary structural violence of the contemporary neoliberal global political economy.

War and political violence is newsworthy, while structural violence is largely invisible. Drawing on John Galtung and Paul Farmer, Jade Sasser explains in her chapter that structural violence is violence that is without a clear victim or perpetrator; it is the slow violence that is built into structures and systems of governance that creates unequal power relations and shapes life chances. It is characterized by the massive unequal distribution of resources and political, economic and discursive power. Sasser states in her chapter (Chapter 11) that 'Rather than direct action taken between individuals and groups, structural violence manifests indirectly, through the impacts of highly inequitable or violent social structures, particularly in the context of bodies' (p. 167). Teresa Healy (Chapter 10) adds that, in Galtung's (1975) idea of structural violence, it is not necessarily the activities of specific institutions that are of interest, but the cumulative impacts of indirect violence that leave individuals' rights to self-realization unmet. She describes structural violence:

> . . . as a complex of socially-embedded and inequitable economic, political, legal, religious and cultural social practices that cause physical and psychological harm to people (Flynn *et al.*, 2015; Bitton *et al.*, 2011) . . . [that] turns large historical and social dynamics into systemic and everyday practices that injure those most marginalized. . . .
>
> (p. 149)

Other contributors to this volume have slightly different takes, with Vanessa Farr, for instance, drawing on Rob Nixon's understanding of slow violence. These are Nixon's (2006–2007) words:

> To confront what I am calling slow violence requires that we attempt to give symbolic shape and plot to formless threats whose fatal repercussions are dispersed across space and time. Politically and emotionally, different kinds of disaster possess unequal heft. Falling bodies, burning towers, exploding heads have a visceral, page-turning potency that tales of slow violence cannot

match. Stories of toxic buildup, massing greenhouse gases, or desertification may be cataclysmic, but they're scientifically convoluted cataclysms in which casualties are deferred, often for generations. In the gap between acts of slow violence and their delayed effects both memory and causation readily fade from view and the casualties thus incurred pass untallied.

(2006–2007: 14)

Taken together, the authors assembled here put forth the case for broadening and deepening our understanding of "health security" beyond the effects and impacts of health and disease on the stability of nation states and the global economy, to the recognition of the impacts of disease, and various forms of violence (military, structural, slow, intimate) on the health and psychological well-being of differently raced, classed, and gendered bodies. There is no one disciplinary perspective or unifying conceptual framework, but what all chapters share in common is the objective to illuminate, to critique, and to disrupt assumed meaning.

The first four contributions to the book apply our collective lens to contexts of war and political violence. In Chapter 2, The invisible tragedy of war: Women and the environment, Patricia Hynes offers a broad brushstroke of the effects of war and political violence on women's bodies, setting the broad context for the chapters that follow. Hynes documents how war and militarism, and the encroachment of military institutions and ends into politics and society, have been normalized by "rites", such as war veterans' parades and "sites", such as monuments to war heroes and the military war dead. The greatest human casualties of modern war are non-combatant civilians, not soldiers, while few have acknowledged that, among civilian casualties, women and girls are deliberately targeted and disproportionately harmed by war and its aftermath. Hynes also illuminates the staggering impacts of war on nature and our lived environment – by the kinds of weapons used, the hazardous waste their manufacture and testing generate, the "shock and awe" intensity of industrial warfare, and the massive exploitation of natural resources and fossil fuels to support militarism. The first effects of war are effects on health, both human and eco-systemic health, and as the other chapters illuminate, those effects are profoundly gendered and racialized.

In Chapter 3, Survivors of conflict and post-conflict sexual and gender-based violence and torture in the Great Lakes region of Africa, Helen Liebling makes the argument that the impact of conflict and post-conflict sexual violence and torture has often been misunderstood in terms of an individual manifestation of psychological trauma and physical injuries, with responses confined to a biomedical approach. Based on research carried out with women survivors of conflict, former child abductees, and women and girls who bore children from rape in the Great Lakes region of Africa, Liebling argues for an alternative understanding that is gendered, recognizes the devastating impact of sexual violence and torture on reproductive and psychological health, as well as on whole communities. Her analysis highlights the resilience of survivors and their ability to reconstruct identities, and argues for a holistic response for survivors with improved professional structures for service providers that are sensitive to gender and culture, informed by a considered understanding of the impact of trauma on survivors, while addressing stigma and shame as barriers to effective service access and response. She emphasizes the need for justice and social support structures, in conjunction with building on the resilience and reconstruction of identities of survivors and their communities.

In Chapter 4, Securing health in Afghanistan: Gender, militarized humanitarianism, and legacies of occupation, Vanessa Farr draws from field research conducted with male and female community health workers in Afghanistan, who, working as unpaid volunteers, form the foundation of the Community Based Health Care pillar of the Ministry of Public Health. The chapter explores how the neoliberal "reconstruction" policies imposed on Afghanistan by donors including the United States military occupiers – now-turned economic advisers – are premised on a highly gendered exploitation of labour, and misuse narratives of women's empowerment even as they seamlessly intertwine with the country's own patriarchal patronage systems. Working from Julie Billaud's observation that in Afghanistan, 'a society torn by violence and war, women's bodies have become the field through which statehood enacts its power' (Billaud, 2015: 18), the chapter argues that an analysis of the health sector, devastated as it is by the "slow violence" of the ongoing conflict, offers eye-opening insights into how contemporary militarized humanitarianism and development approaches function "post"-conflict. The chapter concludes that, far from working towards a "peace dividend" of newly transparent institutions focused on socially inclusive reconstruction, outside forces rely on and reproduce a weakened and unresisting civil society. Ultimately naked profiteers, they collude with and entrench existing male patronage networks, and are both managers and profit-sharers in the violent, divisive, warlike and extractive political economy they maintain.

The next chapter widens national or localized experiences towards the transnational. In Chapter 5, A moving target: Gender, health and the securitisation of migration, Sarah Pugh notes that, with more people on the move than any other time in human history, states are struggling to effectively "manage" the movement of people across borders, navigating deeply emotive and often politically divisive questions of inclusion and exclusion, citizenship and identity, nationalism and human rights. Internationally, many states are responding to migration pressures with an increasingly control-oriented and securitized approach, tightening borders, criminalizing irregular and often low-skilled migrants, and framing migrants broadly as a social, economic, and potentially political threat. The chapter highlights some of the potential health implications of this increasingly securitized approach to migration, applying a gender lens to tease out the ways in which these health implications might be experienced or embodied in different ways by men, women, boys and girls. In particular, the gendered health implications of practices of detention and encampment, access to health care, sexual violence, and mental health are highlighted.

The next chapter speaks to the transnational project to put sexual and reproductive health and rights on the global agenda. In Chapter 6, The global movement for sexual and reproductive health and rights: Intellectual underpinnings, Adrienne

Germain describes the feminist intellectual work, facilitated by the International Women's Health Coalition (IWHC), which first conceptualized sexual and reproductive health and rights (SRHR). The IWHC and their feminist colleagues (most from the global south) recognized SRHR as a vital dimension of women's lives that was widely neglected and undermined by global and national population policies. Those policies aimed to control population growth simply by delivering contraceptives to married women in poor countries, avoiding other aspects of women's health and human rights, and excluding the young and the unmarried. The chapter reflects on IWHC's generation of the intellectual capital needed to challenge such polices, the author drawing on her decades of work with and for women in low and middle-income countries. In the late 1980s, IWHC published the first papers defining SRHR and its components, using a feminist lens and with an emphasis on the policy changes and actions needed. In 1993, with facilitation by IWHC, the emerging global feminist movement for women's health and human rights adopted SRHR as their primary advocacy goal for the United Nation's 1994 International Conference on Population and Development (ICPD), and also elaborated what needed to be done to achieve SRHR. In the decades since their success in the ICPD, feminist health and rights advocates, facilitated by IWHC, have continued work on the conceptual foundation and evidence base for SRHR to use in their countries and in UN negotiations on population, health, women's equality, human rights, and empowerment. Based on her continuing involvement from 1985, the author analyses why and how IWHC and their allies chose to work on SRHR, their collaborative processes, and the contributions this intellectual capital made to international mobilizing for women's health and rights.

Tessa Hochfeld complements this focus on a rights-based approach in Chapter 7, Solving Nandi: the personal embodiment of structural injustice in South Africa's Child Support Grant. Hochfeld's chapter provides a concrete illustration of how social justice and social injustice are structural in origin, yet embodied in the lives of individuals. In multiple ways, the state and society dynamically affect the daily experiences of health and security of individuals and households. Two case studies drawn from narrative research in South Africa illuminate the injustices that can become visible at the interface between the individual and formal/informal institutions. The case analyses focus on the accounts of two women living in a low-income community, both receiving state-funded cash transfers for their children. In their narratives, the two women interact with the state as provider, employer, administrator, and justice agent. They also experience and respond to societal norms and expectations around the relationships between the individual and the state. The stories illustrate how the many-layered interactions can have various beneficial, neutral, and punitive effects, shaping the women's personal trajectories of health and security; how issues of power and lack of power, access and lack of access can tend to disproportionately skew the trajectories downward. Despite an impressive set of laws and regulations protecting the rights of individuals and communities in South Africa, the accounts expose the irony that the actual functioning of formal and informal democracy in times of peace may serve to deny substantive rights, with tangible implications for health and security.

In Chapter 8, Responses to recent infectious disease emergencies: A critical gender analysis, Colleen O'Manique returns to health specifically as a lodestar illustrating structural violence in a transnational focus. HIV/AIDS, SARS, H1N1, and more recently Ebola in West Africa, are infectious diseases that have been constructed by the UN as "threats" requiring biosecurity interventions. The chapter argues that the meanings of health security and the practices to "secure" infectious disease reflect a tension between health as a basic human right linked to broader rights of citizenship and health's social determinants, and health as an instrumental condition for securing geopolitical and economic interests principally of states of the global north. The initial polemic of HIV/AIDS and security was framed within a traditional paradigm that privileged military and economic interests, discursively aligning these with liberal, developmental concerns, while sidelining the crisis at the household level that was experienced largely by women who shouldered the main care burdens and multiple impacts. There are parallels with Ebola: an almost singular attention on containment (with significantly higher levels of female mortality from Ebola) and little focus on the beleaguered state of public health in the West African countries where the virus took hold. The chapter illustrates how global hierarchies of class, gender, and ethnicity shape the environments in which one seeks to secure pandemic infection, and how biosecurity policies and strategies are imprinted on the body.

Continuing the focus on infectious disease and HIV/AIDS specifically, Simon Rushton in Chapter 9, The invisible men. HIV, security, and men who have sex with women, makes heterosexual men his focus. Over the first 20 years of the AIDS pandemic there were regular complaints about the ways in which men, in particular African men, were portrayed in the discourse around HIV transmission. Authors such as Stillwagon (2003) and Watney (1989) examined a range of sources including the media, academic research and policy statements and found that there was a pervasive tendency to attribute the serious epidemics in Sub-Saharan Africa to a hyper-sexualized and primitive culture, frequently (sometimes not even implicitly) constructing Africa as an undifferentiated "deviant continent". Rushton's chapter examines whether the troubling tendencies identified by Stillwagon, Watney, and others are still evident in the global AIDS policy discourse today.

Through a critical discourse analysis of major policy documents from global and national-level AIDS institutions, Rushton argues that this racialized depiction of "African men" has, thankfully, largely been expunged. However, heterosexual men have almost completely vanished from the AIDS discourse – other than as virus transmitters, perpetrators of gender-based violence and exploitation, and as clients of sex workers: essentially through the trail of destruction that they lead. Heterosexual men are not considered a "key population", are not explicitly discussed as holders of rights, and are never recognized as playing important roles such as caregiving. The man himself is seldom anywhere to be seen. The chapter argues that whilst this has the positive effect of avoiding the racially driven over-simplifications of the past, it does not provide a much firmer basis for addressing heterosexual HIV transmission, either in Sub-Saharan Africa or elsewhere.

In Chapter 10, Labouring bodies in the global economy: Structural violence and occupational health, Teresa Healy considers the insecurity of workers whose bodies bear the impact of transnational production processes and privatized social reproduction. Structural violence, intimately felt and socially constructed, relegates workers to the margins of capital accumulation in the twenty-first century. From lessons learned in particular households, workplaces, economic sectors and national social formations, the chapter interrogates how the gendered intersections of global in/security are understood by those who study occupational health and safety. The chapter presents a framework for understanding similarities and differences, as well as absences and promising avenues for a research agenda alive to the embodied, the intersectional, and the diverse impacts of globalized power relations where security is not seen from the perspective of the nation-state, but from that of the embodied worker and (their) collectivities.

In Chapter 11, Public health in the Anthropocene: Exploring population fears and climate threats, Jade Sasser problematizes the structurally violent interplay between gendered public health and climate change. The chapter notes how public health scholars have increasingly demonstrated the wide range of current and possible future health impacts of climate change, through discourses emphasizing the links between public health, environmental instability, and international relations. At the same time, policymakers and NGO representatives have called for greater attention to the links between population growth and climate change, often drawing on discourses that position the fertility and childbearing of poor communities as a threat to local and global environmental sustainability. Sasser explores these parallel approaches through the lens of structural violence. She analyzes the role of public health research in shaping broader anxieties around national security, health threats, and population fears – particularly in the context of global ecological crisis. The chapter argues that the ways policymakers and publics take up and circulate public health research may have unintended consequences in the form of structural and discursive violence. The chapter concludes with a discussion of alternative framings that resist these forms of violence and call for centring social justice in the links between human health and environmental change.

In an ethnographic account exposing the many violent silences surrounding the lived experiences of transgender persons, Chloe Schwenke's Bewitched or deranged: Access to health care for transgender persons (Chapter 12) shows how, in more developed economies, any discussion on transgender health tends to focus on the unique health care needs of this small population, particularly during a process of gender transition. It is simply assumed that transitioning transgender persons (and transsexuals) still obtain unhindered access to routine general health care not associated with the transgender phenomenon. In reality, transgender persons experience significant discrimination in accessing health care services in more developed countries. In the less developed countries of the global south, anecdotal evidence indicates that the level of stigma, rejection, humiliation, and even violence encountered by transgender persons seeking routine health care is both commonplace and extreme, leading to situations where these populations are entirely excluded. However, empirical data remains largely unavailable, with no systematic data collection taking place. Governments in both the north and south are ignoring the discrimination and high levels of insecurity directed at transgender persons, although the degree to which this insecurity is due to governmental intention or ignorance remains unclear. The chapter relies on anecdotal evidence to characterize the structural violence affecting transgender persons in four countries: Jamaica, Kenya, Russia, and the United States, and seeks to make the case for the importance of analytical data collection and analysis by governments and NGOs. The reliance on anecdotal evidence might be considered a weakness, but the reality is that scant evidence of the realities of transgendered people's struggles exists, and we are hopeful that Schwenke's visceral accounts will lead to more attention to, and a deeper understanding of transgendered peoples' lives.

In the final contribution to this book, Development as violence: Corporeal needs, embodied life, and the sustainable development goals, Colleen O'Manique and Pieter Fourie address how the UN Sustainable Development Goals have become the de facto global instrument for "development" from 2016 to 2030, replacing the Millennium Development Goals that were endorsed by the UN in 2001. The chapter analyses the prospects and possibilities of the SDG approach for improving on the MDG record. The analysis is situated in the context of the current global economic and ecological crisis, the rise of religious fundamentalisms, and the ascendancy of private sector solutions to poverty reduction and "empowerment" that are embedded in the outcome document on financing the SDGs endorsed by the UN General Assembly. O'Manique and Fourie ask whether the SDGs serve the project of consolidating the current global neoliberal socio-political and economic order in which corporeal needs (based on the life-sustaining work of gendered social reproduction) compete with the needs of capital, and discuss what this means for the future of genuine health security and gender justice.

All the chapters share a "critical analysis" rather than a unified theoretical or disciplinary framework. Contributors to this volume come from various professions and fields: we include academics, activists, and journalists, who all sometimes wear multiple hats. We view this variety as a particular strength of this volume, as it challenges the often premature attraction of agreement or consensus; it is the disruptive potential of critical feminist lenses that we embrace. What is shared amongst the contributors is the importance of critically analysing how the health and well-being of differently sexed, racialized, and gendered bodies are governed by both the overt and subtle practices of both health governance and governance more broadly. At the foundation of a critical feminist perspective is the understanding that, in the words of Riki Wilchins:

> The instinct to control bodies, genders and desires, may be as close as we have to a universal constant. It is common to cultures rich and poor, left wing and right wing, Eastern and Western, [. . .] And here I mean gender in its widest sense – including sexual orientation, because I take it as self-evident that the mainspring of homophobia is gender: the notion that gay men are insufficiently masculine or lesbian women inadequately feminine. And I include sex, because

I take it as obvious that what animates sexism and misogyny is gender, and our astounding fear and loathing around issues of vulnerability or femininity.

(Wilchins, 2002:11)

We need to acknowledge that most bodies that *need* to be controlled are female. Girls and women are still overwhelmingly responsible for invisible care labour, and this labour is considered the "natural" extension of their role in biological reproduction, which remains across the world, for many girls and women, out of their control. The vast majority of the perpetrators of intimate partner violence are men, and the majority of their victims are women. It is the same with rape and sexual violence during conflict and political violence; whilst men and boys are also the victims of sexual violence perpetrated by other males (and we acknowledge the pressing need to document and analyse this phenomenon), the majority recipients of such violence are female. States Cynthia Cockburn:

> Different feminisms have different slants on this. But there is one constant: the differentiation between and relative positioning of women and men is seen as an important ordering principle that pervades the system of power and is sometimes its very embodiment. Gender does not necessarily have primacy in this respect. Economic class and ethnic differentiation can also be important relational hierarchies, structuring a regime and shaping its mode of ruling. But these other differentiations are always also gendered and in turn help construct what is a man and woman in any given circumstances . . . while formulations of gender show rich diversity from culture to culture a dominance of men and masculinity is pervasive.
>
> (Cockburn, 2001:15)

While feminist perspectives on the "health and security" question are scant, they have much to offer the discussion. It is with this in mind that we hope that this volume contributes to the understanding and practice of "global health security" by expanding the understanding of who and what is being "secured", and challenging the structural/slow violence as well as the overt physical violence inherent to the current gendered global order. We view this book as the beginning of a conversation.

References

Billaud, J. (2015) *Kabul Carnival: Gender Politics in Postwar Afghanistan*. Philadelphia: U Penn Press.

Bitton, A., Green, C. and Colbert, J. (2011) 'Improving the delivery of global tobacco control'. *Mount Sinai Journal of Medicine: A Journal of Translational and Personalized Medicine*, 78: pp. 382–93.

Brodie, J. (2003) 'Globalization, in/security, and the paradoxes of the social' in Bakker, I. and Gill, S. (eds) *Power, Production, and Social Reproduction*. Basingstoke: Palgrave MacMillan.

Cockburn, C. (2001) 'The gendered dynamics of armed conflict and political violence' in Moser, C. and Clarke, F. (eds) *Victims, Perpetrators or Actors? Gender, Armed Conflict and Political Violence*. London: Zed Books.

Flynn, M. A., Eggerth, D. E. and Jacobson, C. J. (2015) 'Undocumented status as a social determinant of occupational safety and health: The workers' perspective'. *American Journal of Industrial Medicine*, 58: pp. 1127–37.

Fourie, P. (2015) 'AIDS as a security threat: The emergence and decline of an idea' in Rushton, S. and Youde, J. (eds.) *Routledge Handbook of Global Health Security*. London: Routledge.

Galtung, J. (1975) *Peace: Research, Education, Action*. Copenhagen: Christian Ejlers. Nixon, R. (2006–07) 'Slow violence, gender, and the environmentalism of the poor.' *Journal of Commonwealth and Post-Colonial Studies*, 13(2)–14(1): pp.14–37.

O'Manique, C. (2015) 'Gender, health and security' in Rushton, S. and Youde, J. (eds) *Routledge Handbook of Global Health Security*. London: Routledge.

O'Manique, C. and Fourie, P. (2010) 'Security and health in the 21st century' in Dunn-Cavelty, M. and Mauer, V. (eds) *The Routledge Handbook of Security Studies*. Oxford: Routledge.

Stillwaggon, E. (2003) 'Racial metaphors: Interpreting sex and AIDS in Africa'. *Development and Change*, 34(5): pp. 809–832.

Watney, S. (1989) 'Missionary positions: AIDS, "Africa", and race'. *Critical Quarterly*, 31(3): 45–62.

Wilchins, R. (2002) 'A continuous nonverbal communication' in Nestle, J., Howell, C. and Wilchins, R. (eds) *Genderqueer: Voices from Beyond the Sexual Binary*. Los Angeles: Alyson Books.

WHO (2007) *The World Health Report 2007 – A Safer Future: Global Public Health Governance in the 21st Century*. Geneva: WHO.

WHO (2008) *Primary Health Care: Now More than Ever*. Geneva: WHO.

2 The invisible tragedy of war

Women and the environment

H. Patricia Hynes

Introduction

The words 'genocide' and 'ecocide' were coined in the latter part of two twentieth-century wars. Raphael Lemkin, a Polish-Jewish lawyer, conceptualized genocide 'to describe Nazi policies of systematic murder, including the destruction of the European Jews' during World War II (Holocaust Encyclopedia, 2016). The scientist Arthur Galston defined 'ecocide' as 'the permanent and willful destruction of the environment in which a people can live in a manner of their own choosing', referring to the methodical chemical warfare the United States employed from 1961 to 1971 against the tropical ecosystems of South Vietnam in order to defeat the National Liberation Front (Zierler, 2011). In 1996 the author Beverly Allen introduced the term 'genocidal rape' to specify the Serbian army's military policy of raping Muslim women for the purpose of genocide (Allen, 1996). In many previous wars the misogynist military strategy of rape was employed to destroy a people, among them the 1937 Japanese 'Rape of Nanking', Pakistani soldiers in the 1971 Bangladeshi Liberation War, and the 1990s civil war in Rwanda.

The twentieth century, one in which conventions and covenants on human rights and environmental protections for all flourished, was also a century of record-breaking death (Ferguson, 2006), human rights violations and ecological destruction perpetrated within wars, both declared and undeclared. The twenty-first century has begun with no less gruesome hostility: the Iraq War (2003–11) culminated with the ensuing disintegration of that society, culture, and country. The year 2014 witnessed more conflicts than any other year in this century, as well as escalating international weapons sales. Some 60 million refugees (the majority being Syrians, Iraqis and Afghanis, and millions of internally displaced people) now suffer from these cumulative wars, the largest number of refugees fleeing war since World War II. Healthcare, public and environmental health (safe food, water, and sanitation), and economic development are casualties of war, such that the costs of conflict in 2014 were US$14.3 trillion, 100 times the official development assistance from rich to poor countries (McCoy, 2015).

All wars, putatively just and unjust alike, and less conventional wars such as 'dirty wars' of repression, low-intensity conflicts within and between countries and political groups, ethnic conflicts, and civil wars are unexamined public health and environmental disasters that leave in their wake humanitarian crises and human rights abuses, aggravated sexual exploitation of women and girls, and extreme and often irreversible environmental degradation (Enzler, 2016; Geiger 2000; Toole, Galson, and Brady, 1993). Early second wave feminist analysis, prominently Susan Griffin's *Women and Nature: the Roaring Inside Her*, explored the identification of women with the earth, both as sustenance for humanity and as victim of male rage. From Plato through Francis Bacon, the world was fatefully breached into spirit and matter, such that patriarchal Western philosophy, science and medicine, religion, industrialization, and politics have used this divide to bolster their power over both women and nature (Griffin, 2000).

This chapter examines, through themes and case examples, the egregious and singular trauma of war for women and the natural world – harm belittled as collateral damage, rarely documented by the perpetrators of armed conflict, and unaccounted for in war reparations. The first narrative focuses on women in war, and the second narrative explores the impact of armed conflict on the environment.

War and women

War has never spared nor protected women civilians. The targets of modern warfare are not primarily combatants; they are the enemy's infrastructure, economy and, thus, civilians. The twentieth century was the most lethal to civilians trapped in armed conflict. Civilian deaths as a percentage of all deaths, direct and indirect, from war rose from between 60 and 67 per cent in World War II to 90 per cent in the 1990s (Renner, 1999; Garfield and Neugut, 2000). The twenty-first century has begun with a similar morbid profile of armed conflict.

In seeking to make explicit the more systemic, sex-based and enduring impacts of war on women, there are many limitations. Women who were assaulted and harmed by martial rape and women who died in childbirth from war-related neglect and trauma, have not generally been documented as civilian casualties of war (Garfield and Neugut, 1991). Moreover, much of the data gathered in conflict and post-conflict situations is not disaggregated by gender, although this is changing with non-governmental organizations (NGOs) conducting independent impact analysis of war and a growing consciousness of documenting violence against women, a result of more than three decades of feminist research, activism and advocacy.

The few recent studies that have examined the death toll of war on females and males have concluded that equal numbers of civilian women and girls die of war-related injuries as civilian men and boys (Reza, Mercy, and Krug, 2001; Murray *et al.*, 2002). This data, however, does not include the morbidity of the spirit and the increased suicide and premature death that directly results from the sexual torture, despair and destitution of women in conflict-ridden and armed societies. To die by a bullet in war is a 'clean death', said one woman refugee and survivor of the war in Kosovo. To lose one's family, home and community in conflict, to be raped by enemy soldiers and then made suspect and shunned by one's husband and community, these are a living death, a social death, marked with acute impoverishment, profound culturally imposed shame and hopelessness (Muska and Olafsdottir, 2002).

In a landmark study of the indirect effects of war (a cross-national analysis of 1999 World Health Organization data on death and disability) researchers found substantial indirect and lasting health effects in largely civilian people who had survived civil wars in the years 1991–97. Of these, women and children were most affected. The lingering war-related disease, disability and death include elevated infectious disease, HIV/AIDS (from rape), cervical cancer (potentially from rape), homicide, and transportation accidents. They concluded, 'overall women and children were the most common long-term victims of civil war' (Ghobarah, Hunt, and Russett, 2001).

Rape, sexual torture, and sexual exploitation

In October 2002, the United Nations Development Fund for Women (UNIFEM) released a commissioned report, written by two independent experts, on the impact of armed conflict on women during and after conflict. The authors, who interviewed women in 14 countries in Europe, Asia, Africa, and the Middle East, found a similar continuum of violence against women in all regions. Some women were deliberately raped in front of husbands, parents, siblings, and children to 'pollute', humiliate, and terrorize the enemy; others were deliberately infected with HIV/AIDS. Soldiers punctured pregnant women with sharp weapons and ripped the foetuses from their wombs. Women and girls were raped and sexually enslaved in war zones; others were trafficked from war zones for sexual exploitation. Women were forced through imprisonment to bear children born of military rape. Soldiers sexually assaulted women for their activism in politics, for relationships with activists, and simply because they were home when the soldiers arrived (Rehn and Johnson Sirleaf, 2002). Women also reported that domestic violence, including rape, dramatically increased during and after conflict, a feature of male domestic abuse of women that was documented during World War II in US civil society, even while rates of negligent manslaughter decreased (Coleman, 2009).

In 2002 the United Nations High Commissioner for Refugees and Save the Children released a report on their investigation into allegations of sexual abuse of West African refugee children in Guinea, Liberia, and Sierra Leone. Their interviews with 1,500 men, women, and children refugees revealed that girls between the ages of 13 and 18 were sexually exploited by male aid workers, many of whom were employed by national and international non-governmental agencies (NGOs) and the UN, and also by UN peacekeepers and community leaders (United Nations High Commissioner for Refugees and Save the Children, 2002).

During the US-led war in Iraq (2003–11), the Organization for Women's Freedom in Iraq (OWFI) observed a sweeping rise in the number of women prostituted in brothels, workplaces, and hideouts in Baghdad, and set up an inquiry that resulted in a seminal study published in 2009, *Prostitution and Trafficking of Women and Girls in Iraq*. Through covert investigation, OWFI learned of the trafficking of women within Iraq for Iraqi men in all regions and for the US military, as well as to nearby countries. In their words, '[t]his industry looked like an octopus with its head in Baghdad while the limbs reached out to Damascus, Dubai, Jordan, and the Emirates'. (And, the organization would later find, also to Saudi Arabia.) 'Trafficking is the hidden face of war, insecurity, and chaos', concludes the study's author (OWFI, 2009).

War refugees

The scale and nature of war in the late twentieth century resulted in unprecedented numbers of people fleeing conflict, such that the displacement of people by war in the 1990s had more severe public health impact, in many situations, than the conflict itself (Toole and Waldman, 1997; Toole, 2000). When the ashes settle on the current war in Syria, the toll will likely be much greater on civilians killed, internally displaced citizens, and refugees who have fled the country than on combatants.

Eighty per cent of the world's refugees and internally displaced persons are women and children (Ashford and Huet-Vaughn, 2000). Being responsible for basic household needs, including procuring food, fuel, fodder, and water and for disposal of waste, women and girls in refugee camps are more likely to be exposed to contaminated water supplies and human waste. They are also more at risk of rape and sexual exploitation than men and boys; a risk heightened by the fact that men can more easily prey upon them in the milieu of conflict-related scarcity.

Child soldiers

More than 300,000 children between the ages of 8 and 18 are trapped as child soldiers in over 30 global conflicts in Africa, Asia, Colombia, and Peru. Further, the number of armed groups exploiting children in war had increased from 40 in 1960 to 57 in 2007 (Morales, 2008).

Few realize how large a percentage of child soldiers are girls, an estimated 40 per cent, who are exploited like boy soldiers as servants, spies, and soldiers. In addition, girls are taken into sex slavery by boy soldiers, adult soldiers, and commanders. Entire generations of children across the world have already been destroyed by this crisis, asserts international affairs and Latin American specialist Waltraud Morales. She adds that armed groups target children for their wars because children, and more so girls because of sex discrimination, are 'obedient, vulnerable, and malleable'. Children can be more easily indoctrinated into being the next generation of armed rebels and terrorists. Child soldiers are cheap because they are unpaid and eat less than adults; they provide functions such as cooking, cleaning, and portering, thus freeing up adult soldiers for more rigorous fighting. With the prevalence of light but deadly weapons, girls as well as boys are trained for combat. In a 2002 survey, nearly half the interviewed girls in armed groups described their primary role as a 'fighter' (Save the Children, 2005).

The 2011 Liberian Nobel Prize Laureate, Leymah Gbowee, wrote recently of her work with ex-child soldiers of Charles Taylor's army during Liberia's civil war. She states that employing children, by whatever means, in armed conflict is a crime that hardens and turns many boys into drug-addicted, almost incorrigibly violent gang members, and torments girls with constant sexual exploitation, severe injury, child pregnancy, stigma, and rejection by their community (Gbowee, 2012). In her autobiography Grace Akallo, abducted at the age of 15 from her boarding school in Northern Uganda by the Lord's Resistance Army, explained that being raped was so extreme and severe a violation that ex-girl soldiers will admit to murder sooner than to having been raped (McDonnell and Akallo, 2008).

Military sexual assault: the other war front for women soldiers

Scholars and investigators who have studied US military culture and attitudes toward women have found that hostility toward women pervades military training, often out of deep antipathy for the presence of women in traditionally male space, sometimes stemming from competition, always linking manliness with sexual dominance, and that such hostility functions like a glue to solidify male bonding over women's status as sex objects (Morris, 1996).

'A woman who signs up to protect her country is more likely to be raped by a fellow soldier than killed by enemy fire', stated Representative Jane Harman in testimony before a July 2008 House panel investigating the military's handling of sexual assault reports (Harman, 2008). Women in the military are raped and sexually assaulted at significantly higher rates than in civilian society. A 2003 study of women seeking healthcare through the Veterans Administration (VA), from the period from the Vietnam War to the first Gulf War, found that nearly 1 in 3 women was raped while serving. This is almost twice the rate in US society, and 8 in 10 women had been sexually harassed during their military service. Rates were consistent through all periods and wars studied. Of those who reported having been raped, 37 per cent were raped at least twice and 14 per cent were gang-raped (Sadler *et al.*, 2003).

Studies have found that military sexual assault contributes more strongly to developing post-traumatic stress disorder (PTSD) than combat-related stress, and that those assaulted sexually suffer more PTSD than those with other trauma. One striking VA study of more than 300 women veterans enrolled in a clinical programme for stress disorders, found that 'sexual stress (stress related to sexual harassment and abuse) was almost four times more influential than duty-related stress in the development of PTSD' (Fontana and Rosenheck, 2007).

The world community must listen to women's voices, during conflict, at the negotiating table, and post-conflict. They must listen in order to grasp war's impact; to strengthen resolve against war and for conflict prevention; to stanch the flow in weapons; and to hold perpetrators of rape, trafficking, and other forms of sexual exploitation accountable for their crimes.

War and the environment

The 'Tragedy of the Commons', Garrett Hardin's 1968 contentious essay, targeted overpopulation as the prime threat to sustainable life on our finite earth

(Hardin, 1968). Population biologists and environmentalists in the North handily picked up his analysis and coined militaristic metaphors for women's reproduction, such as 'population bomb' and 'population explosion', which led to misogynist population control programs forced onto impoverished women of the South (Hynes, 1993).

Ironically, Hardin made his claim at the height of US chemical warfare in Vietnam with dioxin-contaminated herbicides, an assault on nature so catastrophic that scientists coined a new word: 'ecocide' (Zierler, 2011). He, and many who consumed his thesis, failed to single out the very small but politically powerful and protected population responsible for unparalleled environmental impact: the military. Among all institutions, the military worldwide is the most secretive, shielded, and privileged of polluters (Hynes, 2011; 1993).

Environmental destruction has been a methodical weapon of war throughout the history of human hostilities: scorched earth tactics to destroy crops, forest, and infrastructure; polluting water supply; catapulting infected blankets into enemy garrisons; setting oil wells on fire, and so on. During the 10-year American War in Vietnam, the US carried out the largest and most prolonged attempt to destroy forests and mangroves of an ecology-based culture in history – and this in a country of 90 per cent subsistence farmers who had lived on their land for centuries (ECOCIDE, 2014).

Militarism and modern war also breed staggering collateral harm to nature and our lived environment, by the kinds of weapons used (concealed landmines, other unexploded ordnance, and long-lived toxic chemicals), by the 'shock and awe' intensity of industrial warfare, by the growing predilection for air war, and by the massive exploitation of natural resources and fossil fuels to support militarism. By 1990 researchers had estimated that the world's military accounted for 5–10 per cent of global air pollution, including carbon dioxide, ozone-depletion, smog, and acid-forming chemicals. The Research Institute for Peace Policy in Germany calculated that 20 per cent of all global environmental degradation was due to military and related activities (Renner, 1991 and Shulman, 1992).

US military

This section focuses on the US military superpower both as paradigm of and surrogate for international militarism and war. It is a power without precedent in war-making, war-related environmental destruction, and (since the end of the Cold War) global military presence. Consider its naval and airbase centrality in the Middle East, its dominance of NATO in Europe (financing three-quarters of NATO's military spending), and its pivot to Asia, where the US naval presence governs the Pacific as the American Lake (Chomsky, 2016). Moreover, as US military budgets fall and rise, so also do those of the rest of the world, according to the Stockholm International Peace Research Institute. Global military spending fell in tandem with the US defense budget in the late 1980s and 1990s, with the end of the Cold War, and it rose from 9/11 to 2011 by 65 per cent, while the US military budget nearly doubled (Davies, 2016).

To support its strategic full spectrum of power, the Pentagon maintains 6,000 domestic military bases and an estimated 1,000 military bases in more than 60 countries. The US military consumes more oil than any other institution in the world (Smith, 2016), and has been involved in at least 18 military actions since 2000 not including covert actions (Grossman, 2016), all of which intensify its use of oil and natural resources, increase chemical spills, and leave polluted environments. As an example of the ease with which US environmental laws such as the Marine Mammal Protection Act are subservient to the Department of Defense, consider what the West Coast Alliance has tabulated from the Navy's records. Over five years the U.S. Navy is permitted to injure, kill and harass up to 12 million marine mammals, including whales, dolphins, porpoises, sea lions, and seals in the North Pacific ocean, in underwater training exercises using sonar, explosive, drones, ships and submarines (Jamail, 2016).

Consider this categorical profile of US military pollution:

Chemical waste pollution

Nearly 900 of the EPA's approximately 1,300 Superfund sites are abandoned military bases/facilities or manufacturing and testing sites that produced conventional weapons and other military-related products and services, according to the 2008–09 President's Cancer Panel Report (Reducing Cancer Risk, 2009). This figure does not include the full US military enterprise, namely, the Department of Energy's nuclear weapons radioactive waste and the nearly 1,000 US bases worldwide where, with few exceptions, the Pentagon is not accountable for environmental protection (Mitchell, 2016).

The military Superfund sites comprise chemical warfare and research facilities; plane, ship, and tank manufacture and repair facilities; training and manoeuvre bases; and abandoned disposal pits. Common contaminants include metal cleaning solvents, pesticides, machining oils, metals, metalworking fluids, and chemical ingredients used in explosives. Dumped into pits, leaking from corroding containers, buried in unlined landfills, and left on test ranges, military toxics have leached into groundwater and polluted drinking water throughout the country.

Nuclear weapons waste pollution

Since the US exploded the first nuclear bomb in New Mexico, more than 2,000 nuclear weapons have been tested worldwide, in all environments: aboveground, underwater, underground, and in outer space. According to some estimates, the equivalent of more than 29,000 Hiroshima bombs have been tested in the atmosphere, discharging more than 9,000 pounds of plutonium – with a half-life of 24,000 years – into the environment (General Overview of the effects of nuclear testing, 2012).

Most of the uranium mined for the US nuclear program was in or near tribal lands of the Navajo in New Mexico, with more than 1,000 regional mines and mill sites now abandoned, unsealed, and sources of soil and drinking water contamination.

Navajo miners worked without protection from exposure to uranium dust and still live with their families near the contaminated sites. The Navajo and nearby Laguna tribes suffer cancer of the lung, kidney disease, and birth defects at higher than average rates. Even if all nuclear weapons were dismantled tomorrow, the radioactivity of waste from mining, manufacturing, and testing will endure for millennia (Reducing Cancer Risk, 2009).

By 1994, nearly 5,000 contaminated sites at the Department of Energy (DOE) nuclear weapons and fuel facilities had been identified for remediation. Waste from nuclear weapons dwarfs all other hazardous waste in scale, toxicity, and dispersion across the world, as well as in cost to manage the challenge. Moreover, it defies technical solutions for permanent environmental cleanup and environmental security (Alvarez, 2014).

Climate change and the military

In the twenty-first century, climate change is a threat to human security without precedent (Barrett, Charles and Temte, 2014). Only recently has the momentous issue of military fuel use and its massive role in global climate change come to the foreground. Militarism is the most oil-exhaustive activity on the planet, growing more so with faster, bigger, more fuel-guzzling planes, tanks, and naval vessels employed in increasingly intensive air and ground wars and war exercises. At the outset of the Iraq War in March 2003, the Army estimated it would need more than 40 million gallons of gasoline for three weeks of combat, exceeding the total quantity used by all Allied forces in the four years of World War I. A quarter of the world's jet fuel feeds the Air Force fleet (Sanders, 2009).

Researchers at Oil Change International calculated the greenhouse gas emissions of the Iraq war and the opportunity costs involved in fighting the war rather than investing in clean technology, for the years 2003–07. Their key findings are unambiguous about the vast climate pollution of war and the lockstep bipartisan policy of forfeiting future global health for present day militarism:

• The projected full costs of the Iraq War (estimated $3 trillion) would cover all needed investments in renewable power generation between 2007 and 2030 to reverse global warming trends.
• Between 2003 and 2007, the war generated at least 141 million metric tons of carbon dioxide equivalent, more each year of the war than 139 of the world's countries release annually. Further, re-building Iraqi schools, homes, businesses, bridges, roads, and hospitals pulverized by the war, and new security walls and barriers require millions of tons of cement, which is one of the largest industrial sources of greenhouse gas emissions.
• By 2008, the Bush administration had spent 97 times more on military than on climate change. As a presidential candidate, President Obama pledged to spend $150 billion over 10 years on green energy technology and infrastructure – less than the United States was spending in one year of the Iraq War.

(Oil Change International, 2008)

The US military consumes as much as one million barrels of oil per day and contributes 5 per cent of current global warming emissions, according to estimates by researcher Barry Sanders (2009). Given that the military has 1.3 million active duty people (less than .0002 per cent of the world's population) generating 5 per cent of climate pollution, the US military enterprise is far and away the largest single climate polluter and contributor to global warming.

US chemical warfare in Vietnam: a case study of the wages of war on ecosystems

During the ten years (1961–71) of aerial chemical warfare in Vietnam, US planes sprayed nearly 20 million gallons of herbicide defoliants in an operation codenamed Ranch Hand, to destroy enemy forest cover and crops and to clear vegetation around US bases for visibility. Ranch Hand's motto, 'Only You Can Prevent Forests', branded the mission and, like so many military code names, trivialized the tragedy and the crime of chemical warfare. Agent Orange, the dioxin-contaminated and exceedingly toxic herbicide constituted about 61 per cent of the total herbicides sprayed in the war (Agent Orange Record, 2015). Agent Orange, thus, serves as a surrogate for the weaponized herbicidal warfare on the ecology and agriculture of Vietnam.

The ingredients of Agent Orange constituted an equal proportion of 2,4-D and 2,4,5-T, plant growth regulators developed during World War II to target specific plants. Absorption of them by plant life wreaks havoc on the plants' growth hormones and accelerates plant growth. In sufficient strength plants undergo uncontrolled growth until leaves shrivel and fall off within a few days and the plant dies. During World War II, the US government had researched and developed these herbicides for use on Japan's rice crops and forests, but the war ended before they did so. In 1943, government researchers found that arsenic proved more effective against rice than 2,4-D, leading to the development and use of Agent Blue to destroy rice crops in Vietnam. World War II research on weaponized herbicides advanced herbicide use by ten years (as war-related research has done in other technical areas) (Zierler, 2011).

By 1966, over 5,000 American scientists, among them Nobel Prize winners, condemned the use of chemical warfare agents in Vietnam. The US herbicide program ended in 1971 when Nixon's administration was forced to disclose government-sponsored research data that revealed that one of the herbicides in Agent Orange (2,4,5-T) caused extreme birth deformities in lab animals and the other (2,4-D) also caused negative reproductive impacts. The data had been produced in 1966 but the final results were suppressed until 1969 (Lewallen, 1971; Sills, 2014).

Two of the most vocal scientist critics of weaponized herbicides, Dr Arthur Westing and Dr. Egbert Pfeiffer, made five trips to Vietnam between 1969 and 1973 to document the extent of ecological damage and loss from the war, using film, scientific observation, and records. They described what they witnessed as the largest and most prolonged attempt to destroy agriculture and an ecology-based culture in history. Vietnam was a country of 90 per cent subsistence farmers who had lived on the land for centuries. At least 1/3 of the people were forced out of the country-side, leaving graves and ancestor altars as well as agricultural fields, rice paddies, fruit trees, fish ponds and animals, and into cities or planned villages in order to eliminate the rural base of support for the resistance. Fruit trees, they reported, were especially sensitive to the herbicides and easily killed; fish in hand-dug ponds died from changes in their ecosystem. Forty per cent of total useable forest was destroyed from bombing, shrapnel, napalm and herbicides. Ecocide continued to exact a price after the war, given that revival of lost mangrove and hardwood forests would need 'the human hand' to regenerate, as they and others reported (ECOCIDE, 2014).

Ongoing legacy of Agent Orange

Two decades after the war's end, the 2002 Stockholm Environmental Conference on Cambodia, Laos and Vietnam examined the long-term ecological conse-quences of Agent Orange in Southeast Asia. The conference featured American and Vietnamese forestry, botany and coastal mangrove researchers, and practi-tioners who have studied the potential of Vietnam's ecosystem regeneration since the war.

Phung Tuu Boi of the Forest Inventory and Planning Institute in Vietnam reported that the inland forests areas destroyed by Agent Orange were invaded by grasses prone to fire in the dry season and secondary tree species with little value for sustainable development, both of which prevent normal forest regeneration. Furthermore, after Agent Orange eliminated the triple canopy forest, tropical rains eroded and washed nutrient laden soil into downstream rivers and deltas, leaving a depleted, hardened soil base hostile to natural forest regeneration necessary for wildlife recuperation. Even with intense reforestation, the centuries-old triple canopy tropical forests, famed in Asia for the diversity of their wildlife, will take a century or more to restore to pre-war conditions. Complicating recovery, national reforestation programs to return barren land to efficient production, promote sus-tainable development and alleviate rural poverty, are now under pressure from commercial logging (Long Term Consequences of the Vietnam War: Ecosystems, 2002; Ives, 2010).

Agent Orange defoliation of an estimated 40 per cent of mangrove forests caused the irreversible degeneration of Vietnam's marine habitat. Clams disap-peared; giant ferns invaded, trapping sediment and snuffing out mudflats and their marine nurseries, ultimately reducing the fish supply. Researcher Bui Thi Lang described a sequence that trapped locals in a cycle of poverty: overfishing resulted from reduced fish supply, and mangrove trunks were removed for firewood and supplanted with rice cultivation. This has impeded restoring the true wealth of the coastal environment–mangrove forests, with their immense marine nurseries (Long Term Consequences of the Vietnam War: Ecosystems, 2002).

Today a third and fourth generation of children born with horrific birth defects and mental retardation continue to suffer the legacy of US chemical warfare in

Vietnam. Why ongoing toxicity after decades of the war's end? The best studies to date have found that the extremely virulent strain of dioxin in Agent Orange, known as TCDD, persists in the environment of Vietnam, particularly in areas most heavily sprayed and on former US air bases where Agent Orange was stored, loaded into spraying equipment, spilled, and also used liberally to clear the periphery of the bases. Washed into local ponds during tropical rainstorms, dioxin in pond sediment is long-lived with an estimated half-life of 100 years, and bioaccumulates in the food chain, contaminating the fish, fowl, and freshwater mollusks harvested by people living on or near the former bases. Recent studies by the Canadian firm Hatfield Associates have documented the pattern of dioxin soil/sediment and contamination and bioaccumulation in the food chain. Their studies have also found levels of dioxin in the breast milk of women living on these bases that exceed World Health Organization standards for breastfeeding infants (Hatfield Associates, 2000). Thus, a fourth generation of Vietnamese breast-fed children, exposed to dioxin, continue to suffer from the toxic physical and mental effects of exposure to TCDD dioxin.

Many groups, among them the US-based Vietnam Agent Orange Relief and Responsibility Campaign, are working on behalf of the Vietnamese victims, through legislation, policy, funding support for housing, medical services and education (VAORRC, 2016).

Conclusion

The pieces of the 2015 US federal discretionary budget that fund education, energy, environment, social services, housing, veterans services, transportation, science, and new job creation, taken together, receive less funding than the Department of Defense budget, which captured 54 per cent of the discretionary budget (National Priorities Project, 2016). If, as many contend, the principal threat to ecological and human security in the twenty-first century is environmental degradation (through climate change, pollution, soil erosion, habitat loss, and species extinction), then challenging the destruction and damage to the environment and the massive exploitation of oil and metal resources for the military-industrial war machine is paramount in the work for environmental justice, climate justice, and peace.

Finally, engaging women in the peace process, as exacted in the 2000 UN Resolution 1325 on women, peace and security is critical to reversing the masculinist mindset of militarizing conflict (Machel, 2001). Being sexual targets in war, receiving unequal health and food resources in resettlement camps, left out of reconciliation and governance negotiations while being the primary victims of war, women are primed for negotiating peace agreements that redress the impacts gender and human impacts of war, that rid their communities of weapons, and that bring perpetrators of sexual violence to account for their crimes.

References

Agent Orange Record. 'Enough toxic herbicide sprayed to blanket ¼ of the country.' Online. Available HTTP: www.agentorangerecord.com/home/ (accessed 10 May 2015).

Allen, B. (1996) *Rape Warfare: The Hidden Genocide in Bosnia-Herzegovina and Croatia*, Minneapolis, MN: University of Minnesota Press.

Alvarez, R. (2014) 'A primer: US military radioactive wastes', *Bulletin of the Atomic Scientists*. Online. Available HTTP: http://thebulletin.org/primer-military-nuclear-wastes-united-states (accessed 24 February 2014).

Ashford, Mary-Wynne and Huet-Vaughn, Y. (2000) 'The impact of war on women', in Levy, B.S. and Sidel, V.W. (eds), *War and Public Health*, Washington, DC: American Public Health Association, 186–196.

Barrett, B., Charles, J.W., and Temte, J.L. (2014) 'Climate change, human health, and epidemiological transition', *Prevention Medicine*. Online. Available HTTP: www.ncbi. nlm.nih.gov/pmc/articles/PMC4342988/ (accessed 5 January 2015).

Bennoune, K. (2015) 'The women's court: A feminist approach to justice.' Online. Available HTTP: www.popularresistance.org/the-womens-court-a-feminist-approach-to-justice/ (accessed 20 May 2015).

Chomsky, N. (2016) 'American power under challenge masters of mankind.' Online. Available HTTP: www.tomdispatch.com/post/176137/tomgram%3A_noa m_chomsky, the_challenges_of_2016/ (accessed 21 May 2016).

Davies, N.S.J. (2016) 'The science of killing has become an impractical instrument of political domination.' Online. Available HTTP: http://freepress.org/article/science-killing-has-become- impractical-instrument-political-domination (accessed 23 April 2016).

Coleman, P. (2009) 'Does military service turn young men into sexual predators'? Online. Available HTTP: www.alternet.org/story/142942/does_military_service_tu rn_young_men_into_sexual_predators (accessed 21 October 2009).

ECOCIDE: A Strategy of War, A Green Mountain Post & EW Pfeiffer Production Online. Available HTTP: www.gmpfilms.com/ECO.html (accessed 16 August 2014).

Enzler, S.M. 'Environmental effects of warfare.' Online. Available HTTP: www.lenntech. com/environmental-effects-war.htm (accessed 13 May 2016).

Ferguson, N. (2006) *The War of the World: Twentieth-Century Conflict and the Descent of the West*, London: Penguin Press.

Fontana, A. and Rosenheck, R. (2007) 'Duty-related and sexual stress in the etiology of PTSD among women veterans who seek treatment.' Online. Available HTTP: www. ncbi.nlm.nih.gov/pubmed/9603572 (accessed 11 August 2008).

Garfield, R.M. and Neugut, A.I. (1991) 'Epidemiologic analysis of warfare: A historical view.' *JAMA*, 226: 688–692.

Garfield, R.M. and Neugut, A. I. (2000) 'The human consequences of war', in Levy, B.S. and Sidel, V.W. (eds), *War and Public Health*, Washington, DC: American Public Health Association, 27–38.

Gbowee, L. (2012) 'Child soldiers, child wives: wounded for life.' Online. Available HTTP: www.opendemocracy.net/5050/leymah-gbowee/child-soldiers-child-wives-wounded-for-life (accessed 10 June 2013).

Geiger, H. J. (2000) 'The impact of war on human rights', in Levy B.S. and Sidel, V.W. (eds), *War and Public Health*, Washington, DC: American Public Health Association, 39–50.

'General overview of the effects of nuclear testing', Comprehensive Test Ban Treaty Preparatory Commission. Online. Available HTTP: www.ctbto.org/nuclear-testing/

the-effects-of-nuclear- testing/general-overview-of-theeffects-of-nuclear-testing/ (accessed 10 August 2012).

Ghobarah, H.A., Huth, P., and Russett, B. (2001) 'Civil wars kill and maim people – long after the shooting stops.' Online. Available HTTP: www.isn.ethz.ch/Digital-Library/Publications/Detail/?lng=en&id=30056Civil war.pdf (accessed 10 May 2016).

Griffin, Susan. (2000) *Women and Nature: The Roaring Inside Her*, Berkeley, CA: Counterpoint Press.

Grossman, Zoltan. 'From Wounded Knee to Syria: A century of U.S. military interventions.' Online. Available HTTP: https://academic.evergreen.edu/g/grossmaz/interventions.html (accessed 07 January 2016).

Hardin, G. (first published 1968) 'The tragedy of the commons.' Online. Available HTTP: http://science.sciencemag.org/content/162/3859/1243.full (accessed 10 June 2010).

Harman, J. (10 September 2008) 'Female soldiers more likely to be raped than killed in action, says rep.' Online. Available HTTP: http://abcnews.go.com/Blotter/story?id=5760295&page=1#.Tu9 wP2BuHCQ (accessed 10 August 2008).

Hatfield Associates. (2000) *Development of Impact Mitigation Strategies Related to the use of Agent Orange Herbicide in the Aluoi Valley, Viet Nam.* Online. Available HTTP: www.hatfieldgroup.com/wp-content/uploads/AgentOrangeReports/CIDA849/CIDA849_Agent_Or ange_V1_Report_Main.pdf (accessed 15–20 November 2014).

Holocaust Encyclopedia. 'What is genocide.' Online. Available HTTP: www.ushmm.org/wlc/en/article.php?ModuleId=100070 43 (accessed 15 May 2016).

Hunt, S. and Lute, D. 'Inclusive security NATO adopts and adapts', Features, *Prism*, 6, 1: 7–19.

Hynes, H.P. (1993) *Taking Population out of the Equation*, North Amherst, MA: Institute on Women and Technology. Online. Available HTTP: www.readingfromtheleft.com/PDF/IPAT-Hynes.pdf

Hynes, H.P. (2011) See 7-part series on military pollution for more depth and detail, *War and the Tragedy of the Commons*, Truthout. Online. Available HTTP: http://www.truth-out.org/news/item/2491:war-and-the- tragedy-of-the- commons

Ives, M. (2010) 'In war-scarred landscape, Vietnam replants its forests', Environment 360. Online. Available HTTP: http://e360.yale.edu/feature/in_war-scarred_landscape_vietnam_replants_its_forests/2336/ (accessed 7 March 2016).

Jamail, D. (16 May 2016) 'Navy allowed to kill or injure nearly 12 million whales, dolphins, other marine mammals in Pacific', *Truthout*. Online. Available HTTP: www.truth-out.org/news/item/36037-the-us-navy-s-mass-destruction-of-marine-life (accessed 16 May 2016).

Lewallen, J. (1971) *The Ecology of Devastation: Indochina*, Baltimore, MD: Penguin Books.

'List of nuclear weapons tests.' Online: Available HTTP: http://en.wikipedia.org/wiki/List_of_nuclear_weapons_tests (accessed 15 August 2012).

Long Term Consequences of the Vietnam War: Ecosystems. (2002) Report from The Environmental Conference on Cambodia, Laos and Vietnam http://www.nnn.se/environ/ecology.pdf (accessed 20 September 2012). 5–7, 11–13.

Machel, G. (2001) *The Impact of War on Children*, London: Hurst & Company.

McCoy, D. (2015) 'Re-engaging the health community around peace', *The Lancet*, V386, 1005: 1714–1716.

McDonnell, F.H. and Akallo, G.P. (2008) *Girl Soldier: A Story of Hope for Northern Uganda's Children*, Grand Rapids, Michigan: Chosen Press.

Mead, M. Online. Available HTTP: www.nancychristie.com/makeachange/2009/05/we-wont- have-a-society-if-we-destroy-the-environment-margaret-mead/.

Mitchell, J. (9 April 2016) 'Contamination: Kadena Air Base's dirty secret', *The Japan Times.* Online: Available HTTP: www.japantimes.co.jp/news/2016/04/09/national/contami nation-kadena-air-bases-dirty-secret/#.V0SucmNlsnV (accessed May 1, 2016).

Morales, W.Q. (2008) 'Girl child soldiers: the other face of sexual exploitation and gender violence.' Online. Available HTTP: www.airpower.maxwell.af.mil/apjinternational/apj-s/2008/1tri08/moraleseng.htm (accessed 27 February 2010).

Morris, M. (1996) 'By force of arms: rape, war, and military culture', *Duke Law Journal,* 45, 4: 708, 716–20.

Murray, C.L.J., King, G., Lopez, A.D., Tomijima, N., and Krug, E.G. (2002). 'Armed conflict as a public health problem', *BMJ,* 324: 346–349.

Muska, S. and Olafsdottir, G. (2002) *Women, the Forgotten Face of War.* New York: Bless Bless Productions. Online. Available HTTP: https://vimeo.com/19729520 (accessed 15 May 2016).

National Priorities Project, 'Federal spending: Where does the money go?' Online. Available HTTP: www.nationalpriorities.org/budget-basics/federal-budget-101/spending/ (accessed 26 May 2016).

Oil Change International. (2008) *A Climate of War: The War in Iraq and Global Warming.* Online. Available HTTP: http://priceofoil.org/2008/03/01/a-climate-of-war/ (accessed 10 May 2009).

OWFI (2009). *Prostitution and Trafficking of Women and Girls in Iraq* Online. Available HTTP: www.owfi.info/EN/wp-content/uploads/2014/09/ProstitutionandTrafficking_OWFI- report-1.pdf (accessed 17 April 2010).

Reducing Cancer Risk, 2008–2009 Annual Report, President's Cancer Panel, 77. Online: Available HTTP: http://deainfo.nci.nih.gov/advisory/pcp/annualReports/pcp08-09rpt/PCP_Report_08-09_508.pdf (accessed 4 April 2014).

Rehn, E. and Johnson Sirleaf, E. (2002) *Women, War and Peace: The Independent Experts' Assessment on the Impact of Armed Conflict on Women and Women's role in Peace-building,* United Nations Development Fund for Women. Online. Available HTTP: www.unifem.undp.org (accessed 10 April 2007).

Renner, M. (1991) 'Assessing the military's war on the environment', in Brown, L., *State of the World,* New York: W.W. Norton.

Renner, M. (1999) Worldwatch paper #146 Ending violent conflict, Washington, DC: Worldwatch Institute. Online. Available HTTP: www.worldwatch.org/node/844 (accessed 14 October 2015).

Reza, A., Mercy J.A., and Krug, E. (2001) 'Epidemiology of violent deaths in the world', *Injury Prevention,* 7: 104–111.

Rossini, A.O. (2015) 'Sarajevo, the women's tribunal'. Online. Available HTTP: www. balcanicaucaso.org/eng/Areas/Bosnia- Herzegovina/Sarajevo-the-Women-s-Tribunal-161486 (accessed 15 May 2015).

Sadler, A.G., Booth, B.M., Cook, B.L. and Doebbeling, B.N. (2003) 'Factors associated with women's risk of rape in the military environment', *American Journal of Industrial Medicine* 43: 262–273.

Sanders, B. (2009) *The Green Zone: The Environmental Costs of Militarism* Oakland, California: AK Press.

Save the Children. (2005) *Forgotten Casualties of War: Girls in Conflict.* Online. Available HTTP: http://resourcecentre.savethechildren.se/sites/default/files/documents/2717.pdf (accessed 15 January 2010).

Sills, P. (2014) *Toxic War: The Story of Agent Orange,* Nashville, TN: Vanderbilt University Press.

Shulman, S. (1992) *The Threat at Home: Confronting the Toxic Legacy of the U.S. Military*, Boston, MA: Beacon Press.

Smith, G. (2016) 'Global warming's unacknowledged threat – the Pentagon.' Online. Available HTTP: http://warisacrime.org/content/global- warmings- unacknowledged-threat-pentagon (accessed 29 April 2016).

Smythe, A. (2003) 'Women under the law of the gun', News 24 Archives. Online. Available HTTP: www.news24.com/World/News/Women-under-the-law- of-the-gun-20031030 (accessed 21 July 2005).

Toole, M.J. (2000) 'Displaced persons and war', in Levy B.S. and Sidel V.W. (eds) *War and Public Health*, Washington, DC: American Public Health Association, 197–212.

Toole, M.J., Galson, S. and Brady, W. (1993) 'Are war and public health compatible?' *The Lancet*, 341: 1193–1196.

Toole, M.J. and Waldman, R. J. (1997) 'The public health aspects of complex emergencies and refugee situations', *Annual Review of Public Health*, 18: 283–312.

United Nations High Commissioner for Refugees, & Save the Children UK. (2002) *Note for Implementing and Operational Partners by UNHCR and Save the Children UK on Sexual Violence & Exploitation: The Experience of Refugee children in Guinea, Liberia, and Sierra Leone*. Online. Available HTTP: www.unhcr.org/3c7cf89a4.html (accessed 8 March 2008).

VAORRC Vietnam Agent Orange Relief and Responsibility Campaign. 'The Vietnam Agent Orange Relief and Responsibility Campaign is an initiative of U.S. veterans, Vietnamese Americans and all concerned about peace and justice. We insist our government honor its moral and legal responsibility to compensate the Vietnamese victims and *all* victims, of Agent Orange'. Online. Available HTTP: www.vn- agentorange.org. Accessed 26 May 2016.

Zierler, D. (2011) *The Invention of Ecocide: Agent Orange, Vietnam and the Scientists Who Changed the Way We Think about the Vietnam War*, Athens, Georgia: University of Georgia Press. Book Review. Online. Accessible HTTP: www.historynet.com/reviews-the-invention-of- ecocide-agent-orange-vietnam-and-the-scientists-who-changed- the-way-we-think-about-the-victnam-war.htm (accessed 14 July 2015).

3 Survivors of conflict and post-conflict sexual and gender-based violence and torture in the Great Lakes region of Africa

A holistic model of care

Helen Liebling

Introduction

Sexual violence has been part and parcel of war and political violence in all parts of the world, and throughout history. Only recently has it been incorporated into the global security agenda, with the UN Security Council in 2000 formally acknowledging the disproportionate impact of modern warfare and low intensity conflict on women as civilians, and their exclusion from processes of peaceful transition. The UN Security Council Resolution 1325 represented a formal acknowledgement of the ubiquity of sexual violence in modern warfare and political violence, focusing international attention on particular regions of the world where devastating protracted wars shared the systematic feature of sexual and gender-based violence carried out by soldiers, rebel militias and civilians, and even UN peacekeepers (Manjoo & McRaith, 2011). One of the regions most profoundly affected by sexual and gender-based violence in recent times has been the Great Lakes region in Africa comprising: Burundi; Democratic Republic of Congo; Kenya; Rwanda; Tanzania, and Uganda. As Stark and Wessells (2012) argue, the extreme racism and violent masculinity of colonization in the region was the foundation of structural and sexual violence in the post-independence period. Today's situation is complex as the 'formal' end of conflict has carried with it the continuation of the deep impact of sexual and gender-based violence, often with impunity for its perpetrators (Liebling-Kalifani & Baker, 2010a; Peterman, Palermo & Bredenkamp, 2011).

The recognition of continuing human rights abuses, racism and violent masculinity post-conflict has led to increased humanitarian attention and intervention in places of high levels of sexual violence, including in the Great Lakes region (Askin, 2002–2003). Although both necessary and welcome, the impact of conflict and post-conflict sexual violence and torture has often been misunderstood as an individual manifestation of psychological trauma and physical injuries. As a result, subsequent responses have often been confined to a medical approach, thus medicalizing complex problems embedded in contexts of systemic structural violence and insecurities.

The research for this chapter was carried out with women and men survivors of conflict, former girl and boy child abductees, and women and girls who bore children from rape in the Great Lakes region of Africa. Some of the former abductees we spoke with were also forced as children to perpetrate human right abuses including sexual violence, by the Lord's Resistance Army. This chapter analyses the implications of the impact of these atrocities in terms of service and policy improvements required for survivors, arguing for an alternative understanding that is gendered, and recognizes the devastating impact of sexual violence and torture on reproductive and psychological health, as well as on communities. At the same time, it highlights the resilience of survivors and their ability to reconstruct identities. Based on the first-person accounts of those who have experienced human rights abuses including sexual and gender-based violence and torture and its aftermath over a period of five years, it calls attention to a key issue that has been neglected in accounts of 'health and security': the brutal immediate and far reaching gendered physical and mental health impacts on people and communities in situations of violent conflict. It argues for greater attention to the voices of survivors of conflict and post-conflict sexual and gender-based violence and torture in the determination of interventions.

Methodology

All of the research carried out used feminist and participatory methods and were funded by the British Academy, Leverhulme, and the Economic and Social Research Council. Thematic analysis was utilized to analyse the information (Braun & Clarke, 2006). This is a method for identifying, analysing and reporting themes within the information collected. It minimally organizes and describes the interview data in detail and interprets various aspects of the research topic (Boyatzis, 1998). The research was carried out ethically and with sensitivity and ethical approval was obtained from Coventry University and within the respective countries for all of the three projects. Participants were given an informed choice regarding the method of participation they wished to be involved with, which were either in focus groups and/or through individual semi-structured interviews. They were provided the opportunity to narrate their experiences in a way that aimed to be empowering. Focus groups were employed in the light of previous research (Perren-Klinger 1998) indicating that participants might be better able to disclose their experiences of conflict within a supportive network. To minimize the potential for distress and to maximize support for participants, snowballing sampling was utilized. In all three countries, survivors were already supporting each other in groups, and the research utilized these structures for interviews. Participants were also free to withdraw from the research at any time.

Two research projects were carried out in Kitgum and Gulu, northern Uganda and a third in the Eastern Democratic Republic of Congo (DRC). The research team in Eastern DRC included myself (a Clinical Psychologist), Henny Slegh (a medical anthropologist and psychotherapist), Benoit Ruratotoye (Clinical Psychologist and Director of the Institute of Higher Education in Mental Health in Goma), as well as Charlotte and Estelle, two Congolese women interpreters. There were well-established relationships with the Institute of Higher Education in Mental Health in Goma, who trained counsellors in Eastern DRC, and had good links with survivor groups in the area. To maximize support for survivors, volunteer participants were recruited through these existing relationships. Ethical clearance for the project was provided through the administration structures for Goma and Bweremana. In northern Uganda, I worked together with Ms Gladys Canogura, Director, and Mr Geoffrey Ochola at Kitgum Women's Peace Initiative, KIWEPI, for both research projects. KIWEPI are a non-governmental organization based in Kitgum that provide peace-building and conflict-resolution services for survivors as well as reproductive health provision for women and girl war survivors of sexual and gender-based conflict violence. They are well established in Northern Uganda and have excellent relationships with survivors and service providers, which assisted with recruitment and safety structures for volunteer participants. In the research with former child abductees I also worked together with Professor Bruce Baker, Chair of African Security at Coventry University, and for the project investigating the trauma counselling services in Kitgum and Gulu, the research team comprised KIWEPI, Dr Laura Davidson, a barrister from London, and me. Ethical approval was obtained from the Uganda National Council for Science and Technology for both of the projects carried out in Uganda and also from the Peter C Alderman Foundation for the research evaluating the trauma counselling services.

Experiences of survivors of conflict sexual and gender-based violence and torture in the Great Lakes region

Research carried out in August 2011 uncovered women's and girls' experiences of bearing children from rape and the health and justice service responses in Eastern Democratic Republic of Congo (DRC). During a two-week period, we listened to over 110 participants including survivors as well as health and justice professionals, in individual semi-structured interviews and focus group discussions carried out in Goma and rural Bweremana (Liebling *et al.* 2012; Liebling & Slegh, 2012).

Women and girls narrated experiencing sexual violence and rape, including gang rape. Of those interviewed individually, approximately 81 per cent were younger than 18 years when they were raped. Survivors were raped in a variety of locations, for example in a forest, on the family farm, going to the market, travelling to or from work, at home, at an internally displaced persons camp, or going to or from school. Women were also forced to witness violence and torture. Some survivors were abducted and others raped by an armed perpetrator. However, a frequent problem for many survivors we spoke to was not being able to identify the type of perpetrator (military personnel were often plain clothed, and community members sometimes wore uniforms). For those survivors who were 18 years and over, the perpetrators were more likely to be rebels or soldiers and the rapes were mostly carried out as gang rapes in forests. One woman was raped by a civilian while a policeman held a gun to her head. Although most adult women reported being raped by armed personnel, the research concluded that sexual violence had also 'contaminated' communities, particularly for girls less than 18 years old who were assaulted by community members.

The research found that families, relatives, and communities, including other children, 'mocked' the children born from rape. They were stigmatized along with their mothers, considered outcasts, harassed, beaten, and rejected (Ward & Marsh, 2006; Women for Women International, 2010). In the words of Marianne, an 18-year-old survivor of rape interviewed in Goma:

> I am a woman with a bad reputation. I am a woman without value, they look down on me, are disgusted with me. How can I get rid of this bad reputation?
> (Liebling & Slegh, 2012: 3)

Rape survivors reported very conflicting emotions towards the children conceived by rape, wanting to love them and viewing them as helpful for society, but also a constant reminder of the traumatic rape and social rejection they endured. Survivors described their children conceived through rape as 'depressed, not at peace, angry and outcasts' that were unable to attend school due to discrimination as well as poverty, and they therefore lacked skills and were at risk of becoming street children and led into the illegal or informal black economy. Women and girl rape survivors reported extreme poverty leading to an inability to continue with school, therefore lacking a means to earn a living and pay education fees. There were strong feelings that unless survivors and their children were supported, this could lead to serious problems including future violence and instability in Eastern DRC. Key informants expressed their view that the level of anger and rejection of large groups of children born as a result of rape could result in the formation of further rebel groups in the region. This assertion was also noted in previous research with former child abductees and conflict survivors in Northern Uganda (Liebling-Kalifani *et al.* 2008; Liebling-Kalifani & Baker, 2010a).

Survivors narrated the serious impact of sexual violence and bearing a child from rape on their reproductive, gynaecological, and obstetric health. This included developing vesico-vaginal fistula, sexually transmitted diseases, and problems with menstruation including abnormal bleeding, pain (including severe abdominal pain), cysts, HIV infection, AIDS, and long-term disabilities. Longombe *et al.* (2008) describe that genital fistulae are one of the most dreaded outcomes of the trauma resulting from sexual violence. Fistula leads to uncontrollable leakage of urine or faeces (or both) through the vagina. This is a highly stigmatizing condition for survivors who have already endured rejection by their communities. Our research also uncovered the dangers of young girls delivering a child when their bodies were not mature as this could result in rupture of the uterus and death of the baby. Additional gynaecological health risks were associated with illegal abortions. Malnutrition was also a prevalent problem as an indirect consequence of being unable to eat and therefore being unable to breastfeed their children. As a result of being unable to produce milk due to starvation and poverty, survivors' babies and children were undernourished and frequently ill. Sexually transmitted diseases were also prevalent amongst rape survivors, as Faridah, a 29-year-old woman, described during a focus group held in Goma:

> The first effects were that I had sexually transmitted diseases and my health is not good. I am now weak. I am in a state where any disease can affect me and others can recognise I am sick and not strong and it is not possible to look for life. I am in such a state I have to go to the hospital when I am sick and I have to look for life so my children can survive and even myself as my husband rejected me and the children are not studying . . . it hurts inside.

The emotional effects of women's and girls' experiences had a negative impact on their sense of self worth. Due to a lack of trust in others, particularly men, and fear of stigmatization, rape survivors kept their experiences to themselves. They reported psychological effects normally associated with traumatic experiences, including: depression; suicidal behaviours; anger; flashbacks; anxiety; disturbed sleep; withdrawal and avoidance; sexual concerns, and identity problems. The consequences for teenage girls of bearing a child from rape included a premature separation from childhood as they became overloaded with responsibilities. The relationship that rape survivors had with their child was extremely complex, and they described feelings of 'love and hate', which intensified their own and their child's psychological distress.

The poorly resourced health system struggled to respond to the serious physical and mental health needs of rape survivors and their children. The vast majority of survivors failed to access urgent health care within the required 72 and 48-hour timeframe, including emergency contraception and post-exposure prophylaxis, to reduce the risk of HIV infection. For those few who did, it was some time later or during delivery, and they reported a lack of adequate treatment and stated that free treatment stopped after delivery, when women and girls needed the most support. Survivors experienced fear and shame and were reluctant to report assaults, as they lacked trust in services. Others were unable to access treatment, particularly in rural areas because of poverty, lack of transport, and long distances to services. There were a few hospitals treating rape mutilations and fistula for women who were able to prove that they had been raped. Proving the rape placed both survivors and health professionals in an ethically compromised position. At the time the research was carried out, in Goma, government hospitals had no special services for raped women and were only able to provide basic health care. There were two referral hospitals run by non-government organizations (NGOs), Heal Africa and DOCS Hospital, for women who were suffering from injury and infection caused by violent rape. However, key informants told us that funding was strictly for girls who could prove they were raped. In rural areas the health coverage was significantly more limited.

Although some survivors received valuable counselling in Congolese 'listening houses', there was a lack of skilled, co-ordinated and culturally sensitive responses for their mental health needs and those of their children. Despite doing their best, health staff and counsellors described a severe lack of salaries, poor working conditions, and a lack of support and training to support survivors and their children. Many counsellors had in fact experienced rape themselves and were overburdened. They had no protection from the risks that their role entailed or access to support structures for dealing with their own stress and were therefore in danger of burn out.

In the context of such impunity and stigmatization the majority of survivors saw little to be gained from reporting sexual crimes. Adult women in particular preferred to remain silent. Young women frequently did not perceive that a crime had been committed and there was ignorance and confusion about the criminal justice procedure. A culture of sexual exploitation, including frequent rape of young girls, had become normalized. Girls told us that there was social pressure from family and communities to remain silent, although in some cases family members reported on behalf of their daughters due to a desire for financial gain from the perpetrator – if they could be identified. The challenges survivors faced included stigmatization, social rejection, and fear of the impact of reporting. For those in critical poverty, a lack of money to pay bribes limited the success of reporting. In some instances families came to an agreement where the perpetrator paid a fine to the survivor's family. In the worst-case scenario, as also found in Northern Uganda (Liebling-Kalifani & Baker, 2010a), survivors were married off to their perpetrators for a small financial reward to the girl's family. Recent changes in the law deemed it illegal to resolve rape cases through traditional community practices and survivors were encouraged to report through the state, but neither the state nor the community response resulted in a positive outcome for women or girls and the perpetrator was rarely punished.

The police, prisons, and criminal justice system suffered badly from a lack of funding and struggled with overwhelming logistical problems. Even if cases were reported, there were few skilled police and a lack of women officers. For the minority of cases that reached judgement, no compensation or reparation was provided by the government or by the perpetrator. The lack of trust in the process was one of the most important factors that led survivors to be reluctant to report cases. Survivors experienced the criminal justice process as traumatizing, increasing their shame and carrying personal risks, including attacks, death threats, and intimidation.

Similar themes were recorded in research with former girl and boy abductees conducted in Kitgum District in 2010 in Northern Uganda. This research examined the governance of sexual violence, where serious abuses were carried out during the 23-year Lord's Resistance Army rebellion and which was found to have high ongoing levels of local perpetrator sexual violence (Liebling-Kalifani & Baker, 2010a; Liebling-Kalifani & Baker, 2010b; Liebling, 2012). One woman former abductee during a focus group discussion held in Orom explained:

> We all accept that sexual violence during the time we were in captivity was the most common phenomenon. Normally in captivity the person who abducts you is the one who you are forced to accept as your husband until the person

is dead. That is what we experienced as young girls in captivity and this made many of us produce young children during these experiences.

(Liebling-Kalifani & Baker, 2010a: 7)

In total, 51 men and 47 women abductees participated in the research, in groups and individually, in four parishes in Orom sub-county, Kitgum, Northern Uganda, as well as 6 women survivors in Kitgum. Each participant was asked about their experience of sexual violence and of criminal justice and health provision. We also carried out 85 semi-structured interviews with police, justice, and health officials, as well as with non-state providers of health, criminal justice, and policing services that examined their training, facilities, interviewing techniques, deployment of women officials, and success in bringing cases to a conclusion.

The research found that due to a range of factors, the poorly resourced state-health system struggled to respond to the serious health needs of survivors of sexual violence. As a result of inadequate quality and access to health care, survivors reported experiencing fear, stigma, and shame and were reluctant to report assaults. They lacked trust in services to provide confidentiality and support, found health staff absent from clinics, or when referred to the district hospital, were unable to afford transportation and treatment. For those few participants who did manage to access health care it usually comprised basic treatment with post-exposure prophylaxis and/or Panadol for pain. There were no medical doctors at Orom clinic, whilst the district hospital had only one medical superintendent. There were no specialist doctors such as a gynaecologist or surgeon and few survivors received any psychological support. As we had found during the research in Eastern DRC, many of the staff had themselves experienced sexual violence during and since the insurgency. They faced a lack of support, staff shortages, low salaries, and poor working conditions and required trauma counselling for their own experiences.

With respect to justice provision, survivors, criminal justice professionals and key informants were in agreement that the criminal justice system failed to provide justice for survivors of sexual violence in Kitgum. This was partly due to a culture of responding to sexual violence through local negotiation between families of both accused and survivor, which undermined the law's deterrent effect. Though the law regards aggravated rape as a capital offence and less serious cases as liable to life imprisonment, offenders knew that most cases would be settled locally. Should a case enter the criminal justice system, bribes had to be paid to the police, police doctor and magistrate to ensure that the case went unprosecuted. This bypassing of the criminal justice system was further aggravated by survivors' own shame and fear about familial rejection and community stigmatization, the distance and expense of accessing the police, police doctor and court, and by a lack of trust in the police.

Similar to the situation found in Eastern DRC, where cases were actually reported, there were few skilled police officers and a lack of women officers to respond. The police were short of transportation and unable to take survivors (and the accused) to the central police station, police doctor, and the court. Hence cases collapsed due to the failure to obtain a doctor's report within the crucial post-rape 48 hours, or because witnesses and survivors failed to appear in court. There was limited confidential space for interviewing survivors in police stations and officers had received little training in handling cases of sexual violence and were unqualified to gather evidence. Of those crimes reported to the police few ended up with successful prosecution. Some failed as the case was prolonged and survivors gave up, others were dropped due to bribery of officials. Even those that made it to court often failed, as files were lost, witnesses failed to appear and evidence offered by the police was inadequate. The courts suffered from understaffing and normally there was only one senior magistrate to hear 'simple' cases of rape.

A further research project investigated the experiences of survivors and service providers of trauma services in Northern Uganda and examined their implications for mental health policy and legislation (Liebling *et al.* 2014; Liebling *et al.* 2016). In 2008 the Peter C. Alderman Foundation partnered with the Government of Uganda, Makerere Medical School, and Butabika National Psychiatric Referral Hospital, the Catholic Church, and local NGOs to open psychological trauma centres in Tororo, Soroti, Gulu, and Kitgum in Northern Uganda. There were also a few NGOs providing services. This includes Transcultural Psychosocial Organization (TPO), an organization that provides mental health services in conjunction with the ministry of health, particularly for women and children conflict survivors of violence and abuse, providing some short-term counselling. The service facilities where we carried out the interviews were staffed by a small number of social workers, psychiatric clinical officers, psychiatrists, psychologists, and nurses. Psychologists tended in the main to be employed by NGOs rather than in government hospitals.

The research was carried out in June 2013 with the assistance of KIWEPI. In total, the researchers interviewed 35 participants, including 20 survivors of sexual and gender-based violence, torture, and human rights abuses during conflict and/or abduction (10 men and 10 women) that had accessed services for at least one year, as well as 15 key informant providers of trauma services. These were carried out through individual semi-structured interviews in Kitgum, Gulu, and Kampala.

Men and women survivors who attended services had suffered torture including burning and bomb attacks, sexual violence, as well as other conflict-related experiences during abduction by Alice Lakwena in 1986–87 and/or the Lord's Resistance Army led by Joseph Kony. Many were forced to commit and witness atrocities, including the brutal killing of loved ones. Most related understandable traumatic effects, including severe depression and suicidal feelings leading to isolation and loneliness, anger, nightmares, flashbacks, and low self-esteem. Many we spoke to described experiencing severe pain, which they related were sometimes considered by service providers they accessed to be a way they expressed their psychological distress rather than their physical health problems being adequately treated. Several interviewees accessed the support of religious organizations, visited traditional healers and took herbs or engaged in local cultural rituals, prior to accessing trauma services. Prayer was used for ongoing support in conjunction with mental health services. Most had a desire for redress and felt angry and let down by the lack of support, access to justice and social needs. Participants related that since returning from Internally Displaced People's camps, land disputes had dramatically increased, exacerbating traumatic effects, particularly suicide rates among men.

Survivors' access to medication and counselling varied in duration and quality. Antidepressants, sleeping tablets and anti-psychotic medication were frequently prescribed for trauma-related difficulties and insomnia. Interviewees lacked knowledge and understanding about the purpose of the medication. However, it was clear that trauma services served to restore hope in survivors. Counselling extended up to a maximum of 11 sessions, but survivors had to travel for long distances to access them and poverty-restricted regular access. Although a survivor could rarely choose the gender of the counsellor, they voiced the universal appreciation of a listening ear and professional advice. Group counselling tended to be offered after individual counselling, which survivors valued since it helped them realize that their experiences were shared, thus decreasing isolation as they had others to provide them with social support. On occasions in Kitgum staff were unavailable and clinic hours were limited due to a lack of resources and competing demands from Nodding Disease,[1] which had affected large numbers of children in the district. In rural areas it was reported that there was a severe lack of counselling, support and professional expertise, and the outreach provided to rural areas was limited. Stigma and abuse towards survivors in communities negatively affected service access and undermined healing and in some instances, survivors left their communities due to the harassment they experienced.

Survivors expressed a desire for a holistic approach to their difficulties, including the following: regular provision of medication; counselling; vocational opportunities and financial support; school fees for their children. They expressed concern that most organizations that were providing services during the conflict had left the region as it was viewed by them that the emergency had subsided, although there was still conflict in the area as a result of land disputes and attacks by the Karamajong. Alcohol use was common as a way of coping with trauma, especially by men and male adolescents, and this exacerbated levels of domestic violence. Survivors felt medication and counselling in combination with having productive work helped to combat preoccupation with their traumatic experiences and their impact. Key informants and survivors indicated that discrimination and stigma in communities was very high and particularly directed towards those living with HIV/AIDS and former abductees, leading to an exacerbation of trauma. Survivors who were abducted during the LRA insurgency felt let down by the government due to the lack of justice, compensation, and support provided for them. These unfulfilled basic needs limited the progress that could be made through counselling and medication alone. The lack of criminal justice services including policing meant there was very limited provision for investigation and prevention of atrocities and human rights abuses. Criminal justice and police services were also susceptible to corruption and lacked gender sensitivity in their approach to survivors.

Service providers felt that there was a lack of understanding, country-wide, of the traumatic effects of conflict. Those service providers we spoke to felt they were doing their best to rebuild trust between themselves and survivors, but were unable to meet the overwhelming service demand. Service providers indicated that they were doing their best to empower local health services and provide group counselling, including education and problem-solving approaches, but felt that services needed to be extended to cover all the districts in Northern Uganda. There were insufficient numbers of experienced mental health professionals to provide quality trauma counselling services, and it was felt that more psychologists were needed to help build the capacity of village health teams in the rural areas.

Many spoke about the increasing rates of suicide in the region, particularly amongst young men in Gulu. Service providers demonstrated care for clients and experienced feelings of frustration and disappointment when unable to improve survivors' situations and distress. They related dealing with their own traumatic experiences, and as a result, burn out and secondary trauma was common. They expressed a desire for more skills development and training, including more regular refresher training, support, and supervision. They also described several problems that affected service access, including transport difficulties, poverty, stigma, and peer pressure, in addition to a lack of knowledge within the population regarding the value of counselling. It was felt that greater access to logistics and long-term planning was required to carry out their role effectively and that a transport allowance as well as better career development would enhance their motivation. On the whole the service providers felt rewarded by positive responses to their individual and group interventions, and described their services as leading to a reduction in depression, greater empowerment and return to engagement in productive activities by survivors.

Although our study found that survivors and providers valued the services provided, it revealed that the medication supply for survivors with trauma-related problems was erratic with insufficient information given to service users regarding their function. There was no psychiatrist in Kitgum district and the coverage for Gulu was insufficient for the population, particularly given the increasing levels of suicide reported. Counselling was provided mainly in the town, with a limited number of sessions available. There was inconsistency in the meaning of 'counselling' and no accreditation of counsellors.

At the time when the research was being carried out, there was a national mental health policy in draft form, but with no specific policy for those with trauma-related difficulties. The mental health legislation had not been properly implemented due to a lack of infrastructure. Participants felt there was a lack of effective influence of knowledgeable mental health professionals, service users and providers, and legal policy makers. Some we spoke to felt there was a need for a greater understanding and political will to recognize the importance of trauma services and provision in Uganda. They voiced a need to improve ethical practice and professional boundaries in trauma counselling as well as the accreditation of professionals. There was an urgent need for justice and police services to increase prevention, investigation and prosecution of those who committed atrocities and abused survivors' rights, as well as a need to manage corruption and increase gender sensitivity.

What can we learn from the voices of people living the conflict?

Interviews carried out with survivors of conflict and post-conflict sexual and gender-based violence and torture, and with service providers provided several significant themes relevant to service provision. The research highlighted the devastating impact of sexual violence and bearing a child from rape, on the reproductive, obstetric and gynaecological health of survivors. Chronic and degrading health consequences including fistulae and HIV infection further stigmatize survivors and impact whole communities. Health provision requiring proof of rape in DRC negates the rights of survivors to make informed choices and puts health care staff in difficult ethical situations. The illegal status of abortion in this region of Africa restricts service access and limits informed choice and improvements in this area, and remains a key priority. Access to reproductive and mental health services could be provided in rural areas through donor funding of mobile clinics. If safe abortions were made available to survivors, it would provide informed choice regarding decisions about their futures. However, this issue is very sensitive within African cultural contexts and it is recommended that this debate could helpfully include recognition of a survivor's mental and physical health difficulties following rape. Some former male abductees in Northern Uganda also disclosed they were rape survivors, and this subject requires further sensitive research and attention by policy makers and service providers (Liebling-Kalifani & Baker, 2010a).

It is argued that the diagnosis of post-traumatic stress disorder (PTSD) is not a meaningful way to understand the effects of survivors' experiences in an African context, and it is therefore contested. PTSD is a medical, non-gendered concept that does not effectively account for the social and cultural realities of the survivors we listened to. Previous research in Uganda and Eritrea found that services for conflict survivors tend to be based on the 'medicalization of distress' rather than a considered understanding and approach based on conflict survivors' own views, experiences, and needs as well as their strengths and resilience (Almedom & Glandon, 2007; Liebling-Kalifani, 2010). Although our research suggests that conflict survivors may have psychological effects that could be partly understood within what has been termed a 'complex Post Traumatic Stress Disorder' model (Herman, 1992), it is argued that trauma arising from exposure to such human rights violations is 'normal', not 'pathological' (Tal, 1996; Summerfield, 1997; Liebling-Kalifani, 2009). Some survivors in our study described long-term traumatic effects, which we therefore argue also requires recognition as 'normal' by service providers and policy makers (Liebling-Kalifani, 2010; Summerfield, 2000). Analysis of research data demonstrated that the effects of conflict, sexual violence, and torture are gendered, that is, although men, women and children endure these experiences, their responses are different. For example, suicide rates and substance use particularly amongst young male former abductees in Northern Uganda were found to be a significant concern (Liebling *et al*. 2014; Liebling *et al*. 2016). In contrast we found that women conflict survivors reconstruct their identities following violence and torture experiences. However, the enduring impact of conflict experiences on women and girls are equally valid as those on men and boys, and are therefore also deserving of compensation and facilities for recovery, as has historically been awarded to male soldiers (Liebling-Kalifani, 2009).

The research carried out demonstrates that beyond the individual's trauma, the impact of conflict, sexual violence and torture affects whole communities and identities. The types of sexual violence and atrocities carried out caused destruction of cultural norms and respectability codes that are important within the communities. Women and girls, as carriers of ethnic and community knowledge, values and practices and bearers of honour for men, were targeted for sexual dishonour and cultural disruption. However, women and girls, who were the main objects of attack, resisted the breakdown of their cultural identity, not only physically and militarily, for example in Luwero by taking up arms to protect themselves from rape, but also socially, psychologically, and culturally, by educating their children born from rape, supporting each other through activism and income-generation groups (Liebling-Kalifani & Baker, 2010b).

The atrocities carried out in Luwero caused a destruction of social capital where social devastation had dramatic effects on gender roles. Death, sickness, injuries and torture of relatives, friends and neighbours caused a social absence of men (Liebling-Kalifani, 2009). Samuel, a worker in a non-government organization, described how the war changed relationships between women and men:

> The situation has left women as breadwinners because many men died. As the social structures have been destroyed the family head traditionally should be the man but now the woman takes over the role. Even if the man is there he does not have the moral authority to give direction to the family, as he cannot provide for them. He could not defend his own children and family, many of who were abducted, in front of his own eyes. That is quite dehumanising for a man and has a lot of psychological effects.

It was found that during conflict in Luwero, men were targeted in particular for annihilation by torture and murder. Significantly greater numbers of men died leaving behind widows and orphans (Liebling-Kalifani, 2009). Young male abductees interviewed in Northern Uganda were forced to carry out acts of sexual violence and some were also subjected to sexual violence. Boys were forced to take girls as wives after proving themselves as soldiers and some reported being raped themselves, as this man narrated during a focus group in Orom:

> The LRA [Lord's Resistance Army]) was full of sexual violence and harassment particularly of young girls. They also forced us as young men to loot

food and we were sent to Arabs [Sudanese soldiers] where the Arabs demanded sex in exchange for food.

(Liebling-Kalifani & Baker, 2010a: 7)

Liebling-Kalifani and Baker (2010a: 7) found that disclosure of sexual violence by men is an extremely sensitive issue in Africa and there are particular cultural influences that affect reporting, as a psychologist interviewed in Kitgum described:

The factors that affect men reporting are as follows. Firstly, cultural factors in our communities; men are supposed to be resilient and not weak; secondly, they may not be aware that they can be helped and they feel there are no solutions to their problems, and finally it is an abomination within our community to be raped as a man; it is not manly and the survivor would be 'cast out'.

Research in Eastern DRC (Liebling *et al.* 2012) argued that it was important to note that sexual violence occurred against men and boys in the region and that interventions should be sensitive to this (Christian *et al.* 2011). Following our research, groups for male perpetrators were established to promote changes in attitudes and behaviour towards male victims and these are producing encouraging results (The International Bank for Reconstruction Development/The World Bank, 2014).

The research highlights the resilience of survivors and their ability, even after highly traumatic experiences, to reconstruct new identities. In Luwero, the use of drama, links with international women's groups, and income-generating schemes were found to contribute positively to the development of collective empowerment and positive growth (Liebling-Kalifani, 2010). In Kitgum those who became pregnant as a result of sexual violence focused on securing work to educate their children and this helped them to manage their depression and suicidal feelings (Liebling & Baker, 2010a). Girls in Eastern DRC who became pregnant from rape were brought together by women's organizations to form support groups that assisted in reducing suicidal feelings and distress (Liebling *et al.* 2012).

What also emerges from our research is a strong desire for justice among survivors. Despite the gross level of human rights abuses and torture of women, men, and children during conflicts, there has been a failure to address the injustices, and attempts to seek justice is fraught with risk and complexities and rarely results in a positive outcome for survivors. Despite their suffering, women have been active campaigners for peace and active in presidential elections. Their role in national liberation struggles, in guerrilla warfare or in the military has varied, but generally international research has still tended to view them in a supportive and nurturing relation to men, even when they have taken most risks (Yuval-Davis, 1985). Feminist analyses of women's roles by Anthias and Yuval-Davis (1989), Lovell (2003), Liebling-Kalifani (2010) and Liebling-Kalifani and Baker (2010b) enable us to view women's contributions during and following conflict as active agents. This research argues that conflict survivors demonstrate resilience, resistance and power. It is therefore important that researchers, policy makers and service providers promote conflict and post-conflict responses that enhance the resilience and agency of survivors and communities, in order for them to be most effective (Summerfield, 2000).

There is a pressing need for a holistic response for survivors with improved professional structures for service providers. In order to be successful, services need to be rights-based, and in addition to providing sexual and gynaecological health services and psychosocial support, they also need to facilitate access to criminal justice and social support structures whilst at the same time building resilience and assisting with the reconstruction of the identities of survivors and their communities. There is growing evidence that this model of post-conflict reconstruction promotes healing in communities (Summerfield, 2000). As our previous research with women conflict survivors in Liberia argues:

> It requires health and justice service provision that conceptualises conflict sexual violence as gendered, incorporates a resilience framework for under-standing survivor's needs. The most appropriate developmental approach to the delivery of health and justice in post-conflict conditions is one that recog-nizes the differing nature of states and the presence of multiple providers whose services are layered to meet differing contingencies.
>
> (Liebling-Kalifani & Baker, 2010b: 196–97)

Conclusion

I argue for the importance of placing the voices of survivors of conflict and post-conflict related human rights abuses central in the security debate. The research carried out has highlighted that atrocities including sexual and gender-based violence continue once conflict ends and protection of communities at this critical time is often lacking. Humanitarian service provision may also have ceased, to the detriment of survivors. In research carried out with former abductees in Northern Uganda the authors investigated 'health and justice' provision together as:

> Sexual violence was experienced simultaneously as a violation of the survi-vors' body and rights. It left the survivor in need of both a health and a justice response. As the two are connected in the experience of the survivor so they go hand in hand in terms of service responses required. We therefore argue that there is real value in promoting increased collaboration between local health and justice services.
>
> (Liebling-Kalifani & Baker, 2010a: 52)

This chapter argues that it is imperative that the needs of survivors and their children born as a result of sexual violence are addressed holistically in line with their wishes; with provision of gender-sensitive physical and psychological health care including regular provision of medication and counselling if desired, opportunities for employment, meaningful 'justice', safety and financial support, especially school fees for the children. Our research found trauma services served to restore hope and reduce depression for survivors in Northern Uganda, and group counselling helped survivors realize their experiences were shared and decreased isolation. However, it is also argued that there is a limit to the progress survivors can make without meaningful 'justice'. Continued reconciliation processes in order to transform society following conflict are important here. Indeed, Rimé *et al.* (1992) argue that describing experiences to others can transform its representation so that it takes a less emotive form. This process assists survivors to gain a better sense of coherence, and social support and coping are also invaluable where a person's basic security is undermined (Liebling *et al.* 2014: Liebling *et al.* 2016).

Specialist reproductive health services with access to emergency contraception and post-exposure prophylaxis is required within the correct timeframe – as well as specialist fistula repair provision. It is important for service responses to be sensitive to gender differences, as well as addressing cultural influences, stigma, and shame as barriers to effective service access and responses. As Ahmed and Braithwaite (2006) argue, social relationships and shame management are central to the processes of restorative justice. In Eastern DRC, for example, girls spoke about social rejection by communities being particularly distressing. It is essential that all organizations treat survivors of sexual violence and children conceived from rape with respect, and increase their involvement in programmes. This would empower survivors and encourage acceptance whilst assisting communities to realize the issues are everyone's responsibility whilst combating social rejection and improving service responses. It is important that a model of care is developed for service providers, including effective professional supervision, counselling, and support to prevent compassion fatigue. Finally, service and policy developments would benefit from involving the expertise of survivors in all stages and put them at the very heart of their design and implementation.

Note

1 Nodding Disease or Nodding Syndrome is a little-known disease that emerged in Sudan in the 1960s. It is a mentally and physically disabling disease that only affects children, typically between the ages of 5 and 15. It is currently restricted to small regions of South Sudan, Tanzania, and Northern Uganda (WHO, 2016).

References

Ahmed, E. & Braithwaite, V. (2006) Forgiveness, reconciliation, and shame: Three key variables in reducing school bullying. *Journal of Social Issues*, 62, 2, 347–370.
Almedom, A. M. & Glandon, D. (2007) Resilience is not the absence of PTSD any more than health is the absence of disease. *Journal of Loss and Trauma: International Perspectives on Stress & Coping*, 12, 2, 127–143.
Askin, K. D. (2002–2003) The quest for post-conflict gender justice. 41 *Colum. Journal of Transnational Law*, 41, 3, 509–522. Available at: http://www.peacewomen.org/sites/default/files/reconpb_the_quest´_for_post-conflict_gender_justice_askin_2003_0.pdf

Boyatzis, R. E. (1998) *Transforming Qualitative Information: Thematic Analysis and Code Development*. Thousand Oaks, London, and New Delhi: Sage Publications.

Braun, V. & Clarke, V. (2006) Using thematic analysis in psychology. *Qualitative Research in Psychology*, 3, 77–101.

Christian, M., Safari, O., Ramazani, P., Burnham, G. & Glass, N. (2011) Sexual and gender based violence against men in the Democratic Republic of Congo: Effects on survivors, their families and the community. *Medicine, Conflict and Survival*, 27, 4, 227–246.

Herman, J. L. (1992) *Trauma and Recovery: The Aftermath of Violence: From Domestic Abuse to Political Terror*, New York: Basic Books.

Liebling, H. (2012) Experiences of a young girl abducted by the Lord's Resistance Army, Northern Uganda. *Psychology of Women Section Review*, 14, 1, spring, 44–48. British Psychological Society. Leicester.

Liebling-Kalifani, H. (2009) *A Gendered Analysis of the Experiences of Ugandan Women War Survivors*. Saarbrucken Germany: VDM Verlag Dr. Muller.

Liebling-Kalifani, H. (2010) Research and intervention with women war survivors in Uganda: Resilience and suffering as the consequences of war, in H. Bradby. & G. Lewando-Hundt (Eds) *War, Medicine and Gender: The Sociology and Anthropology of Structural Suffering*, Farnham Surrey: Ashgate Books.

Liebling-Kalifani, H., Ojiambo-Ochieng, R., Marshall, A., Were-Oguttu, J., Musisi, S. & Kinyanda, E. (2008) Violence against women in Northern Uganda: The neglected health consequences of war. *Journal of International Women's Studies*, 9, 3, 174–192.

Liebling-Kalifani, H., & Baker, B. (2010a) Justice and health provision for survivors of sexual violence in Kitgum, Northern Uganda. *African Journal of Traumatic Stress*, 1, 1, 22–31.

Liebling-Kalifani, H., & Baker, B. (2010b) Women war survivors of sexual violence in Liberia: Inequalities in health, resilience and justice. *The Journal of International Social Research: Woman Studies Special Issue*, 3, 13, 188–199.

Liebling, H. & Slegh, H. (2012) *Bearing Children through Rape in Eastern Congo: Community and State Responses*. Addressing Inequalities: The Heart of the Post-2015 Development Agenda and the Future We Want for All. Global Thematic Consultation. UNICEF.

Liebling, H., Slegh, H., & Ruratotoye B. (2012) Women and girls bearing children through rape in Goma, Eastern Congo: Stigma, health and justice responses. *Itupale Online Journal of African Studies*, IV, 2012, 18–44.

Liebling, H., Davidson, L., Akello, F. G., & Ochola, G. (2014) Improvements to national health policy: Mental health, mental health bill, legislation and justice. *African Journal of Traumatic Stress*, 3, 2, 55–64.

Liebling H., Davidson, L., Akello, G. F., & Ochola, G. (2016) The experiences of survivors and trauma counselling service providers in northern Uganda: Implications for mental health policy and legislation. *International Journal of Law and Psychiatry*, 49, 84–92. AVilable at: http://dx.doi.org/10.1016/j.ijlp.2016.06.012.

Longombe, A. O., Claude, K. M. & Ruminjo, J. (2008). Fistula and traumatic genital injury from sexual violence in a conflict setting in Eastern Congo: Case studies. *Reproductive Health Matters*, 16, 31, 132–141.

Lovell, T. (2003) Resisting with authority: Historical specificity, agency and the performative self. *Theory, Culture & Society*, 20, 1, February 2003, 1–17. London, Thousand Oaks, and New Delhi: Sage Publications.

Manjoo, R. & McRaith, C. (2011) Gender-based Violence and justice in conflict and post-conflict areas. *44 Cornell International Law Journal*, 11. Hein Online. Available at:

http://heinonline.org/HOL/LandingPage?handle=hein.journals/cintl44&div=7&id=&page=

Perren-Klinger, G. (1998) *Self-Empowerment: Psychosocial Work by, with, and for Women: Work Hypothesis and Experiences*. Paper presented at a consultative meeting on gender leadership and trauma management for African women, Hotel Equatoria, Kampala, 16–19 November 1998.

Peterman, A., Palermo, T., & Bredenkamp, C. (2011) Estimates and determinants of sexual violence against women in the Democratic Republic of Congo. *American Journal of Public Health*, 101, 6, 1060–1067.

Rimé, B., Philippot, P., Boca, S. & Mesquita, B. (1992). Long-lasting cognitive and social consequences of emotion: Social sharing and rumination. *European Review of Social Psychology*, 3, 225–258.

Stark, L. & Wessells, M. (2012) Sexual violence as a weapon of war. *Journal of the American Medical Association*, 308, 7, 677–678.

Summerfield, D. (1997) Trauma is a dangerous label for a normal reaction. Challenging Western wisdom, *Recovery*, Jan/Feb, 1, 9–10.

Summerfield, D. (2000) War and mental health: A brief overview. *British Medical Journal*, 22, 321, 232–235. http://www.ncbi.nlm.nih.gov/pmc/articles/PMC1118225/

Tal, K. (1996) *Worlds of Hurt: Reading the literatures of Trauma*. Cambridge: Cambridge University Press.

The International Bank for Reconstruction Development/The World Bank. (2014) *Living Peace Groups Implementation Manual and Final Project Report: GBV Prevention and Social Restoration in the DRC and Burundi*. Prepared by Promundo-US for LOGiCA.

Ward, J. & Marsh, M. (2006) *Sexual Violence against Women and Girls in War and its Aftermath: Realities, Responses and Required Resources*. Briefing Paper presented in Brussels, Belgium.

Women for Women International, WFWI. (2010) *Briefing on Women's Status in DRC: July 2010. The Democratic Republic of Congo Survey: Stronger Women: Stronger Nations*.

World Health Organization. (2016) Nodding Syndrome (NS). Available at: http://www.who.int.onchoceriasis.symptoms (accessed on 13 November 2016).

Yuval-Davis, N. (1985) Front and rear: The sexual division of labour in the Israeli army. *Feminist Studies*, 11, 3, 649–676.

Yuval-Davis, N. (1989) National reproduction and 'The Demographic Race', in Israel in N. Yuval-Davis and F. Anthias (Eds) *Woman-Nation-State*, London: Macmillan.

4 Securing health in Afghanistan

Gender, militarized humanitarianism, and the legacies of occupation

Vanessa Farr

Introduction

This chapter reflects on the Polio Eradication Initiative (PEI), a long-term humanitarian intervention aimed at under-five-year-old children in Afghanistan, and teases out some of the implications of the lack of space in this well-funded initiative for the cadre of female Community Health Workers (FCHWs) who have been in place since 2003 to deliver Community Based Health Care (CBHC) services that, theoretically at least, form the foundation of the Basic Primary Health Services (BPHS) package, housed within the Ministry of Public Health (MoPH).[1] Brought in on two consultancies lasting from a few weeks to a few months to support the Ministry to better understand how CHWs might help advance the emergency programme's goal of permanently interrupting the transmission of the polio virus, I was able to undertake some travel beyond Kabul and could interview ordinary Afghan women and men about both the PEI and their overall access to health services – a level of exposure to daily life that is unusual for an outsider in the ongoing insecurity of Afghanistan.[2] This access gave me rich opportunities to observe, as a feminist peace activist with nearly two decades of experience in war-torn countries, how Afghanistan's gender-exclusionary social and political conditions, exacerbated by the civil wars and foreign military occupations that have ravaged the country for decades,[3] are implicated in the political economy of perpetual war. In what follows, I argue that this entwining of social and political conditions unfavourable to women, and their children, is an exemplary instance of what Rob Nixon identifies as 'slow' violence: that which, although it is hidden by the more spectacular and attention-commanding aspects of war, 'is not just attritional but also exponential, operating as a major threat multiplier' that 'fuel[s] long-term proliferating conflicts in situations where the conditions for sustaining life become increasingly but gradually degraded' (Nixon, 2009: 3).

Afghan religious and cultural norms and beliefs play an important part in either enabling or inhibiting good health practices, and families make decisions to prevent illness, maintain health or care for the infirm based on what they think is important and affordable. While healthcare decision-making may appear to be highly personal, it is in fact embedded in larger, although sometimes invisible or difficult-to-assess, social structures. These are inflected by gender ideologies, ethnicity, social class and other variables, and are influential on how decisions are made, and by whom. The emphasis placed in Afghanistan on women's confinement to the private sphere of the family is itself a form of slow violence against public health:[4] because of it, educational messages on children's health often target male decision-makers rather than women caregivers, with an unstated hope that mothers will also get the message along the way, probably through the mother-in-law.[5] In a country as geographically and politically complex as Afghanistan, the success of the BPHS depends on both community participation and support, and a partnership between community and health staff. On the ground, however, the reality is that the formal health apparatus is generally poor or inaccessible, so families and communities, as much as possible, look after their own health. From this perspective, the bedrock of the PEI is mothers, who are the primary caregivers of young children across Afghanistan.

Women, however, are largely excluded from the PEI. They represent a tiny minority of frontline workers who deliver pro-vaccination messages and administer the Oral Polio Vaccine (OPV) door-to-door; and they are nowhere to be found in the decision-making structures that have been set up to manage this complex health intervention. Their exclusion is particularly noticeable because the PEI has persistently failed to overcome the poor quality and low level of commitment of national health workers, which translates into a failure to reach its target of 100 per cent coverage of under-fives – thus constituting the kind of 'slow moving and long in the making' disaster Nixon is alert to (Nixon, 2009: 3). Those currently in charge are part of an entrenched cadre of permanent, salaried polio personnel – virtually all male – working in the national and provincial PEI structures, who in turn contract temporary, volunteer workers to support polio efforts such as National Immunization Days (NIDs) on an *ad hoc* basis. The success of Afghanistan's polio programme is compromised due to the overall poor performance of this team, and after decades of effort, the goal of reaching every child every time the OPV is offered, in every household, marketplace, shrine, health centre or transit station, has never been fully realized. This failure, too, is gendered: the common practice of sending pairs of young men door-to-door to deliver health messages and administer the OPV is fraught with cultural complexities. Women cannot open the door to or admit non-kin males into the family compounds where small children live; newborn babies may not be seen by anyone other than immediate family for 40 days after birth;[6] insecurity is high and there is general suspicion about strangers, and male household heads, who are the public decision-makers, sometimes hear oppositional messages to vaccination in the mosques, market places and when crossing the border into and out of Pakistan.[7]

Beyond a discussion of the impacts of the patriarchal social exclusion that shapes intimate life, a gendered political economy analysis of Afghanistan's health services is also crucial. Because of the vital importance of polio eradication for global health, PEI has attracted a steady, and significant, amount of funding; but such financial commitment carries a price tag of its own. Over the years of polio eradication efforts in a steadily deteriorating economy, some of the senior officials involved in the programme have used its resources to promote their own power. One reason for the lacklustre performance of polio workers, therefore, is that the selection of all levels of personnel suffers from interference from men in a position to influence appointments for personal gain. As a result, women – who are the best candidates for the job of communication, house-to-house OPV delivery and other key functions – have generally not been those who do the work or enjoy the accompanying incentives. For its part, the international community, funders of the PEI, has done little beyond a vaguely articulated rhetoric of 'consulting' or 'including' women', to challenge their obvious absence from the programme's delivery. The jarring inconsistency between the aims of this particular health intervention and its delivery, then, are no coincidence. Women, who have the highest chance of being able to enter households to find every child and support caregivers in making the choice to vaccinate all their children, neither gain from the financial opportunities working in the PEI brings, nor contribute in any systematic way to achieving its goals. From this perspective, the PEI is exemplary of neoliberal 'post-war' reconstruction efforts 'assailed', Nixon would observe, 'by coercion and bribery that test [a community's] cohesive resilience' (Nixon, 2009: 4). Rhetoric aside, such interventions do nothing to enhance women's ability to assess the circumstances in which they are living, extend their level of control and other influence over decision-making spaces and approaches, or improve their lives in a way that is consistent with promises made in the passage of United Nations Security Council Resolution (UNSCR) 1325 in 2000.[8]

Gendered exclusion and its impacts on community health

Efforts to improve the efficiency of the PEI draw from occasional surveys to identify how Afghans receive and understand the initiative's work.[9] Among the insights of a 2015 survey is that individuals are concerned and distrustful because the PEI sends strangers into their community. This is problematic because people most trust polio prevention and other health messages given to them in a form already familiar to them, by people they already know (family, friends and community members including those working at local health centres). Indeed, the approach taken for the delivery of both polio prevention messages and vaccines is often antithetical to the stated intention of promoting family health. While those who benefit financially from the PEI's over-reliance on men as frontline workers argue that it is appropriate and culturally responsive to send men out to vaccinate children, in reality, this practice enables powerful men to maintain and strengthen their patronage networks, and to dominate and misshape the PEI's purpose for their own ends. The distortion may be said to originate at MoPH level because of an intentional misalignment with the BPHS health pillar. As a result, the internationally driven[10] PEI programme has overlooked CHWs, an established, female-dominated health workforce that is managed by the BPHS and, theoretically, operates in communities across the country. Not only are already-mobilized and trusted CHWs not being supported to deliver the PEI, but leaving them out has negative ramifications well beyond polio eradication, undermining routine immunization and other related aspects of an already weak healthcare system rather than promoting sustainable, holistic repairs to it that would contribute to security and improved well-being in the future.

To phrase this problem differently, in the example of the PEI, gender-blindness on the part of the international community colludes in disconcerting ways with Afghanistan's own patriarchal praxis to undermine health delivery, in this instance, by bypassing mothers and those who can most effectively reach them, as the most reliable vectors of access to children. As this chapter discusses, PEI might be likened to one of 'the largely opaque collusions between transnational and national forces' driving slow violence (Nixon, 2009: 160). The challenges (both real and perceived) of working in Afghanistan appear to combine with an exagger-ated commitment to 'respect local culture' that enables donors to blindly endorse the approaches vouched for by men in authority, who argue, against the evidence, that giving a role to women would not be well-received. Rather than taking the time to investigate systems that were already in place, if largely invisible and often degraded as a result of localized corruption and mismanagement, and working judiciously to enlarge and strengthen them by developing a programme delivery format useful for basic healthcare as a whole, the PEI in Afghanistan has reinforced male dominance and patronage networks at every turn. Programme planners in the United Nations (UN) system have tried to deliver the PEI as a parallel humani-tarian intervention that can remain untethered from national development goals. Because of its importance and ability to attract sustained funding, the PEI could have played a central role in advancing long-term health-promotion and left a positive legacy from its spending that would continue to contribute to communities once the disease has finally been eliminated. This connection to the 'human secu-rity' aspects of delivering healthcare in highly unstable political conditions is insufficiently made, however; and as a consequence, UN entities appear complicit in undermining the Security Council's stated commitment to promoting peace by non-military means. The goal of increasing women's inclusion in conceptualizing new forms of security, as invited in SCR1325, should create practical opportunities for delivering interventions, including in the health sector, that are based on an 'ethic of care' capable of addressing 'the root causes of all unequal (not just gender) relations and biases . . . founded on the relations of care that exist at community level and through the actions of women and others as caregivers' in communities desperate to recover from, and find alternatives to, endless war (Hudson, 2012: 80–105).[11] In Afghanistan, however, such opportunities seem repeatedly to be overlooked and lost.

An overlooked opportunity: Female Community Health Workers

The earliest reports on maternal-child well-being that were prepared during the brief window of stability that followed the United States-led military intervention into the country in 2001, which then precipitated the (temporary) dislocation and rearrangement of Afghan warring factions including the Northern Alliance and the

Taliban, observe the 'staggeringly' high costs paid by women and children over decades 'of conflict, drought, political instability and isolation'.[12] One solution offered was to upgrade the capacities of existing Traditional Birth Attendants (TBAs) by re-skilling them with a broader portfolio and redeploying them as CHWs, while implementing urgent measures to improve institutional healthcare for women during pregnancy and in childbirth, and safeguarding their newborns. It is a nationally implemented approach intended to reach the poorest, most marginal and most precarious in the population. While men play a crucial support role, the system's focus is squarely on women and their children. In other words, the design of the CHW system exactly matches the goals of the PEI: it is intended to provide families with access to a very basic type of community-based healthcare that starts before birth, and therefore operates at the level needed if the PEI is to reach all Afghan children.

The CHW system has to function inside Afghanistan's severely constricting patriarchal system with its core emphasis on women's seclusion and constricted public movement. As a result, it has been built in such a way that it can get around some of the problems associated with accessing women and their children. It makes sense in its context and is trusted by Afghans, including in the very conservative parts of the country. As such, it provides an effective, if very basic, method to respond to the critical situation in women's health (and in the well-being of their children) that results from entrenched restrictions on their access to any public space, even including community-based health services. As such constraints continue to affect women's health-seeking behaviours today,[13] the household-level CHW programme remains unusual in operating through mobilizing female capacities to work in women's interests.[14]

To overcome limitations on women's freedom of movement, the structure calls for a *mahram* male and female CHW (MCHW and FCHW) pair,[15] elected by the village *shura* (council), to serve the community's basic health needs on a voluntary basis.[16] Women had long been able to serve community health needs as TBAs; so when Afghanistan followed WHO guidelines and disallowed TBA work in 2003, a large number of them elected to become CHWs. They could only do this only if they were able to convince a male family member to act as *mahram*. In the early days of the CHW programme, then, recruitment appears to have been driven through *women* with some community reputation for dealing in family health concerns, not through men.

Numbering in the tens of thousands, CHWs were never intended to become official, salaried, or in any other way regulated workers within the MoPH. This factor remains crucial today: the system's inclusion of women seems to be possible because theirs was always conceived of as a voluntary role, and while FCHWs do gain community recognition and status, it accrues to them privately as positive role models and influencers in their families and village networks, not through elevating them into publicly visible leadership roles – which, requiring an accumulation of wealth and influence beyond the immediate family, would mark them out as highly unusual women.[17] Ironically, what was originally a financially prudent decision in a system that simply cannot afford to pay health workers, has proven to be an important factor in keeping women engaged and CHW work firmly focused on women's well-being. Women-to-women health service delivery, as humble as it is, remains possible not only because women can be comfortably associated with the care-giving aspects of health-related service, but because voluntary work is regarded as an appropriate expression of piety. Its vital practical importance to women and their children aside, CHW work is a low-status enough social activity to keep attention off its practitioners.[18] The CHW system is also unlike other interventions that try to focus on promoting women's well-being, because it recognizes that men can be encouraged to support women and children if they can do so in ways they accept as culturally appropriate. Men's dominance can remain unchallenged because the MCHW's backing is essential for the FCHW to do her work, and he remains in control of the public aspects of CHW service such as writing reports and negotiating with other men when women need help beyond what the village health post can deliver. Within the constraints of the patriarchal political economy of Afghanistan, therefore, it can be argued that the existing CHW system offers an ingenious indigenous response to the problem of enabling women, and through them children, to access a basic level of healthcare service.

Whatever successes the CHW system has achieved are possible because it is highly localized and draws on the voluntary support of community members who enjoy a good level of respect. The importance of this fact cannot be over-estimated given Afghanistan's decades-long history of armed conflict, which has destroyed basic education, produced deep levels of suspicion of outsiders and underlies hyper-vigilance about messages that try to instil new behaviours. The household level of their work is made possible because of the *mahram* pair approach, and communities highly appreciate that they are served by both a woman and a man in matters of basic health decision-making.[19] As a health official in put it in a field interview in a basic health post on the outskirts of Jalalabad:

> . . . *a scared, hungry, poor, uneducated person forgets messages easily. What people do remember is house-to-house visits from familiar people. Routine contact is good.*[20]

Given the tightly knit structure of Afghan society and suspicion resulting not only from direct experiences of conflict but also encounters with conflict-related disinformation, rumours, moral panics and propaganda, it is unsurprising that communities want to receive healthcare within structures and through formats they trust. However, contrary to what communities recognize and endorse, PEI work conducted to date has only peripherally engaged with the CHW system and failed to recognize the pitfalls of using predominantly male social mobilizers as well as male-only pairings of vaccinators to build community support for polio eradication. This challenge aside, there are other complex difficulties affecting the success of the PEI that entrench women's exclusion from decision-making about child health.

Economic uncertainty and PEI as an 'income-generating activity'

The majority of Afghans, caught as they are in both local and 'international feedback loop[s] of corruption and repression' (Nixon, 2009: 81), face extreme impoverishment and very limited legitimate income-generating opportunities. In this economic reality, the PEI's use of regular NIDs, through which a wide network of people are paid to deliver the OPV, has become regarded as a fairly predictable income source. Afghans jokingly talk of 'polio and poppies' as the two economic activities available to them, and refer to NIDs as 'National Income Days', but this apparent levity disguises an uncomfortable set of practices that have arisen around the PEI as a well-resourced health initiative. Because money changes hands in the course of NID campaigns, complex patronage networks appear to have evolved around who gains access to PEI assets.[21] As a result, some of those who are invited to 'volunteer' for NIDs may assume that their closeness to their employer makes them unaccountable. Indifference to the need to reach every child with OPV every time it is offered, and inefficiency in recording either a successful vaccination process or why some children are missed – which are crucial factors in designing revisit strategies – are system-wide. Distressingly, in fieldwork interviews the suspicion was raised that obstructing the goal of eradicating polio is acceptable in order to keep the money associated with the PEI flowing.

Culturally sanctioned and justified exclusions

Because patronage networks may be over-determining recruitment and remuneration policies, the inefficient delivery of OPV can be easily excused as a 'necessary evil' rooted in cultural constraints on women's participation in public economic activity; unsurprisingly in Afghanistan, gender inequalities play a fundamental role in undermining the eradication of polio. Men, protecting male patronage networks, argue that women cannot be deployed for NIDS for reasons they ascribe to Afghan culture. Yet it is demonstrably inefficient to send male-only pairs from household to household to deliver the OPV: men outside the family kinship network, who cannot enter the private space of an Afghan compound, cannot always determine the number and age of children in the household, and rely instead on what an older child at the doorstep can tell them about his or her younger siblings. As (predominantly male) vaccinators are currently paid per number of households reached and try to achieve a daily quota, the evidence shows that inadequate effort is being made to reach children who are not obviously around. Sleeping, sick, absent or newborn children, the children invisible to non-kin males, are missed in every campaign. There are relatively elaborate checks-and-balances to record which children do not receive their OPV dose, and these go some way to ensuring that revisit strategies in the days after a NID are successful. But when the overall emphasis is on speed and numbers rather than the thoroughness that would come from actually going inside a compound to talk to mothers and meet all their infant children, missed households may not even be properly revisited after campaigns.[22]

It is difficult not to conclude that opportunities for better practice have been ignored because changes might undermine male patronage networks, especially because there is good evidence that women, when they have been included, make a worthwhile contribution to advancing PEI goals. In those urban areas in which women are working during NIDs, there are extremely positive reports of their efficiency and determination to reach every child in every household, including accounts that they take time to win over reluctant caregivers and diligently revisit households in which children were missed. A re-thinking of the PEI approach from an informed gender analysis of the conditions for delivering an effective programme is therefore a necessity, not an external imposition, a distraction or an irrelevancy, as both male Afghan officials and UN-contracted doctors and other personnel interviewed in the course of fieldwork often tried to imply.

Trust-building and positive caregiving

An extremely high child mortality rate (a tragedy with multiple causes) may have produced a fatalistic approach to children's well-being in Afghanistan.[23] Yet attitudes surveys indicate a profound mistrust in a stressed population that any formal or government-backed interventions are positively intended, especially when those delivering them are remunerated. People find it difficult to believe that help is available without codicils or hidden prices, which is not surprising given reports that some corrupt health officials insist on payment for free services, and even accounts that people are allowed to die if no payment is forthcoming. While such distrust is unsurprising in a generationally war-torn society, the lesson is that health delivery has to be as much a psychological, or perhaps spiritual and philosophical endeavour, as it is a practical, scientific effort to eradicate diseases such as polio in Afghanistan. Yet little thought is given to how to build trust and optimism through a health delivery approach that demonstrates to caregivers that their children are more than numbers on a list, and have the right to health.[24]

Women in the BPHS

At the time of writing, the female-focused structure of the BPHS appears to be both entrenched and delivering – to a greater extent than any other form of intervention – access to health to women and their children across the country. At this point, then, female CHWs are the largest (if unregulated) mobilized group of women working for a public system in Afghanistan. Can their influence be preserved and enlarged, and their status and efficacy as basic deliverers of community health be enhanced, without endangering individuals or their work as a whole?

A question raised in the field research for this analysis is whether the delicate balance in which the CHW system currently operates is beginning to change and might be too radically or rapidly modified as UNICEF, the WHO and other organizations become more interested in working with CHWs. In particular, there are important concerns to consider before deciding how (and whether) to change the remuneration or incentives CHWs receive, or to scale up CHW work. At the base of the CHW system is equilibrium between what women and men do, and how their inputs and knowledge are valued. Given how patriarchal exclusion operates in Afghanistan, there is a very real danger that placing too much emphasis on CHWs, or appearing to overly enlarge the space they currently occupy, might in fact distort and undermine the purpose of CHW work, and even lead to women's exclusion from it in future.[25]

It appears that some shift away from women at the centre of the CHW system has already begun. As is remarked earlier, while the earliest female CHWs were recruited from the ranks of women who had served as TBAs, i.e., had some pre-existing status in community life as health workers, it seems that some new FCHWs enter the system not through their own established interest in working on health issues, but because a male with whom they are *mahram* is elected by the village health *shura* as the MCHW. MCHWs, in this new paradigm, receive their appointment because of their relative literacy or because they are in some way distinguished (a successful farmer or businessman), or merely because they are linked in a patronage relationship with the village headman and their CHW service enhances existing hierarchies of power.

In interviews, it was clear that more recently appointed female and male CHWs bring very different value systems to their work. Males see themselves as the authoritative member of the CHW pair because they are both male and literate. The fact that non-literate women have to report information for them to pass on, in the view of these men, appropriately places and maintains females in a deferential role. Even if they are not the primary contact point for women asking for health advice and support, the fact that a male CHW records any information that needs to be written down entrenches his sense of superiority: in the prevailing masculinist value system, being able to record data is prized, but not the collection of the information itself, which is merely 'women's work' involving FCHWs talking to other women.

A similar dismissal of women as having agency in knowledge production and use is seen when male CHWs are asked to express their views on women in their role as caregivers of children. Asked why they thought children were being missed in PEI NIDs, they tended to blame women for 'being too ignorant' to avail their children of healthcare services. Even beyond MCHWs, men in official roles gave little consideration to whether the messages or the approach of the campaign were improperly calibrated to reach all caregivers, and seemed surprised when they were asked whether ineffective methods of communications might be a factor in the PEI's failure to reach its goals.[26]

Female CHWs, by contrast, give very different answers to these questions. They defer to men's role as scribes but proudly report on their capacity to remember the names and ailments of people they treat, and value their memory for detail and their ability to recall and apply the information they learn in training courses. They appear to place little value in the written reporting that male CHWs do – this is just a detail for them; knowing what to do to help someone in distress is more important.

Asked about what makes caregivers miss getting their children vaccinated through campaigns, they were much more interested in interrogating the process than in blaming any individual responses. They tended to believe that caregivers (especially women) had simply not had enough time to internalize PEI messages or were not being helped to influence other decision-makers. Their insight is supported by reflections made by female frontline workers in the PEI campaign, who observed that some caregivers are simply not receptive to health interventions unless they are convinced through patient, time-consuming face-to-face dialogue about why they should subscribe. They saw this interaction as an important part of their workload and reported it as a successful tactic when facing vaccine refusal from a parent.[27]

Volunteerism under threat?

The growing prominence of MCHWs – if perhaps only, at this point, discursively – is leading to questions about whether the 'voluntary' basis of the CHW system should be maintained in the future. It is difficult to gauge the extent to which the monetized approach of PEI NIDs – which pay people for their campaign work but continue to describe them as 'volunteers' – has brought about a changed perspective on the delivery of healthcare as a whole, but it was clear from their responses that both male and female CHWs know that working for the PEI, as a specific health intervention, brings in regular money. They feel confused, excluded and slighted because they are told that they should not expect remuneration for the work they do, beyond the tiny stipend they receive for attending training workshops. Then they find themselves excluded from earning the money available through NID payments. MCHWs were clear that they lacked access to patronage networks that allowed some men to benefit from paid PEI work, while FCHWs seemed not to know how the system worked, beyond recognizing that it excluded them.

There are gendered differences in how they perceive and articulate the disparities between working full-time as unpaid volunteer CHWs, and the temporary paid work associated with the PEI. In interviews, MCHW made it clear that they, too, expected better and more regular remuneration for their contributions. They stated that the low status associated with 'voluntary work' makes it a burden for them to facilitate what FCHWs do, especially since they work with the least valuable members of society.[28] Their opinion was shared by men in the more formal parts of the health system (within NGOs, at DoPH level and even at the MoPH), who took every opportunity available to urge the author to encourage remuneration for CHW work.[29] By contrast, female CHWs did not dwell to the same extent on money and were more likely to comment on the value of regular training and properly supplied health kits as incentives for their work.[30] They spoke of feeling respected as women with learning and reported satisfaction with their work as an expression of their active piety. Women's response is quite possibly an expression of their satisfaction at somehow evading the severe limitations within which Afghan women can operate; but the gendered differences in the sense of the value of this work, as reported here, should also be read as a warning that if CHW positions do become formalized or salaried, it may become increasingly difficult for women to be drawn into this work, or to operate with any of the autonomy they currently seem to enjoy.

With the introduction of attractive technologies such as *Zaranj*,[31] which are fully in the control of MCHWs even though their sole purpose is to transport women and their children to health facilities, and as more opportunities for remunerated/ incentivized CHW work are put in place to enlarge and improve basic healthcare delivery, it should be anticipated that men will try to find ways to dominate the CHW system that are not available to them at present. Because there are no socially acceptable avenues for women to move up in the CHW system (currently, all paid supervisory positions within the CBHC are held by men), there is a major risk that women's central role will become diminished and compromised. This fact has to be kept at the forefront of any efforts to expand or further systematize CHW work and it must remain the central focus of any new interventions that the CHW system delivers to women.

Family health programmes in Afghanistan will always have to be devised in such a way that they remain focused on and accessible to women. This means, as I have shown, that planners need to keep finding the best ways to deliver services *through* women, with men offering important and socially necessary support but not dominating every aspect of the programme. My focus will now turn to some of the specific concerns facing Afghanistan's FCHWs in the future.

Afghan women and access to the economy

For Afghan women, the slow violence of decades of war, and the ongoing instability caused by armed insurgents and exaggerated by foreign military occupation, shape every aspect of life from birth to death. While a small group of elite women in Kabul and provincial capitals may have begun to experience incremental gains in status,[32] overall, and despite millions of dollars in aid and much rhetoric about 'post-war reconstruction', the situation for women and many men has failed to improve. Indeed, in areas still dominated by armed groups and their subterranean and illicit war economies, the lives of the most impoverished women (and men) remain bleak. Security remains erratic in the provincial capitals and Kabul and the pendulum threatens to swing back, in 2017, to all-out armed conflict.[33] In such an uncertain environment, access to paid work remains severely restricted even for men. The impacts on women are profound because they are disproportionally excluded from paid work, not only because of 'cultural' as well as pragmatic and security-focused constraints that keep them in seclusion, but because decades of poor or non-existent schooling for females both re/produces and reinforces women's subordination.[34]

On a positive note, for both religious and social reasons, women in Afghanistan do have limited rights to health-seeking behaviours and can claim such support as is available when the conditions for their access are calibrated correctly.[35] In this framework, working as a FCHW appears to give women who have the personality and opportunity to take it, a space in which to make a social contribution that does not disrupt cultural/social norms. Much less than the MCHWs interviewed for this research, FCHWs emphasized that the value they derive personally from their work is cultural and/or religious, and is therefore very rewarding to their sense of themselves as 'good Muslim women' and 'good wives, mothers, daughters and sisters'. While they liked receiving some payment for attending trainings, they placed far less emphasis on their CHW work as a potential source of income than MCHWs did. This does not mean that FCHWs should be unpaid or differently paid from men for what they do, but it exhorts us to look beyond money as the only reward system in which any value can be placed.

Also, lessons from other efforts to economically empower Afghan women teach that it is important not to overestimate the extent to which they can function as 'autonomous economic agents' given that 'investments in and loyalty to the family and community matter for the security they can provide' in the absence of a functioning state or regulated markets (Grace and Pain, 2011: 263). FCHWs never function outside of their *mahram* relationship and it is therefore important to calibrate any recognition they receive for their contributions within parameters that make sense to male family members and men in the broader community. To do otherwise would be to put them, and the work they do, at risk.

With this in mind, it becomes clear that monetizing CHW work, while it may be advocated for by men and even appear to provide a good avenue to improve and regulate delivery of basic health services, may produce more than one negative effect. First, finding the resources to provide salaries to a currently voluntary work force will be costly and will prove unsustainable if, or rather, when current levels of donor funding decline. Second, paid work has greater status: being paid more, and paid more regularly, probably would benefit men and enhance their social standing – but risks taking the focus off community health work as primarily a women's health initiative. This problem is made likelier because voluntarism is seen as an enactment of personal religious convictions, and offers a contribution to family honour and community well-being that is appropriate for women to make. It is likely to be much more difficult for women to occupy salaried roles without being constructed as competing with men for scarce jobs or moving into space that men see as belonging exclusively to them. Overall, the greatest loss incurred by monetizing this work may be to the currently uncontested fact that working as a FCHW is rewarding to the women who do it. Losing FCHWs would stop whatever contributions they make to reversing the slow violence evident in Afghanistan's extremely poor maternal-child health statistics.

Understanding women's motivations

There are some questions to consider. What rewards lie beyond money for FCHWs (and this question can also be extended to PEI's female frontline workers) – why do they do what they do? What motivates this small cadre of women to become exceptional in their culture as actors and public servants beyond the confines of the extended family, to be as visible in the public sphere as ordinary Afghan women can be? And simultaneously, how is it possible to continue to motivate the men who support them, without ending up with a male-focused system which would ultimately fail to deliver to the target group?

In the severely demarcated social and cultural space open to humble, impoverished and non-literate female Afghans, it should be postulated that access to interventions that afford women who can take them up a modicum of freedom of movement and thought, authority, the potential for personal expansion and intellectual growth, are *as gratifying and valuable* as the small contributions to economic security that are currently being considered as a measure to recognize CHWs for their work. Despite the dominant neoliberal insistence on monetizing every aspect of human life, offering cash incentives is not always the best way to proceed, perhaps especially in the extended aftermath of war under the guise of 'post-conflict reconstruction'. With this caution in mind, future interventions with CHWs should be designed not so much to accommodate, but also to carefully stretch, deeply embedded patriarchal norms about how a good Afghan woman should behave. This cannot be done without also acknowledging how these norms are regulated, often through less 'spectacular' forms of violence – those 'layered predicaments of apprehension' to which Nixon alludes (Nixon, 2009: 14) – that so easily become invisible in the broader spectacle of war-torn Afghanistan.[36] Non-monetized work might offer itself as a surprising means to shape a different kind of security altogether – one whose rewards are seen in how individual women access public space and resources, and contribute to enhancing one another's quality of life, through an ethic of care that they themselves control and extend.

'Culture' as a rationalization for women's exclusion

The fieldwork conducted for this analysis suggests that asking feminist-inflected questions about the design and implementation of humanitarian and development initiatives in Afghanistan is important, despite the difficulties of the working environment and the shared resistance to considering gender that is demonstrated by both national and international actors. A very broad commitment to identifying the greatest possible means to achieve social inclusion, which is a necessary precursor to sustainable peace (Schnabel and Farr, 2012) can lead, then, to an apparently narrow and context-specific discussion about remuneration or incentives for ordinary people to participate in the field of healthcare, such as the one presented here. In this analysis of CHWs and other social mobilizers who have been drawn into the ongoing work of the PEI, an important disjunction was noticed: arguments, put forward by men, that participation in the paid, public work of NIDs is suitable only for men, do not tally with the actual on-the-ground presence of a number of women, particularly in urban areas, participating in implementing polio campaign goals. What men in male-dominated societies say is happening, or should happen, is excessively inflected by their self-interest and may, in reality, obscure opportunities for positive changes away from maintaining ideologies that do little to sustain human well-being. In other words, FCHWs can be seen as a tiny building-block in the vast enterprise needed to stop the militarized destruction of Afghanistan.

In addition to discussions with female and male CHWs, interviews with PEI frontline workers confirmed that women from a wide variety of backgrounds can, and do, find ways around apparently insurmountable obstacles if they see an opportunity to do something that is interesting, and beneficial to them and their family. Respondents said they were working for polio because they had found opportunities to negotiate with male family members, because mothers-in-law were no longer exerting undue influence on them, or because they were from relatively open families (usually as refugee returnees) and were educated. Many of them identified their family's relative poverty (and men's unemployment) as the reason they were allowed to do work that demands them to operate in public space: their families were simply too poor not to mobilize everyone who could find paid work. What this shows is that apparently entrenched Afghan social and cultural practices, can, in reality, 'be transgressed by various factors, one of which is poverty' (Grace and Pain, 2011: 265). Indeed, evidence from research on women's livelihood practices shows considerable adaptability in how extended families interpret social norms in order to earn much-needed resources. Women's roles change continuously as family fortunes rise and decline – despite rhetorical efforts to claim that they are set in stone.

When it is clearly understood than even an apparently immobile cultural sphere is in fact endlessly in motion, it also becomes evident that there is considerable elasticity in how men and women mobilize arguments about the 'cultural' reasons for women either to remain secluded or to enter public space.[37] It becomes crucial, especially as opportunities are sought to enhance FCHW's authority and presence in the broader CBHC system, to look beyond what men tend to say about what women can and should be allowed to learn and do; to be appropriately cautious about 'culture' as a legitimate reason for exclusion or marginalization; and with existing gendered structural inequalities in mind, to proceed carefully in determining how incentives for CHW work should be calculated and dispersed, including by focusing on ways to provide non-monetized forms of recognition for work well done.

Conclusion

Women's interests and debates about their capacities are, as Julie Billaud puts it, 'the field through which [Afghan] statehood enacts its power' (Billaud, 2015: 18); but foreign rhetoric about the central importance of women as beneficiaries of peace dividends, including through participation in advancing the nation's health and wellbeing, has also produced little coordination, poor monitoring of the impacts of existing initiatives and lack of accountability for spending on 'women's issues'. Afghanistan is frequently described as 'the worst place in the world to be a woman'. This sobering aphorism is an important reminder that ongoing efforts to eradicate polio cannot take place in a vacuum: the surrounding context of this initiative is one of the highest maternal and under-five mortality rates in the world, an iteration of slow violence caused and maintained by women's inferior social position and the dominance of militarized forms of masculinity in both Afghanistan, and in international interactions with the country.

Like polio itself, the majority of these deaths are preventable, requiring comparatively simple – unspectacular – and coherent basic health interventions to safeguard mothers and their children. Above the ground-level catastrophe of women's lack of access to basic health lies a complex superstructure of exclusions, which combine to ensure the 'woman is doubly in shadow' (Spivak, 1988: 84), unable to represent her interests or properly safeguard those in her care. From a polio eradication perspective, arguably the most important negative impact of the international community's exaggerated respect for Afghan patriarchal politics – in itself a thin guise for the lucrative opportunities of ongoing militarization – is that the primary caregivers of under-five-year-olds have never been regarded as the initiative's most important allies. Unless this foundational error is corrected and ways are found to bring women to the centre of PEI outreach, the goal of achieving universal vaccination to eradicate polio or indeed, sustainably advocate for any other child or women's health initiative, will remain as elusive as the much bigger goal to stop the decades of war in which the country is mired.

When Nixon warns that attention must be paid to the unquantifiable signs of slow violence – the attrition of basic well-being and support for life – he joins a chorus of voices that have been calling for a re-definition of security focused not on militarized approaches, but on ending the 'repeated cycles of political and criminal violence that cause human misery and disrupt development, [and] contribute to instability and conflict' (Schnabel and Farr, 2012: 3). If the core goal of security is to 'give back societies' ability to meet their own welfare and development needs' (Schnabel and Farr, 2012: 5), even the humblest woman in the remotest community is an important participant. To refocus the security lens with her in view is a goal every bit as important as breaking the chain through which the deadly polio virus passes. In truth, as measures of human safety, they are one and the same.

Notes

1 The BPHS was initiated in 2003. It is intended to provide a comprehensive interaction between the public health system and the communities it serves. Structurally it is intended to work at the very baseline of community health, through a system of associations between provincial Departments of Public Health (DoPHs) and the health NGOs they subcontract, which manage thousands of unpaid CHWs (around 20,000 of them). If priority really was given to improving development indicators such as the Millennium Development Goals or the new Sustainable Development Goals, it would make sense, given the country's very low development indicators, if the BPHS received the most significant funding and attention of any health sector in Afghanistan. In reality the BPHS is a marginal, under-resourced and often unreliable system of health delivery, highly variable from province to province, and stronger in areas closer to urban centres than in the rural peripheries. Up-to-date published information on the BPHS and CHWs is hard to come by, but see Najafizada, Labonté and Bourgeault for useful account of the system and its challenges (2014, 8).

2 Fieldwork from which research conclusions in this chapter are derived was conducted in 2015 and 2016 for the MoPH and supported by UNICEF Afghanistan, which is

technical co-lead with WHO Afghanistan on the PEI. I work as a gender specialist with two decades of experience in conflict zones, and I draw on my PhD in Women's Studies as I undertake research for agencies that hire me. In Afghanistan, all interviews are accompanied by Afghan colleagues who are my interpreters and co-interviewers, and I am always accompanied by a woman so that I can talk to women unaccompanied by men. Interviews are set up, under tight security controls, through NGO or government partners. We ask the approval of those who speak to us to use their words in our analysis and undertake, for security reasons, never to identify informants. I am fully responsible for all analysis in this account and none of the conclusions are to be attributed to other individuals or any institution.

3   An excellent account of the gendered dimensions of this history is found in Stabile and Kumar (2005: 765–82).

4   Across the country, Afghans practise a form of female seclusion called *purdah*. Some families still enforce this seclusion so completely that women never meet anyone outside their kinship network throughout their lives.

5   Literacy rates of both men and women are extremely low. In fieldwork I was told that there is usually one male child in the household who can read sufficiently well to translate health messages to others. Nonetheless, the MoPH continues to rely, among other methods such as radio, on written banners in public places and leaflets to let communities know when a mass health intervention is planned. These may have more impact as a visible signifier that work is being done than in actually enhancing community knowledge; more discussion of health communication is beyond the scope of this chapter.

6   Official Afghan health policy opposes home births, in line with the WHO's dictates. In reality, especially in poor and inaccessible areas, women cannot always reach public health stations. If they do, they often cannot pay fees that are demanded (against policy) for services. As a result, large numbers of babies are born at home and miss their zero-dose of OPV, which is administered minutes after birth. Afghanistan is said to have the second-highest rate of maternal mortality in the world, although how this figure is arrived at, in the absence of reliable data or a national census, is difficult to assess. More information about women's access to pre-and post-partum services can be found online at http://www.unicef.org/afghanistan.

7   Afghanistan and Pakistan are the last two states in the world to interrupt transmission of polio, and thus share responsibility for implementing a unified and synergistic approach to the problem of virus transmission across their long and porous border. Vast numbers of people cross between the countries daily with their children, sharing their personal space, beliefs and concerns as well as information. Consequently, there is a crucial need for a coherent and complementary communication and OPV delivery strategy across the borders; but managing this process is difficult for larger geopolitical reasons that this analysis will not discuss. More details can be found in the resources section of the Global PEI website, http://polioeradication.org/.

8   Passed only ten months before the US/NATO invasion of Afghanistan in 2001, the first ever Security Council Resolution driven by civil-society, SCR1325, was intended, by the feminist community that wrote and promoted it, to challenge women's exclusion from all aspects of security-related decision-making and usher in a new era of peacemaking. It was intended to redefine 'security' in such a way that the gendered devastation of the social fabric during and after war could be overcome. In reality, it took nearly a decade for any uptake of the Resolution in Afghanistan. Feminist analysis of the consequences of the Security Council's failure to implement SCR1325 in Afghanistan is still ongoing. For more on the UN's 'women, peace and security' agenda, see http:www.peacewomen.org..

9   A recent source of information, in 2015, took the form of an unpublished 'Knowledge and Practices' (KAP) survey, designed and conducted by Harvard University's Opinion Research Program in partnership with UNICEF. Data from this survey helped shape the field work approach from which conclusions in this chapter are formed.

10 In Afghanistan, the PEI receives donor funding from, among others, The Gates Foundation and national governments such as the UK and Canada. UNICEF and the WHO are tasked with technical assistance to the MoPH. There is also significant influence and oversight from a Technical Advisory Group (TAG) that comprises international experts on polio eradication, which meets biannually to discuss progress and problems.

11 It would be impossible to summarise the torrent of commitments to 'peace in Afghanistan' that have been issued by the USA, its latest military invaders, since US President George W. Bush declared in October 2001 – on the eve of the military exercise named, without apparent irony, Operation Enduring Freedom – that the 'fight against terrorism is also a fight for the rights and dignity of women'. For more see Stabile and Kumar (2005).

12 One such report is the 'Assessment of Services and Human Resource Needs for the Development of the Safe Motherhood Initiative in Afghanistan', cited here. Unpublished report from field visits conducted between 24 March to 2 May 2002 on behalf of UNICEF, by Suraya Dalil, MD, Mark Fritzler, BA, Denisa-Elena Ionete, MD, ScD, Noel McIntosh, MD, ScD, Judith O'Heir, RN, RM, Patricia Stephenson, ScD. This report offers intriguing glimpses, usually in its footnotes, of a rudimentary women-focused healthcare system having survived the civil war in some rural areas.

13 It is important not to exaggerate the extent to which CHWs can reach such women, but the point is that those who can become direct beneficiaries of some healthcare are more easily reached by FCHWs than through any other means.

14 At least at the delivery level where voluntary work is done. Women do not easily or often ascend the hierarchy into public, paid positions.

15 In Afghan culture, a woman leaving her house must be veiled (in many parts of the country, she must be completely covered by a *chadari* or *burka*) and accompanied at all times by a male family member (father, brother, son, husband). The Taliban made attempts to curtail women's freedom of movement well beyond what was already considered culturally appropriate. Even since their retreat from power, ongoing insecurity and conservatism maintain a backlash against external efforts to 'liberate women' from this seclusion.

16 CHWs are not entirely unremunerated, as will be discussed in greater detail below.

17 FCHWs tend to be very humble, mostly illiterate women. MCHWs, by contrast, tend to be literate men already in a public role such as school teacher.

18 This point is important in a context in which levels of targeted violence against women in public space are high. It is not always possible to ascertain whether such attacks are against women for their public participation, or whether elite women are simply a more visible target because of their intimate association with prominent men in the complex war/criminal economy of the country. Regardless, threats against professional women began to escalate in earnest in 2013 when two chiefs in the directorate of women's affairs were murdered one after another, a woman parliamentarian's daughter was killed in an attack aimed at her mother and a top woman police officer in Helmand was assassinated as she left her home. Similarly, in 2014, parliamentarian Shukria Barakzai narrowly escaped death in a bombing that killed three others and in February 2015, Angeza Shinwari, a provincial councillor in eastern Nangarhar province, died of injuries sustained in a targeted car bombing. In March 2016, Farkhunda was beaten to death by thirteen men in the streets of Kabul after being falsely accused of burning the Qur'an. For updates and ongoing analysis of public violence against women, see http. www.rawa.org.

19 The Knowledge and Practice (KAP) survey conducted for UNICEF by Harvard University in early 2015 revealed that CHWs are the most highly trusted source of health information, with religious leaders and neighbours coming close behind them. This tells us that it is the *localization of the messenger* as much as the localization of the message that promotes better health-seeking behaviours.

20 Field-level research for this report was conducted in Jalalabad, Kandahar and Kabul in August and September 2015 and between January and May 2016. Findings were corroborated with key informants in Kabul.

21 These resources are primarily a small daily wage for the five days of each NID campaign, although the 'big money' appears to be attached to payments made for the use of private vehicles to do campaign work.

22 In Afghan culture, it is not unusual for parents and sons, and their wife or wives, to share a compound. Families visit one another regularly, for days at a time. This means that a single door can open onto many young children, or that missing only one household could leave a lot of children unvaccinated. The risk of transmission is, of course, increased, when these children are then moved back to their household of origin.

23 In field discussions, childhood death is often presented as a regrettable instance of 'the will of Allah' rather than something preventable through better healthcare practices. The practice of taking sick children to 'healers' at shrines rather than to medical personnel, is another piece in the puzzle of poor child health.

24 More than one key informant, and several Afghans engaging in casual conversation with the author, commented that engagement with children themselves seems to be missing from the campaign. There are no efforts to draw them in through activities, songs, making the finger marking they receive to show they have been vaccinated an appealing colour, etc. Slightly older children appear to be quite proud of their finger mark and like showing it off, but one of the problems unearthed during fieldwork is that marks are given in black, a colour Afghans associate with death. Once this was observed, the author's suggestion of marking in bright colours was taken up with great success. Simple changes like this indicate that it might in fact be helpful to create a demand and interest in the work of NIDs among children themselves, especially since it is often an older child, in the absence of a senior male, who answers the door when frontline workers do their rounds.

25 Drawing attention to any system that is working well appears to be fraught with pitfalls: the author's first report on working more closely with CHWs in PEI, delivered in October 2015, led not to the implementation of the report's suggestions, but to a distorted, expensive, ill-conceived and still male-dominated 'pilot' project designed by two male officials in the MoPH that produced an entirely new set of problems that now have to be managed. That this eventuality was predicted in the report was still not enough to prevent it from happening.

26 In fieldwork, the author was told that men were unhappy with a recent campaign (conceived by an all-male international communications unit, at great expense) that had tried to use the still nascent Afghan cricket team to spread pro-PEI messages. In particular, they objected to fliers featuring handsome young athletes giving the OPV dose to children: they did not want such pictures in their household where women could look at them. Nonetheless, the association with the national team carries on.

27 Refusal is considered to be a significant factor in failing to reach the 100 per cent coverage goal. It is usually ascribed to oppositional messages from mosques and seen as part of a disinformation campaign coming from Pakistan, which has a violent history of opposing polio vaccinations – in other words, a problem of male information networks and values. As a result, significant resources are spent on encouraging Mullah-Imams to support positive messaging. The author's fieldwork could not, however, verify that this is the most pressing problem, turning up much more evidence that poor messaging and a lack of patience with sitting talking to caregivers were important factors in refusal. Changes are needed in communications strategies, based in recognizing the differences between how women and men receive and act on information.

28 Focus group discussions with MCHWs were conducted separately from those with FCHWs and a female interpreter assisted in taking with women in the hopes that women-only spaces would allow for a freer exchange of information.

29   Of course, this solidarity has much to do with men trying to expand opportunities for paid work with all the opportunities this brings to those who find ways to control who accesses the jobs. It was carefully explained to anyone who made this suggestion that formalizing CHWs into the MoPH's paid labour force would be both unsustainable, as there are so many of them and funding cannot be provided by the MoPH; and undesirable, because it would be likely to challenge women's currently central position in the system.

30   CHWs are supposed to receive a limited supply of simple medications and supplies every few months. Being able to disburse these is a significant source of status and is regarded as the best reward for being a volunteer; but the supply of these kits seems highly variable based on how efficient and committed each BPHS NGO is.

31   *Zaranj* are small three-wheeler ambulances to be used by CHWs to bring pregnant and labouring women, or children needing vaccinations or other healthcare, to medical centres. UNICEF is currently piloting them in five provinces.

32   This claim still needs to be read in light of the ongoing and apparently unpunishable violence against women who try to move into public spaces, including government institutions or the education system.

33   The deteriorating situation led to US bombing raid against Kunduz, a Taliban stronghold, in April 2016 that destroyed a trauma hospital managed by Médecins Sans Frontières. Up-to-date information on the political and material consequences of this airstrike is available online at http://www.msf.org/en/topics/kunduz-hospital-airstrike. In 2017, Afghanistan was assailed by the GBU-43/B Massive Ordnance Air Blast (MOAB) dropped by the USA in Nangahar Province on 13 April and the deadliest terror attack ever against Kabul on 31 May. Lethal assaults across the nation, especially in cities, are making this the deadliest year on record since 2001.

34   This problem is central to Afghanistan's very poor record on maternal and child health, and its impacts on individuals and communities complicate every aspect of health delivery, from nutrition to sanitation to protection to medical access.

35   Some of this calibration, at family level, implies better understanding how mothers-in-law control their sons' wives. In field discussions, young women often complained that older women prevent them from accessing community health clinics, fearing that young women want to escape the confines of the home to gossip and relax; whereas young women themselves want to parent better than their mothers did. This problem is not exclusive to Afghanistan, but feminist insights on how societies as a whole create and collude in upholding patriarchal exclusion, a problem long accounted for in women-and-development literature, appear to have had little impact in on-the-ground programming there.

36   That interpersonal violence against Afghan women is endemic is fairly well documented, but my implication here is that there is a scale of the 'spectacular' in this violence, to use Nixon's phrase, which means that national and international attention tends to focus on the most extreme instances and overlook how threat and fear operate in daily life to control and shape women.

37   Such elasticity is already visible in how female Social Mobilizers (SM) are identified and retained in the long-term PEI programme, although women have participated predominantly in urban centres to date.

References

Billaud, J. (2015) *Kabul Carnival: Gender Politics in Postwar Afghanistan*. Philadelphia, PA: U Penn Press.

Dalil, S., Fritzler, M., Ionete, D., McIntosh, N., O'Heir, J. and Stephenson, P. (2002) 'Assessment of services and human resource needs for the development of the safe motherhood initiative in Afghanistan'. Unpublished report for UNICEF.

Grace, J. and Pain, A. (2011) 'Rural women's livelihoods: Their position in the agrarian economy', in Jennifer Heath and Ashraf Zahedi (eds) *Land of the Unconquerable: The Lives of Contemporary Afghan Women*, Berkeley, CA: U California P. 262–75.

Hudson, H. (2012) 'A bridge too far? The gender consequences of linking security and development in SSR discourse and practice', in A. Schnabel, and V. Farr (eds) *Back to the Roots: Security Sector Reform and Development*. Geneva: Democratic Centre for the Control of Armed Forces. 77–114.

Najafizada, Said Ahmad, Labonté, Ronald and Bourgeault, Ivy Lynn (2014) 'Community health workers of Afghanistan: A qualitative study of a national program'. *Conflict and Health* 8:26. Online. Available: www.conflictandhealth.com/content/8/1/26 (accessed 15 September 2015).

Nixon, R. (2009) *Slow Violence and the Environmentalism of the Poor*. Cambridge, MA, and London, England: Harvard UP.

Schnabel, A. and Farr, V. (eds) (2012) 'Returning to the development roots of security sector reform'. *Back to the Roots: Security Sector Reform and Development*. Geneva: Democratic Centre for the Control of Armed Forces. 3–28.

Spivak, G. C. (1988) 'Can the subaltern speak?' In Cary Nelson and Lawrence Grossberg (eds) *Marxism and the Interpretation of Culture*. Urbana, IL: University of Illinois Press. 82–83.

Stabile, C. and Kumar, D. (2005) 'Unveiling imperialism: Media, gender and the war on Afghanistan'. *Media, Culture, and Society* 27(5): 765–82.

5 A moving target

Gender, health, and the securitisation of migration

Sarah Pugh

Introduction

Recent flows of people into Europe from conflict-ravaged countries such as Syria, Afghanistan, and Iraq have cast into the global spotlight a set of competing pressures faced by modern states in navigating the complex dynamics of contemporary international migration. One set of pressures calls upon states to uphold international humanitarian and human rights obligations towards migrants, particularly through upholding the protections afforded by the global asylum regime. However, in doing so, states risk opening themselves up to the potentially intense domestic political, economic, and social migration-related pressures that large movements of people across borders can evoke.

For decades, states have been defining and redefining their migration strategies and policies in keeping with the social and political imperatives of the day. Bureaucratic and administrative tools, such as requirements around finances or skills, have long been imposed by states to keep out the "wrong" kind of migrants. While such administrative strategies continue to shape state responses to migration management, migration has also emerged in recent years as a new object of securitisation, with migrants themselves as new subjects of security. Internationally, many states are responding to migration pressures with an increasingly control-oriented and securitised approach, tightening or attempting to close borders, criminalising irregular and often low-skilled migrants, and framing migrants broadly in the language of social, political, and economic threat.

While the term "migrant" may refer to anybody moving from one place to another, this chapter focuses on those who are either forced, or choose, to leave their countries of origin due to (often inter-related) issues beyond their control, such as war, insecurity, famine, climate change, environmental disaster, or lack of economic opportunity. While some such individuals may meet the formal administrative criteria of an "asylum seeker" or a "refugee", others may not. Given the contemporary nature of mixed migration flows, it has become increasingly difficult for officials to disentangle and categorise what are often the multiple, complex motivations of individuals who leave one country in search of a better future in another. What unites such a diverse group is not a label, or a particular administrative categorisation, but the fact that the state in their preferred destination would, most often, prefer to keep them out. It is the asylum seekers, the "economic migrants", and those without legal documents who represent for states the biggest perceived security threats.

This chapter draws on insights from the field of feminist security studies to interrogate migration as a field in which state security practices and the rights and well-being of such migrants collide, with profound embodied and gendered implications for individual migrants' lives and health. Guided by feminist insights into the importance of articulating connections across what are often distinct literatures (Wibben, 2014: 743), the chapter attempts to forge some initial connections between the literatures relating to migration, securitisation, gender and health. It also attempts to draw attention to often neglected sites of violence and insecurity, which can result both directly and indirectly from states' migration policies. In this way, feminist security studies can offer a different lens from conventional approaches to International Relations (IR), which tend to focus on "high politics" issues such as "war" and "peace", and often neglect the politics of everyday violence (Shepherd, 2009: 208). Such violence is not necessarily active in its shape and form, but can also be evoked more passively through state practices of denial, such as denial of belonging, of citizenship, or of access to services and care, as illustrated in this chapter. As Shepherd (2009: 208) notes, feminist security scholarship pushes conventional IR boundaries in asking *which* violences are considered worthy of study, and *when* these violences occur.

After positioning migration within contemporary securitisation debates, the chapter explores how the health implications of a securitised approach to migration may be experienced or embodied in different ways by men and women, traced through various sites of a migrant's potential journey. The first section highlights some of the potential gendered health implications of migration during transit, where the impacts of securitisation are acutely felt by many migrants, and particularly women, far beyond the political borders of the destination country. The second section interrogates gender as a factor in access to care for migrants within host countries, teasing out the potential impacts of securitisation on this access. Finally, this chapter looks at the gendered health implications of increasingly utilised state practices of detention, one of the most striking modern manifestations of the securitisation of migration. The chapter draws on the concept of intersectionality, first coined by Kimberlé Crenshaw (1989), to highlight the ways in which securitised migration policies and practices contribute both directly and indirectly to negative health outcomes for migrants, with the most severe impacts being felt by those who exist at the intersection of multiple determinants of vulnerability and exclusion, including gender, disability, age, race/ethnicity, social class, and migration status.

Migration and security: security for whom?

With the post-Cold War broadening of security theory and the development of securitisation theory as advanced by the Copenhagen school, the attention of many security scholars in recent decades has expanded from a traditional state-centred focus on issues of conflict and war, towards a much wider range of security subjects, objects and practices, including migration. Processes of globalisation, including enhanced information and communication technologies and the intensification of international travel routes, have contributed to the development of new and shifting global flows of people, while the entrenchment or widening of global inequalities in an age of neoliberal economic hegemony has intensified regional and global migration push and pull factors. In addition, a powerful discourse linking migration to the fear of Islamic extremism and terror attacks emerged in the wake of the 9/11 attacks in New York and Washington, and through the ensuing narrative of a "war on terror". This has been exacerbated by the emergence of extremist groups such as Boko Haram and ISIL, and by events such as the attacks in November 2015 in Paris, March 2016 in Brussels, June 2016 in Nice, and December 2016 in Berlin. Recent dramatic flows of people into Europe from areas of prolonged civil and regional conflict have further combined to position migration firmly as a focus of state security agendas.

Drawing on the work of the Copenhagen school, the term "securitisation", for the purposes of this chapter, refers to the outcomes of a process in which an actor (or group of actors) of sufficient credibility and authority is able to successfully convince an audience of the existence of a specific, existential threat, real or perceived, and to similarly convince this audience that an exceptional response and mobilisation of resources is necessary to address this threat. Incorporating the insights of McInnes and Rushton (2010: 244), the approach to securitisation used here also recognises that 'securitization is not a binary condition: there is a spectrum from failed, to partial, to successful securitization processes. Nor are the results of a securitizing move homogenous'. The successful securitisation of migration exists along such a spectrum, but is evident in both ideational and material spheres, whether through the framing of migrants as carriers of disease and blatant threats to public safety, or through the building of walls, barbed-wire fences, and detention facilities to keep migrants out.

The securitisation of migration necessarily entails an approach to migration primarily based upon the deterrence and exclusion of those migrants deemed by states to be unwanted. It largely positions the migrant-receiving state as the referent; the state is considered to be the primary risk-bearer in relation to the (real or perceived) threat presented by migration. In this framing, the historical roots and embeddedness of structural and systemic inequities, many of which continue to contribute to the various forces that motivate global and gendered movements of people, are set aside in favour of an approach that paints migrants largely as economic opportunists, potential threats to public order, and a collective burden that is best to be avoided. In preventing the arrival of migrants, member states are able to avoid the responsibilities, expenses, and complications associated with assessing individual migrants' situations or asylum claims, and with ensuring the provision of housing, education, health care, and other ongoing basic needs, and social protections. However, while the securitisation of migration may deflect the costs and risks associated with migration from the potential host state, it exacerbates the costs and risks for individual migrants, with the highest costs often paid by those who are most vulnerable. This outcome is deeply at odds with the protection of the health and human rights of migrants, and with global public health agendas more broadly.

Gender, securitisation, and health in transit

The impacts of the securitisation of migration may be felt by migrants far beyond the political boundaries of destination countries, mediated by factors such as race/ethnicity, social class, and gender. The policies and practices of securitisation heighten the risks and potential exposures to harm for precisely the kinds of individuals that international refugee law aims to protect, highlighting what Gerard and Pickering (2014: 338) have called the "structural contradiction" in international migration policies and practices. Many migrants' journeys involve the navigation of hazardous routes and forms of travel, including interactions with smugglers or traffickers who may have little regard for the safety of those paying for passage. Especially for those individuals attempting to leave behind some combination of conflict, poverty and lack of opportunity, migrant journeys may present multiple, and often gendered, risks to health and safety. Exposures to risk and physical harm in transit can take various forms, with studies from across international migration routes pointing to experiences of extortion and violence, including sexual and gender-based violence, as well the risks associated with increasingly dangerous and clandestine methods and routes of travel.

Many migrants, particularly the most vulnerable, face significant risks of violence, including sexual and gender-based violence, in transit. One study exploring migrant women's experiences of transit from North Africa to Malta, for example, documents evidence of both direct and indirect violence against women, including sexual violence, perpetrated by a mix of state and non-state actors (Gerard and Pickering, 2014: 5). Some women reported the insistence by gatekeepers of sexual services in exchange for assistance in border crossing, while some male partners of women were reported to have faced threats of harm or even death if they objected or attempted to intervene (2014: 9). Elsewhere, in many Mexico/US border towns with high migratory flows, irregular migrants face a host of threats from '*polleros*' (migrant smugglers), gangs, armed forces, local police, and immigration agents (Infante *et al.*, 2012: 2). For irregular migrant women (many of whom are travelling from Central America), travel through Mexico is ridden with gender-based risks. While abuses against migrant women are seldom reported, they are nonetheless widespread, with some estimates suggesting that as many as six in ten women and girl migrants experience sexual violence during the journey (Amnesty International, 2010: 5). For those fleeing violence or unrest, violent and traumatic experiences in transit are often compounded by violent and traumatic experiences in the country of origin, adding to both physical and mental health risks faced by people in these circumstances.

The securitisation of migration has contributed to migrants' usage of increasingly dangerous routes and means of travel, heightening risk of harm not just from traffickers, smugglers, officials and others, but also from environmental factors and injuries. Irregular migrants may be profoundly vulnerable in spaces of transit, as they are 'funnelled into increasingly clandestine routes that make their journeys more dangerous, time-consuming and costly' (Vogt, 2013: 765). For example, when US migration policies have been tightened or border monitoring increased along traditional points of entry, migrants may also search for points of entry with less monitoring, but where they encounter even more dangers, including increased risks of environmental exposure and injury. To illustrate, Infante *et al.* (2012: 2) point out that since 2001, over 100 irregular migrants have died every year in southern Arizona due to heat stroke alone, while unknown numbers of US-bound Central American migrants, usually amongst the poorest, have died or lost limbs attempting to ride the notorious freight train through Mexico known as "*La Bestia*", or "The Beast" (Vogt, 2013: 771).

Currently, the images and narratives of migrants crossing the Mediterranean by boat into Europe are perhaps most often in the media spotlight, highlighting the costs and risks of transit to migrants' health, well-being and lives. While these Mediterranean crossings are associated with a range of risks to health, from disease to dehydration (a particular issue for pregnant women), they also provide some of the most visible and dramatic contemporary examples of migrants paying for their journeys with their lives. The International Organisation for Migration's (IOM) Missing Migrants Project, which attempts to track migrant deaths along global migration routes, estimates more than 60,000 migrant fatalities in the last two decades alone, noting that due to the methodological challenges of documenting migrant fatalities globally, this number represented the minimum number of global migrant deaths in transit. In a foreword to a recent IOM report, William Lacy Swing notes that the 'real number is unknown, as many deaths are never registered, especially in more remote regions of the world', nor is the capturing of such data a priority for most states (Brian and Laczko, 2016: iii).

The securitisation of migration is closely linked to the restriction of opportunities and the deterrence of human mobility, often through the explicit goal of keeping unwanted migrants out of their preferred countries of destination. The tightening of borders and increasing restrictions on legal avenues for migration has led many migrants into undertaking risky and sometimes life-threatening journeys. The period of transit represents an important and often overlooked site of potential risk, ill-health, and violence for migrants, and especially the most vulnerable groups.

Access to care: exclusion and barriers in host countries

For those who reach their destination, the securitisation of migration continues to have an impact on migrants' health and well-being. In many host countries, securitisation discourses contribute to a climate in which issues of migrants' entitlements to services and social protections, including health care, are politically sensitive and highly emotive; regardless of their legal status, migrants are often presented as undeserving and illegitimate recipients of host state resources (Huysmans, 2000: 767; Willen, 2012). Securitisation also contributes to the production of irregularity, in which migrants with no other perceived options become or remain undocumented in a host country, a status that may have serious ramifications for health-seeking behaviour and ultimately, health outcomes. Importantly, these outcomes may be experienced and embodied in different ways for men and women, again intersecting with other potential determinants of discrimination and exclusion, including race, sexuality, disability, age, and access to resources.

For many states, the issue of migrants' access to health care creates a dilemma. On one hand, through securitisation practices and policies, states both create and respond to wider public narratives or fears of migrants as competitors for limited state resources, including health care. In the face of cutbacks to social welfare and services since the 1970s and 80s, many states must navigate a citizenry that largely views migrants as rivals in the labour market, and as illegitimate competitors in the distribution of social goods (Huysmans, 2000: 768). States may be unwilling to provide what they perceive to be incentives for new migrants; in other words, the restriction of entitlements to health may be a state practice of immigration control to discourage the entry of new migrants (Rechel *et al.*, 2013: 1240; Cuadra, 2012: 267). Yet, on the other hand, many host states are bound, at least in principle, by domestic law or international human rights commitments to uphold at least a basic standard of health care for all those within their borders. Policy-makers are also faced with the reality that whatever the political implications, the denial of access to health care and health services for migrants may have broader negative public health impacts within the country and potentially beyond.

Currently, migrants' legal access to health care differs significantly across and even within states and regions, as states seek ways to manage this dilemma. In the EU, for example, migrants' access to health care is varied and inconsistent amongst different states, and amongst different administrative categories of migrants. As Rechel *et al.* (2013: 1239) note, 'one of the most fundamental barriers for migrants in accessing health services in Europe are inadequate legal entitlements and, where entitlements exist, mechanisms for ensuring that they are well known and respected in practice'. In 2010, emergency care was effectively inaccessible to undocumented migrants in nine of the 27 EU countries, and access to health services beyond the level of emergency care was available to undocumented migrants in only five EU member states (though one of them, Spain, substantially reduced such entitlements in 2012) (Rechel *et al.*, 2013: 1240). In the United States, the provision of care for undocumented migrants also varies both between and within states, while in Israel, the state's policy of 'temporary collective protection' legalises the stay of asylum seekers from countries such as Eritrea and Sudan, but denies these asylum seekers access to work permits, the national health care system (aside from emergency care) and other social services.

The securitisation of migration can impact not just the legal framework regulating migrants' access to health services, but it can also have important impacts for migrants' actual usage of health services. The securitisation of migration has been accompanied by less opportunity for legal entry particularly of unskilled migrants and asylum seekers, along with the design and implementation of more rigorous state mechanisms for detecting, detaining and deporting irregular migrants.

Given this, irregular migrants may shy away from public spaces to avoid detection. While the gathering of information about migrant health in host countries is complicated by factors such as conceptual and methodological challenges around who constitutes a migrant, and difficulties in accessing many migrant populations, research bears out that the legal or administrative status of migrants does have an impact on access to health services and care (Rechel *et al.*, 2013: 1237; Gushulak, Weekers and Macpherson 2010: 6). Unauthorized migrants and some foreign-born women have been shown to utilise health services less than the local population, health services may be out of reach for migrants without health insurance coverage, and even where services are available, accessible and affordable, migrants may also be unaware of their rights and entitlements in terms of access (Gushulak, Weekers and Macpherson, 2010: 6).

The diversity of migrant populations in host countries makes it difficult to generalise about migrant health outcomes, yet there are important distinctions to be made in health outcomes between those migrants from high-income countries and those from more deprived states, where decisions to migrate may be forced or take place in the context of broad structural economic and social inequities between the countries of origin and the countries of destination (Malmusi, Borrell and Benach, 2010: 1611). The health status of migrants who enter a country as asylum seekers or irregular migrants may be particularly vulnerable when subjected to 'the unequal distribution of socio-economic determinants [of health], including income status, housing and accommodation, education, nutrition, sanitation, and employment' (Gushulak, Weekers, and Macpherson, 2010: 8). Migrants who are subjected to legal, social or economic isolation and deprivation may develop levels of ill health much different from those seen in the local or host populations (Gushulak, Weekers, and Macpherson, 2010: 5).

Migrant women, who are often at the intersections of multiple determinants of vulnerability and exclusion, may face particular challenges. For example, Llácer *et al.* (2007: ii4) highlight migrant women's 'heightened vulnerability to situations of violence, as well as important gaps in our knowledge of the possible differential health effects of factors such as poverty, unemployment, social networks and support, discrimination, health behaviours and use of services'. They note that immigrant women face a higher risk of sexual violence and abuse at workplaces, particularly if they are undocumented or working in the sex industry, and that they may also be at a higher risk of domestic abuse, with fewer potential resources and social networks to rely upon for assistance (Llácer *et al.*, 2007: ii7). A range of negative health outcomes in the EU in terms of migrants' access to sexual and reproductive health rights have also been noted, with studies that show migrant women from outside of the EU are screened less often for cervical and breast cancer, have less access to family planning and contraception and have a lower uptake of gynaecological care (Keygnaert *et al.*, 2014: 216). Further, they are more at risk of unintended pregnancies, pay fewer and later visits to antenatal care facilities, experience poorer pregnancy outcomes, and have higher infant and maternal mortality rates. They also note that both migrant men and women are more at risk of sexual violence, and of sexually transmitted infections, including

Hepatitis B and HIV (Keygnaert *et al.*, 2014: 216). Migrants from outside of the EU also access general and sexual and reproductive health service far less than EU citizens (Keygnaert *et al.*, 2014: 216). While these outcomes and health-seeking behaviour will differ across various contexts, the social and economic exclusion and vulnerability of migrants, and particularly migrant women and children, is a common theme globally, raising important questions about the role of the securitisation of migration in contributing to poor health outcomes not just for migrants, but for all.

The deterrence and exclusion that characterises the securitised migration practices of states must be scrutinised for their impact on the health and well-being of those migrants, particularly asylum seekers and undocumented migrants, who do reach a destination country. Securitisation, which ties together ideas of migrants with notions of criminality and threat, contributes to attitudes around the entitlement or deservingness of non-citizens to access care, and to policies that seek to limit that access, in which the denial or restriction of health care becomes an indirect tool of immigration control. Securitisation also contributes to the construction of illegality or irregularity, leaving many migrants undocumented and potentially unwilling to seek health care for fear of detection. These practices and their impacts vary across different contexts, and across different migrant groups, but may be compounded for those who exist at the axes of various determinants of vulnerability and exclusion.

Detention, gender, and health

Perhaps the most obvious manifestation of the securitisation of migration is the increasing use of migration detention as part of the state's arsenal of migration control tools. As Tabak and Levitan (2014: 10) note, the impact of immigration detention as a deterrent for migrants is far from clear, and it appears that despite the best efforts of governments to secure their borders, irregular migration is on the rise globally. In the United States, Department of Homeland Security data shows that in 1994, an average of 6,785 migrants were detained across the country on any given day, while by 2012, this number had risen to 32,953 (Tabak and Levitan, 2014: 10). European Union member states have also acknowledged that they have significantly expanded their use of detention as a response to the arrival of asylum seekers and irregular arrivals, though numbers are unclear (Tabak and Levitan, 2014: 10). Migrants with legal documents are generally able to avoid detention, but for many irregular migrants, the risks of detention are omnipresent, raising important questions about the ways in which interlacing factors (such as gender, race, and class) contribute to the creation and structuring of irregularity, as well as the embodied impacts of that irregularity. The detention of migrants is associated with a well-documented range of both direct and indirect health risks, including adverse mental health outcomes, exposure to violence and disease, and nutritional and sanitation risks. There are also particular risks for women, including maternal health risks and increased risk of sexual violence, and for children, who can face long-term adverse impacts from detention.

In many parts of the world, the gathering of reliable data regarding immigration detention, both in terms of numbers and conditions, is hampered by a lack of accurate records, or the denial of access by researchers to those records. A recent two-year investigation by the Global Detention Project and Access Info Europe, for example, sought basic statistics and details about such detention practices in 33 countries across Europe and in North America, but concluded that information is frequently unavailable, and many countries do not answer freedom of information requests. Further, when information is released or publicly available, it is often incomplete or unclear, and does not fully reflect realities on the ground (Global Detention Project, 2015: 3).

Australia's offshore immigration detention centres are also notoriously difficult for researchers or human rights monitors to access, while in other countries, irregular migrants, including asylum seekers, are often simply jailed alongside criminal prison populations, with few or no reliable records kept. While such data is difficult to access, there is, nonetheless, significant data regarding the potential health risks of detention, though many of these risks can vary significantly according to the specific location and conditions of detention.

A growing body of evidence emerging from detention sites in various parts of the world, indicates that the detention of migrants, combined with what is often an indefinite period of detention, can both create and exacerbate mental illness in migrants (Tabak and Levitan, 2014: 40). Even short-term detention has been shown to contribute to high levels of depression and post-traumatic stress disorder, while longer-term detention further aggravates symptoms (Cleveland *et al.*, 2012: 3). For example, a recent report by the *Guardian* in Australia has revealed that people held in immigration detention are suffering from rates of severe mental distress nearly four times that of the general population of Australia, and that detainees' mental health is deteriorating dramatically the longer they are detained (Doherty and Evershed, 2016). Documented cases of self-harm by migrants in detention represent another disturbing phenomenon; Cleveland *et al.* (2012: 3) for example, note that from 2010 to 2011, there were 1,100 documented cases of self-harm by migrant detainees in Australia (including 6 suicides), for a population of 6,000, most of whom had been detained for less than a year. Detention has the potential to cause damage not just to mental health, but also to family relationships, and it can exacerbate existing health concerns, which, as Askola (2010: 174) notes, is of particular import given the fact that many irregular migrants face barriers to accessing health care due to their immigration status even before detention. In April 2016, the World Bank co-hosted a high-level meeting with the World Health Organisation, highlighting the negative global developmental impacts of mental health issues, in particular depression and anxiety. Importantly, the World Bank notes that the issue of mental health 'is becoming ever more urgent in light of the forced migration and sustained conflict we are seeing in many countries of the world' (World Bank, 2016). The increasing recognition of the prevalence and the impact of mental health issues, particularly in relation to migration, stands in stark contrast to the increasing use of detention as a tool of immigration deterrence and control.

Aside from mental health implications, the overall health of detainees may be adversely impacted by a range of factors, including overcrowding, lack of ventilation, poor nutrition and sanitation, along with verbal and physical violence and abuse from detention or prison facility staff, as well as other detainees. Inadequate access to general health care in detention facilities is another commonly cited issue across various contexts, including countries as diverse as the US, Libya, Australia, and South Africa (Kalhan, 2010: 47; Gerard and Pickering, 2014: 11; Sanggaran, Haire and Zion, 2016: 2; de Wet, 2014). Other issues include disruption of treatment, a lack of continuity of care, and the ethical and health implications of detaining those who may already be victims of torture and abuse (Harper and Raman, 2008: 16). Further to this, there are indirect health impacts of detention policies and practices, such as migrants' avoidance of health care and other social services out of fear of detection and detention.

The detention of migrants can have important, though often overlooked, gendered impacts for health. In the context of some predominantly male migration flows, it is young, male migrants who are most at risk of detention and the associated adverse health impacts. For example, hundreds of young Ethiopian men, most with ambitions of reaching South Africa, are currently detained indefinitely in overcrowded, unsanitary prisons in Malawi; though many have already served time and paid fines for illegal entry, they remain imprisoned due a lack of funding from the Malawian government to repatriate them (Mponda, 2015). Unfortunately, widespread associations of young, undocumented migrant men with notions of threat and criminality may contribute to perceptions that detention is a deserved and appropriate response to immigration infractions. As Askola (2010: 174) writes, 'irregular migrants are "dangerous men", and thus automatically seen as potentially violent and in need of a brutally repressive regime'. For women, risks of sexual violence may be higher in detention, and the mental health implications can be particularly severe for women who have previous experiences of psychological and physical abuse (Askola, 2010: 174). Cleveland *et al.* (2012: 3) note that the detention of women who are pregnant, or have recently given birth, 'may have particularly serious consequences because of the negative impact of maternal depression on the child's physical and mental health'. Research is also now beginning to highlight the largely overlooked issue of the specific health needs of LGBTI migrants in detention. While all detainees are vulnerable to human rights abuses, LGBTI detainees are particularly at risk to heightened levels of both mental and physical abuse, including targeted violence and sexual assault, lack of access to appropriate medical care, and subjection to solitary confinement as a means of controlling or preventing violence against them from other detainees (Tabak and Levitan, 2014: 3).

Practices of detention illustrate how a securitised approach to migration can both directly and indirectly affect the health and well-being of some of the most vulnerable groups of migrants. The mental health impacts of detention, along with risks of disease, poor nutrition, and violence, including sexual violence, showcase some of the ways in which individual migrants bear the embodied consequences of state practices and policies of securitisation.

Conclusion

The policies and practices of securitisation may be blatant, such as the building of fences, or they may also be subtler, such as a host states' restriction of the rights or entitlements associated with asylum. However, they share a common goal of preventing and deterring migrants, particularly asylum seekers and irregular migrants, from entering a host country in the first place. Yet, global structural social, economic and political inequalities continue to contribute to the conditions of poverty, insecurity, and conflict that underscore the movement of millions of people globally.

The securitisation of migration is both ideational and material, from the framing of migrants as criminals and threats, to the building of walls, fences and detention centres to keep migrants out. Drawing on insights from feminist security studies and the concept of intersectionality, this chapter has highlighted the very real, embodied impacts of these policies and practices on the mental and physical health and well-being of migrants, noting how these impacts may be especially negative for those who exist at the crossroads of various determinants of vulnerability, such as race/ethnicity, social class and gender, as well as migration status. These impacts are felt across various phases of migrants' experiences, including exacerbating the threats and dangers involved in migrants' journeys, including sexual and gender-based violence, and affecting migrants' access to health care and services in host countries. The health and well-being of migrants may also be significantly impacted by state practices of detention, and particularly prolonged detention.

As Gerard and Pickering (2014: 16) write, '[t]he securitization of migration contributes to the conditions in which mobility comes at a higher price, literally and metaphorically'. Currently, it is individual migrants, and often the most vulnerable amongst them, who are paying that price with their health and with their lives.

References

Amnesty International. (2010) *Invisible Victims: Migrants on the Move in Mexico*. 28 April 2010, AMR 41/014/2010, Amnesty International Publications.

Askola, H. (2010) 'Illegal migrants', gender and vulnerability: The case of the EU's returns directive', *Feminist Legal Studies*, 18(2): 159–78.

Brian, T., and Laczko, F., eds. (2016) *Fatal Journeys Volume 2: Identification and Tracing of Dead and Missing Migrants*. Geneva: International Organisation for Migration.

Cleveland, J., Rousseau, C., and Kronick, R. (2012) 'The harmful effects of detention and family separation on asylum seekers' mental health in the context of Bill C-31: Brief submitted to the House of Commons Standing Committee on Citizenship and Immigration concerning Bill C-31, the Protecting Canada's Immigration System Act.' Available at: www.cssssdelamontagne.qc.ca/fileadmin/csss_dlm/Publications/Publications_CRF/brief_c31_final.pdf.

Crenshaw, K. (1989) 'Demarginalizing the intersection of race and sex: A black feminist critique of antidiscrimination doctrine, feminist theory and antiracist politics', *University of Chicago Legal Forum*, Vol. 1989, Article 8. Available at: http://chicagounbound.uchicago.edu/uclf/vol1989/iss1/8.

Cuadra, C.B. (2012) 'Right of access to health care for undocumented migrants in EU: A comparative study of national policies', *The European Journal of Public Health*, 22(2): 267–71.

de Wet, P. (October 10, 2014) 'Waiting for change at Lindela.' *Mail & Guardian*. Online. Available at: http://mg.co.za/article/2014-10-09-waiting-for-change-at-lindela (accessed 15 June, 2016).

Doherty, Ben and Evershed, Nick. (2016) 'Immigration detainees four times more likely to suffer severe mental distress', *The Guardian*. 18 January 2016. Accessed at: www. theguardian.com/australia-news/2016/jan/19/immigration-detainees-400-percent-more-likely-to-suffer-severe-mental-distress.

Gerard, Alison and Pickering, Sharon (2014) 'Gender, securitization and transit: Refugee women and the journey to the EU', *Journal of Refugee Studies*, 27(3): 338–359.

Global Detention Project and Access Info Europe. (2015) 'The uncounted: The detention of migrants and asylum seekers in Europe.' Available at: www.globaldetentionproject. org/the-uncounted-the-detention-of-migrants-and-asylum-seekers-in-europe.

Gushulak, B., Weekers, J. and Macpherson, D. (2010) 'Migrants and emerging public health issues in a globalized world: Threats, risks and challenges, an evidence-based framework', *Emerging Health Threats Journal*, 2(10): 1–12.

Harper, I. and Raman, P. (2008) 'Less than human? Diaspora, disease and the question of citizenship', *International Migration*, 46(5): 3–26.

Huysmans, J. (2000) 'The European Union and the securitization of migration', *Journal of Common Market Studies*, 38(5): 751–77.

Infante, C., Idrovo, A.J., Sánchez-Domínguez, M.S., Vinhas, S. and González-Vázquez, T. (2012) 'Violence committed against migrants in transit: Experiences on the Northern Mexican border', *Journal of Immigrant and Minority Health*, 14(3): 449–59.

Kalhan, Anil. (2010) 'Rethinking immigration detention', *Columbia Law Review Sidebar*, 110: 42–58.

Keygnaert, I., Guieu, A., Ooms, G., Vettenburg, N., Temmerman, M. and Roelens, K. (2014) 'Sexual and reproductive health of migrants: Does the EU care?', *Health Policy*, 114(2): 215–25.

Llácer, A., Zunzunegui, M.V., Del Amo, J., Mazarrasa, L. and Bolûmar, F. (2007) 'The contribution of a gender perspective to the understanding of migrants' health', *Journal of Epidemiology and Community Health*, 61(Suppl 2): ii4–ii10.

Malmusi, D., Borrell, C. and Benach, J. (2010) 'Migration-related health inequalities: Showing the complex interactions between gender, social class and place of origin', *Social Science & Medicine*, 71(9): 1610–19.

McInnes, C., and Rushton, S. (2010) 'HIV, AIDS and security: Where are we now?' *International Affairs*, 86(1): 225–45.

Mponda, Felix. (October 14 2015) 'Dreams turn sour for Ethiopian migrants jailed in Malawi', *Mail & Guardian*. Online. Available at: http://mg.co.za/article/2015-10-14-dream-turns-sour-for-ethiopian-migrants-jailed-in-malawi (accessed 13 June 2016).

Rechel, B., Mladovsky, P., Ingleby, D., Mackenbach, J.P. and McKee, M. (2013) 'Migration and health in an increasingly diverse Europe', *The Lancet*, 381(9873): 1235–45.

Sanggaran, J.P., Haire, B. and Zion, D. (2016) 'The health care consequences of Australian immigration policies', *PLoS Med*, 13(2): e1001960.

Shepherd, L.J. (2009) 'Gender, violence and global politics: Contemporary debates in feminist security studies', *Political Studies Review*, 7(2): 208–19.

Tabak, S. and Levitan, R. (2014) 'LGBTI migrants in immigration detention: A global perspective', *Harvard Journal of Law and Gender*, 37(1): 1–45.

Vogt, W.A. (2013) 'Crossing Mexico: Structural violence and the commodification of undocumented Central American migrants', *American Ethnologist*, 40(4): 764–80.

Wibben, A.T. (2014) 'Researching feminist security studies', *Australian Journal of Political Science*, 49(4): 743–55.

Willen, S.S. (2012) 'Migration, "illegality", and health: Mapping embodied vulnerability and debating health-related deservingness', *Social Science & Medicine*, 74(6): 805–11.

World Bank. (2016) 'Out of the shadows: Making mental health a global development priority'. Online. Available at: http://live.worldbank.org/out-of-the-shadows-making-mental-health-a-global-development-priority (accessed 16 June 2016).

6 The global movement for sexual and reproductive health and rights

Intellectual underpinnings

Adrienne Germain

Introduction

Women's sexuality, fertility, health and protection of their human rights, especially freedom from violence and discrimination, are pivotal to their security. While it should be obvious that failure to invest in SRHR jeopardizes not only women but also the health and security of their families, communities and nations, SRHR was largely ignored in global policies until 1994. Until then, population control was a dominant goal of governments and others who believed that rapid population growth, especially in the South, was the pivotal obstacle to national development, poverty reduction and environmental preservation. Many believed that rapid population growth also constituted a threat to national and global peace and security. From the late 1960s onward, women around the world expressed deep concern about the limitations and harms of single-minded population control programs and, in 1994, catalyzed an international policy paradigm shift at the UN International Conference on Population and Development (ICPD). There, 179 governments responded to women's demands for SRHR, and for prevention and mitigation of the structural factors, such as women's inequality, sex discrimination in education and employment, violence against women, and harmful practices such as child marriage, among many others, that threaten their health and violate their human rights.

What were the population and health policies that women wanted to change? The international 'population establishment' aimed to limit population growth through policies and programs that persuaded and enabled married women of reproductive age in the South to use modern contraception. Many of the resultant national family planning programs were of poor quality. They delivered only a few of the increasing range of effective contraceptives, emphasizing long-acting and permanent methods, and neglecting condoms, the one method that protects against both unwanted pregnancy and sexually transmitted infections (STIs). Many failed to consistently provide full information on contraceptive safety and side effects, and to respect every client's right to informed and free consent to contraception. By definition, these programs excluded women younger and older than reproductive age, and those who were not married.

During this time, a separate global 'health establishment' initiated maternal and child health (MCH) policies and programs, which focused on children, provided only minimal antenatal and delivery care, and reached only a fraction of the women who needed them. Instead of augmenting services for pregnancy and delivery, seen as expensive and hard to deliver in countries with weak health systems, many in the MCH community promoted family planning services to reduce the number of pregnancies. Safe abortion services were hardly available, even where laws allowed them, and STIs as well as violence against girls and women were ignored. Finally, until the mid-1970s, most countries and the international community made little to no effort to change the wider structural conditions that jeopardized girls' and women's health and violated their human rights.

Women recognized that these early contraceptive and health services provided vital services to many, but protested that they fell far short of protecting women's health and human rights, and they began to demand action on the structural factors that contribute women's ill health and unnecessary death. In 1975, the UN convened the first world conference on women during which governments for the first time identified these structural factors and their consequences for all aspects of women's lives. Simultaneously, some leaders of the population and health fields were realizing that their programs and policies would have to be modified to achieve their goals, and women's health advocates, part of an emerging women's movement worldwide, demanded better quality services.

From 1970 to 1985, I worked in two leading agencies, first The Population Council and then The Ford Foundation, to develop programs for women's development and rights in Southern countries, and to reduce the shortcomings of the population and health programs they supported. By the late 1970s, both organizations had begun making significant program changes and had increasing impact on other institutions, as well as some governmental and UN policies and programs. In 1985, therefore, I left the 'insider' role in order to advocate more widely from 'outside' the establishment, as Vice President and later President of the International Women's Health Coalition (IWHC).

Drawing on my earlier work inside mainstream institutions, IWHC originated a new framework for population and health policy, namely 'sexual and reproductive health and rights' (SRHR), and began to create an evidence-based case for significant investment in the SRHR of all women and girls ages 10–49, particularly those living in the South.[1] IWHC marshaled evidence and arguments, identified allies in the women's movement especially in the South, and cultivated supporters inside the health and population establishments. We pioneered collaboration between feminists who were mobilizing for women's reproductive rights, and population and health researchers and leaders whose work validated women's concerns about poor quality family planning services, lack of access to safe abortion, and sex-based biases in pivotal disciplines such as demography, among others (Presser, 1997; Dixon-Mueller and Germain, 2000). This work emphasized girls' and women's health, human rights and agency, as persons not as instruments of population control and public health.

Predictably, most leaders of the population establishment rejected the SRHR concept as an existential threat, fearing that combining family planning with other sexual and reproductive health services, and applying a women's rights lens, would hamper the progress of single-focus contraceptive services. They further believed that broadening their clientele beyond married women of reproductive age, addressing adolescents' sexuality, and providing safe abortion would fuel political opposition to contraception. Health leaders similarly asserted that providing comprehensive services for pregnancy prevention, abortion, maternity care and STIs was beyond the capacity of weak health systems; and that addressing abortion and STIs would undermine political support for their 'maternal and child health' initiatives. Neither sector wanted even to promote, let alone implement, programs and policies to address wider structural factors inhibiting women's health and human rights, although they did recognize and promote attention to girls' education and women's literacy.

This chapter illuminates work by IWHC and its partners, beginning in 1985, to generate evidence and propose actions that would position SRHR at the center of global population and health policies and programs. The chapter documents how the original concept of SRHR, and also in-depth knowledge on selected components if it, were created. IWHC's and partners' use of this substantive work to secure major United Nations agreements on SRHR has been chronicled separately (Corrêa, Germain and Sen, 2015). The chapter concludes with reflections on progress to date as well as the need for today's vibrant SRHR movement to deepen the foundational work created by IWHC and its partners, while holding governments and the UN accountable for implementation of hard won international and national commitments to the human rights, health and wellbeing of all (see also Sasser, this volume, Chapter 11).

Defining the SRHR concept

In the late 1980s, prior to the 1994 UN ICPD, IWHC defined basic parameters for SRHR:

*   Values: women's equality and human rights are necessary for securing their SRHR, and vice versa, and all three are essential for wider social and economic justice;
*   Goal: policies and programs addressing population, health, development and human rights in the South have women's health and human rights at their center;
*   Objectives: health systems deliver a minimum package of four services (contraception, maternity care, safe abortion, and STD/HIV prevention, diagnosis and treatment), while other sectors provide comprehensive sexuality education, help protect sexual and reproductive rights, and redress the structural factors underlying poor SRHR, such as sex discrimination, violence, other harmful practices;
*   Implementation: women must be actors in, not simply subjects of, policies, services and programs; service quality must meet both public health and human rights standards; and governments must be held accountable.

IWHC's collaborative intellectual initiatives on SRHR in the 1980s and 1990s tackled several tasks simultaneously: building the evidence base, using both qualitative information from women and demographic and public health data; assessing the adequacy of national and international population and public health policies, funding, research frameworks, and service design and monitoring; making recommendations on which the population and health sectors could reasonably be expected to act, separately and together; and creating evidence-based tools for policy advocacy.

Late in 1992, several of IWHC's international colleagues suggested that feminists mobilize a 'women's voice' for ICPD. With IWHC support, 24 women from 18 countries, most from the Global South, met to draft a 'Women's Declaration on Population Policies.' The Declaration built on earlier work by IWHC and by a global South-based feminist network of researchers and activists 'Development Alternatives with Women for a New Era' (DAWN). The 1992 Declaration adopted a holistic approach, linking SRHR to wider enabling environments. It set out 'minimum program requirements' to support women as whole persons; identified the socio-economic conditions necessary for women to 'control their sexuality and their reproductive health' and to 'exercise their reproductive rights'; and defined 'ethical principles' to guide population and development policies. Within six months, the originators of the Declaration secured additional signatures from over 2,500 individuals and organizations from about 110 countries – testimony to women's exceptional networking capacity before the Internet.

Because official UN preparations for ICPD showed little support for SRHR, IWHC and feminist allies decided early in 1993 to engage a larger, representative group of activists in preparing a final women's platform for the ICPD and, in so doing, identify a core group to advocate throughout the ICPD process. In January 1994, IWHC, CEPIA (a leading Brazilian women's rights organization) and an International Steering Committee co-organized a meeting of 215 broadly representative women from 79 countries in Rio de Janeiro. The resultant women's platform encompassed the content of the 1992 Declaration and expanded further on structural factors that affect women's SRHR (poverty, development and 'gender power relationships,' including their expression through myriad forms of violence against women and girls); 'fundamentalisms' (social and political, not only religious, conservatisms that include, as a central tenet, the control of women's sexuality and their bodies); accountability, and the need to invest in women's organizations (Reproductive Health and Justice International Women's Health Conference for Cairo 1994, 1994). Simultaneously, IWHC continued work to legitimize SRHR in influential population and health circles. For example, with DAWN and Harvard University, IWHC commissioned international specialists and Southern feminists to produce a book on the significance of SRHR for population and development policy (Sen, Germain and Chen, 1994). Seventeen chapters address population growth, women's health and human rights, ethics, youth, the women's health movement, sexual rights including violence against women and girls, gender and household dynamics, biomedical research, and financing, all topics that IWHC and DAWN wanted governments to address at the ICPD.

The 1994 UN ICPD outcome, a Programme of Action agreed by 179 governments, is widely recognized as a 'paradigm shift' in population policy (United Nations, 1995). The Programme commits to securing the equality, empowerment and SRHR of women and adolescents, especially girls, in their own right, and also acknowledges for the first time in a UN population conference that SRHR are essential for fertility reduction. The agreement includes almost all of the women's Reproductive Health and Justice platform: expansive definitions of reproductive and sexual health and reproductive rights (SRH+RR), the supply side of SRHR (provision of good quality, comprehensive SRH services), and also the demand side (socio-economic conditions and human rights protections that enable women and girls to access and use SRH information and services).[2] The agreement encompasses other vital issues never before addressed in intergovernmental population agreements, including access to safe abortion where not against the law, sex education, adolescents' right to SRH services, violence against women, STIs prevention and treatment, and infertility and reproductive cancers (Germain and Kyte, 1995).

Before the ICPD, women's health and rights advocates had been pursuing improvements in population policies and programs in countries as diverse as Brazil, Nigeria and the Philippines (Dixon-Mueller and Germain, 1994). The ICPD Programme of Action provided a powerful new tool for such advocates everywhere, but examples of actual implementation of SRHR were needed. IWHC helped create a major example in Bangladesh when the government decided to transform its national family planning program, widely considered a 'success,' into a 'health and population' program using the ICPD SRHR approach. The Swedish government, a donor to the Bangladesh program, asked IWHC to help ensure that the new program would include, at a minimum, expanded access to early abortion services; skilled obstetric care; the first national STD and HIV prevention initiative; and improved service quality. They also provided vital political support for IWHC's engagement of Bangladesh civil society, especially women, as central stakeholders in the design process (Jahan, 2003). After five years of program implementation, contrary to pessimistic forecasts by most donors and the population establishment, contraceptive prevalence, already high compared with other high fertility countries, remained so, while maternal mortality, among the highest in the South, dropped 25 percent (Jahan, 2007). The Bangladesh initiative thus demonstrated that the SRHR approach is feasible and highly beneficial at national scale (Jahan and Germain, 2004).

Post-ICPD, IWHC and some of its ICPD allies also created an informal international association called HERA (Health, Empowerment, Rights and Accountability) to produce advocacy materials containing definitions, evidence and actions for central elements of SRHR, including reproductive rights, reproductive health, sexual rights, sexual health, adolescents' sexual rights and health, abortion, men's roles and responsibilities, gender equality and equity, women's empowerment, and advocacy (HERA Secretariat and IWHC, 1996). HERA members helped ensure that the 1995 UN Fourth World Conference on Women ('Beijing Conference') reaffirmed the ICPD's SRHR commitments, and strengthened several of them.

Remarkably, although the conference agreement did not use the term 'sexual rights,' it defined the content of these rights for the first time in a UN agreement (Dunlop, Kyte and Macdonald, 1996; United Nations, 1996).[3]

In the following decades, IWHC facilitated the creation of many fact-based advocacy tools for UN intergovernmental negotiations on SRHR, including myriad UN-mandated reviews of implementation of the ICPD and Beijing Conference commitments and of UN agreements on ending HIV and AIDS. IWHC also contributed substantively to the follow up of the UN Millennium Development Goals (MDGs) 2000–15, and to the creation of the Sustainable Development Goals (SDGs), 2016–30, aiming to make SRHR and gender equality a priority. The MDGs included a goal on gender equality and another on reduction of maternal mortality, but fell notably short of SRHR in concept and in implementation. IWHC, its colleagues and many other advocates thus worked intensively with governments and UN agencies during SDG negotiations to ensure stronger attention to SRHR. IWHC also published articles and advocated with specialists contributing to technical aspects of the MDG and the SDG health and gender equality goals and targets, including health system strengthening and universal health coverage (Germain and Dixon-Mueller, 2005; Sen *et al.*, 2015; Germain and Liljestrand, 2009). In these technical debates, IWHC asserted that prioritizing provision of an integrated package of SRH services, with an emphasis on quality and accountability, would build a strong foundation for strengthening health systems overall. The resultant SDGs, while not ideal, especially in regard to adolescents' sexuality, health and rights, contain more robust targets than the MDGs had and address most of the central elements of SRHR, including universal access to SRH services, recognition of reproductive rights, ending violence against women, and achieving gender equality, among others.

In-depth work on specific elements of SRHR

Coincident with work on the comprehensive SRHR concept, prior to and following ICPD, IWHC and its partners worked intensively on four of the central components of SRHR: safe abortion; contraception; prevention and control of sexually transmitted infections (STIs), including HIV; and the sexual and reproductive health of adolescents.[4] All of this work took into account both a core SRHR goal – access to comprehensive, preferably integrated, SRH services that meet human rights as well as public health standards – and also the constraints faced by health systems. It aimed both to elevate SRHR in debates about health and population sector priorities and to make recommendations that were actionable in prevailing circumstances.

Abortion

The central premise of IWHC's substantive work on abortion was established at the 1985 UN Third World Conference on Women. There, IWHC and allies, leaders in national women's movements in the South, countered anti-abortion 'right to life' polemic with a women's definition of the 'right to life' that includes women's rights to protect their own health and lives, to control their bodies, and to have only the children they want. A pressing task following that conference was to design and document abortion services suitable for scaling up by governments that face legal, health system and resource constraints.[5] The main elements of these exemplary services were training and equipment for manual vacuum aspiration (MVA), an inexpensive and also the safest abortion technique, which was not then widely known in Southern countries; the provision of contraception and other SRH services with abortion care; other improvements in service quality; and expanded outreach to women, especially young women (Dixon-Mueller, 1993). Coincident with these investments, in 1987 IWHC designed and led an International Symposium in which over 200 members of the International Federation of Obstetricians and Gynecologists (FIGO) discussed global and national actions to reduce high levels of maternal morbidity and mortality due to unsafe abortion, particularly in the South. The Symposium papers, grounded in country experiences including IWHC-supported services, were written by physicians, experts on law and ethics, service providers and policy makers (Rosenfield *et al.*, 1989). Invitations to write papers, IWHC collaboration with authors during drafting, and the Symposium itself introduced both authors and participants not only to improved abortion practices but also to SRHR.

Over the years, to face down international anti-abortion activism and create a foundation for advocacy in both national and UN forums, IWHC continuously developed and refined a multi-faceted, data-based case for access to safe services. These publications helped disseminate evidence that women throughout the world commonly resort to abortion; that the procedure is exceptionally safe when provided by trained providers (doctors and mid-level professionals such as nurses) in hygienic conditions; that access to safe abortion is essential for reducing maternal mortality and morbidity; and that abortion access is also a fundamental right, the fulfillment of which is essential for women's empowerment and the realization of their other human rights.

Perhaps most significantly, IWHC adopted and promoted a new perspective for advocacy. Most advocates referred to abortion as 'illegal,' believing that eliminating legal restrictions was necessary for expanding access. Knowing that legal change would take many years during which thousands of women would die or be severely injured by unsafe abortion, IWHC promoted safe abortion services for all women who are 'eligible under existing laws.' Almost all national laws allow abortion to save the life of the woman and on one or more additional grounds (e.g., health, rape, incest, severe fetal anomalies). Using this perspective, IWHC asserted that all but four or five countries are obligated to train and equip health care workers to provide safe services (Germain and Kim, 1998).

In response to strong advocacy for this premise by IWHC and allies, the 1999 UN intergovernmental review of ICPD implementation significantly enhanced the ICPD agreement (abortion should be safe where allowed by law) by specifying that health care providers should be trained and equipped to serve women eligible under law (United Nations General Assembly, 1999). Following this agreement, IWHC persuaded the World Health Organization (WHO) to produce guidance for countries, which addressed both clinical practice and also strategies to address policy barriers (WHO, 2003).[6] Many recommendations and examples of action in the Guidance are based on IWHC-supported services and advocacy for legal, policy and regulatory reforms.

Contraception

Substantive work on improving the quality of contraceptive services, like the work on safe abortion access, faced complex political challenges. Many conservatives recognized contraception as a way to reduce the need for abortion or as a means to population control, but opposed adoption of a women's health and rights perspective. Women's health activists, concerned about contraceptive safety and abuse of women's rights, distrusted contraceptive researchers and providers. IWHC believed that dialogue among these parties could facilitate inclusion of women's health advocates in contraceptive research and development processes, and also help to revise key assumptions underlying demographic research and training, population policies, and the design and monitoring of SRH services.

In 1990, when the head of WHO's Special Programme of Research on Human Reproduction (HRP) asked for insights on women's perspectives, IWHC proposed co-convening a meeting between HRP's worldwide contraceptive researchers and IWHC's feminist colleagues to determine where they could agree, and where more dialogue was needed. The meeting report describes the process – equal leadership and participation by both groups throughout – as well as the substantive outcomes (WHO Special Programme of Research, Development and Research Training in Human Reproduction and IWHC, 1991). Significant collaborative work between WHO and women's health advocates flowed from this landmark meeting (Germain and Faundes, 1994). A notable global effort was an international symposium convened by HRP and the Government of Mexico prior to the ICPD, whose final Declaration reflects the emerging willingness of some scientists to listen to and address women's concerns about contraceptive research, policies and programs (Van Look and Pérez-Palacios, 1994; Marcelo and Germain, 1994). WHO also made significant staffing and program changes in the years after the original meeting that had lasting impacts on their work agenda, processes and outputs (Cottingham, 2015).

Complementary substantive work by IWHC challenged the population sector to revise its core planning tool, 'unmet need for family planning,' to include not just married women who wished to avoid pregnancy but also unmarried women including adolescents, those dissatisfied with their contraceptive method, and those who had discontinued use for remediable reasons such as poor quality services (Dixon-Mueller and Germain, 1992). IWHC challenged the field to improve family planning program indicators and to pay attention to the connections among contraception, sexuality and reproductive health (Dixon-Mueller and Germain, 2007a; Dixon-Mueller, 1993). IWHC's and other feminists' advocacy secured attention to these issues, and others such as consent to contraception, improving the technical quality of services, and ensuring that family planning clients are treated with respect, in the 1994 UN ICPD agreement.

Sexually transmitted infections, HIV and AIDS

In response to women's expressed concerns, in 1991 IWHC organized the first meeting of academic researchers, UN and government experts, and women's health advocates to discuss the health and social consequences of STIs and HIV for women. Participants agreed that STIs are preventable and most are treatable at reasonable cost, and also framed specific recommendations for integrating STI prevention, diagnosis and treatment into public health and family planning programs that serve general populations of women in the South. Using its subsequent position paper, IWHC invited leading scientists, STI/HIV clinicians and family planning/MCH practitioners, social scientists, and national experts from Brazil, India, Kenya, Nigeria and Mozambique to review current research and policies and propose actions to reduce women's vulnerability to STIs and HIV (Germain *et al.*, 1992).

Though significant, these papers did not fully address the determinants of women's vulnerability to infection and, from a women's health and rights perspective, their recommendations were incomplete. IWHC and the Women and Development Unit, University of the West Indies, therefore convened 44 feminists from 22 countries in 1992 to review factors (such as poverty, violence, men's sexual behaviors, age differences and unequal gender power between partners) that make women vulnerable to STIs and HIV. Recognizing the limitations of condoms, participants called for creation of one or more fully women-controlled STI prevention technologies. They identified the essential characteristics such methods should have, named these potential methods 'microbicides,' and urged IWHC to promote research and development of female-controlled vaginal protection (Antrobus, Germain and Nowrojee, 1994).

IWHC identified a biomedical scientist at The Population Council; raised funds to hasten his work; persuaded the Council to collaborate with feminists on the research (a major innovation at the time); and convened Women's Health Advocates on Microbicides (WHAM), whose members represented, among others, communities of sex workers in Asia and women and girls in Sub-Saharan Africa. WHAM worked with The Population Council to identify which of the method characteristics that women desired could be pursued. It also helped to develop research approaches and ethical standards to protect women's rights during clinical trials, which, for technical reasons, were conducted among highly vulnerable women; to create processes for including women's health advocates in data analysis; and to share findings early and often with participating women and communities. As interest grew, IWHC, WHAM and the Council encouraged other researchers to engage women in their work, including by convening an unprecedented, multi-agency symposium of researchers and women's health advocates (Heise, McGrory and Wood, 1998).

Throughout this period, it was becoming clear that mushrooming global HIV and AIDS policy, funding, and institutions were ignoring girls and women in the general population, despite their disproportionate vulnerability to infection compared with men. One reason for neglect was the core premise that communicable disease control is best achieved by focusing on the groups most likely to transmit infection. In the HIV case, these groups are men who have sex with men, IV drug users, and sex workers and their clients, not women in the general population. Further, the global AIDS sector did not address the other SRHR needs of women living with HIV and AIDS, or women's roles as caregivers. To address these gaps, IWHC and its allies realized they would have to secure an HIV and AIDS policy paradigm shift analogous to the earlier one in population policy.

This work challenged the core premise of the lead discipline, epidemiology, and sought a strong voice for Southern women in global and national policy making and advocacy. The work promoted two premises. First, protecting the SRHR of women and girls in the general population is necessary to end HIV and AIDS. Second, HIV and AIDS information and services would best serve women when integrated into other SRH services. The HIV and AIDS sector disagreed with the first, and felt the second threatened the sector's autonomy and resources. Nonetheless, feminists, including women living with HIV and AIDS, persisted in their promotion of three priorities: actions to address the determinants of girls' and women's vulnerability and to provide services to women in the general population; protections for women's rights in negotiations of intergovernmental agreements on HIV and AIDS; and modifications of global HIV and AIDs policies, funding and institutions to encompass women's SRHR.

IWHC and allies proposed that HIV and AIDS be addressed as part of a broad SRHR agenda for girls and women; countered simplistic assertions about prioritiz-ing HIV over other SRH causes of premature death and disability in women; and promoted greater emphasis on men's and women's ethical responsibility to inform partners of their HIV status (Germain, Dixon-Mueller and Sen, 2009; Germain, 2009; Germain and Dixon-Mueller, 2010; Dixon-Mueller and Germain, 2007b). As data emerged on vertical (parent to infant) transmission, HIV and AIDS invest-ments in pregnant women were introduced, but policy attention to non-pregnant women in the general population remained largely rhetorical (Joint United Nations Programme on HIV/AIDS, 2010).

Though they neglected women in the general population, the HIV and AIDS sector, unlike the population sector, was open to working on two aspects of SRHR that had been widely avoided: sexuality and sexual rights, and adolescents' SRHR. On sexuality and sexual rights, in the early 2000s, a WHO expert group, including IWHC and allies, produced a 'working definition' of sexual health and rights that reflected feminists', including HERA's, intellectual work since the late 1980s, and elaborated on the pivotal agreement on sexual rights secured in the 1995 Beijing Conference mentioned above. IWHC also proposed an ethical framework for sexual partnerships (Dixon-Mueller *et al.*, 2009). In 2015, WHO published a touchstone technical paper on sexual health, human rights and the law that drew on decades of work by feminists, among others (WHO, 2015b).

Adolescents' sexual and reproductive rights and health

Violations of adolescents' health and human rights are widespread and include many forms of violence, such as child and forced marriage, female genital mutilation (FGM), crimes in the name of honor, and sexual violence and trafficking. School-based sex education is still not offered in many countries in the South and unmarried adolescents are typically excluded from SRH services by law or by the attitudes and practices of health care providers, families and community leaders. In the early 1990s, colleagues, in Brazil, Cameroun, Indonesia and Nigeria, asked IWHC to support SRHR programs with and for adolescents aged 10–19. IWHC staff and consultants worked with these colleagues to develop program strategies and curricula.

Based on years of experience with these programs, IWHC published evidence-based lesson plans and program guidance on sexuality education suitable for local adaptation by policy makers, educators and others across the South (Irvin, 2004). These addressed not only standard topics (puberty, contraception, HIV) but also topics that were rarely addressed (relationships, sexual behavior, sexual rights, STIs, sexual orientation, abortion, violence and harmful practices). Program guidance emphasized securing community and parental support, and training facilitators to respond nonjudgmentally and accurately to adolescents' needs and concerns. Drawing on these and other such programs, feminists persuaded delegations to the 1994 ICPD to recognize adolescents' rights to sex education and to SRH services in 42 paragraphs of the Program of Action.[7] These commitments have been reaffirmed, with intensive advocacy, in most UN negotiations since, and the lead UN agency for education, United Nations Educational, Scientific and Cultural Organization (UNESCO), has produced technical guidance that addresses many though not all of these topics (UNESCO, 2015; Dixon-Mueller, 2010). In the last decade, some 25 years after IWHC and allies first called for attention to adolescents' SRHR, most global population and public health institutions, leading journals and professional associations now address adolescents' SRHR at least to some extent, undergirded by a vital young people's movement.

Conclusions: where are we today?

Achieving sexual and reproductive health and rights requires fundamental changes in how girls' and women's bodies and personhood are situated in social norms, laws and policies, and in the attitudes and practices of educators and health service providers. As challenging, achieving SRHR requires seismic shifts in the balance of power between men and women in intimate relationships, families, and throughout all aspects of social life. In 2018, is the SRHR glass half full or half empty? After nearly 50 years of work both inside and outside the population and health establishments, and considering the rock-bottom base from which SRHR started, I suggest that this huge glass is at least half full.

Progress is suggested by global indicators such as lower rates of maternal mortality and adolescent pregnancy, and higher contraceptive prevalence (United

Nations, 2015). Less measurable, but no less important, progress can be seen in the rhetoric and actions of influential health and population institutions, such as the Population Council. Potentially game-changing innovations have been made in birth control technologies – notably, emergency contraception and medications to induce abortion – and in training standards for provision of safe abortion (WHO, 2015a). Microbicides researchers are on the verge of producing the first woman-controlled protective methods suitable for wide distribution (International Partnership For Microbicides, 2016). UNFPA and others have significantly increased the number of skilled midwives in countries with the weakest health systems, while WHO has improved methodologies to track maternal morbidity (long ignored) not only mortality (Chou *et al.*, 2016). Significant global initiatives have been launched, notably 'Every Woman Every Child' (Every Woman Every Child, 2015; The World Bank Group, 2016). In 2016, the World Health Assembly adopted the first global plan of action to prevent and mitigate violence against women and girls not only through direct services and legal protections but also by addressing the underlying structural conditions that allow and perpetuate violence (WHO, 2016). National actions on abortion access include progressive revisions in abortion laws, which far outnumber regressive ones, and robust abortion rights campaigns by both advocates and governments (Asuagbor, 2016).[8]

In recent years the UN Human Rights Council has held numerous governments to account for sexual rights violations and urged states to decriminalize abortion, provide sexuality education, and protect reproductive rights (International Planned Parenthood Federation and Sexual Rights Initiative, 2012). Other UN human rights bodies have issued official statements on adults' and adolescents' right to the full range of quality SRH services including safe abortion, and to comprehensive sexuality education (Committee on the Rights of the Child, 2013; Committee on Economic, Social and Cultural Rights, 2016).

Despite such progress, the SRHR glass is still half empty. About 300,000 women die each year in pregnancy and childbirth, almost all of them from preventable causes in Southern countries. At least 225 million women in the South still have an unmet need for family planning (using a definition somewhat closer to that desired by SRHR advocates). Rates of unsafe abortion remain high in the South, even where laws are liberal (Sedgh *et al.*, 2016). Globally, women and girls are still the most affected by the AIDS epidemic, and about 270,000 women die annually of cervical cancer, reflecting continued neglect of STI and HIV prevention for girls and women in the general population (Office of the High Commissioner of Human Rights, 2016). An estimated one in three women ages 15–49 worldwide experience physical and or sexual violence either within or outside the home (Every Woman Every Child, 2015). Severe inequities remain within and across countries by income, urban vs. rural residence, and ethnicity. Furthermore, addressing disparities in the realization of the SRHR of the LGBTQ population, with which IWHC has increasingly worked in solidarity, is only in its infancy (see Schwenke, this volume, Chapter 12).

The challenge today is to implement the full array of SRHR commitments, including but not limited to those contained in the UN SDGs 2016-30. It is estimated that $39 billion is needed annually to deliver SRH in the global South, but far less than that has been allocated (Singh, Darroch and Ashford, 2014; Anderson *et al.*, 2016). Of equal concern is disproportionate use of available funds for particular elements of SRHR despite the known benefits of investing in SRHR as a whole and in other program and policy changes (Singh, Darroch and Ashford, 2014; Cottingham, Germain and Hunt, 2012; Family Planning 2020, 2016).

Feminist activists have brought SRHR a long way since 1980 – farther than most thought likely in our lifetimes. We secured the moral high ground at ICPD by giving voice and political weight to women and adolescents as primary constituents with the most at stake. By continuously analyzing evidence, fostering exemplary programs, and strengthening relationships with governments and other gatekeepers, the movement has secured intergovernmental and national commitments to SRHR, profound shifts in population and health policy paradigms, and transformational changes in many population and health sector institutions. The feminist health and rights movement itself has proven resilient in the face of setbacks and increasingly able to hold governments and other actors accountable for the implementation of their commitments.

Nonetheless, in 2018, the movement faces the persistent challenge to change structural factors that work against women's health and human rights, factors significantly exacerbated by global retreat from the feminist and democratic values that underlie SRHR. With the 2016–17 changes in the US government, the world's women and girls have not only lost one of their foremost champions but also now face a powerful, likely intractable, opponent. Continuing progress toward full implementation of global and national SRHR agreements, and protection of the agreements themselves, will require continuing, skilled engagement of, and investments in, the feminist SRHR movement as part of and in collaboration with wider social movements for social and economic justice (Corrêa, Germain and Sen, 2015; Germain *et al.*, 2015; Sen *et al.*, 2015).

Notes

1 This chapter uses 'SRHR' throughout, in conformity with general usage after the 1994 ICPD. IWHC's early materials used 'SRRH' so that 'rights' preceded 'health' and would be associated directly with both 'sexual' and 'reproductive.' Many today use truncated terms, such as 'reproductive health,' especially in intergovernmental negotiations, because they do not agree with all elements of the SRHR concept, particularly sexual and reproductive rights, and/or with the comprehensive approach implied by 'SRHR' (Girard, 2009).
2 SRH+RR separates 'rights' from 'sexual,' reflecting insurmountable opposition to 'sexual rights' by some government delegations in the ICPD and in many negotiations that followed.
3 The facilitator of this negotiation, one of several HERA members who served on government delegations, masterfully navigated extremely conflicting views among delegations.
4 IWHC promoted, but did not elaborate to the same extent, two vital SRHR elements, maternity care and violence against women, which were addressed by other NGOs, UNFPA, and WHO among others. IWHC and partners worked from the premise that health is a human right, and requires comprehensive health care for all, but our substantive work aimed to make visible, and to identify remedies for, the specific neglect of SRHR.

5 Bangladesh, Brazil, Cameroun, Colombia, India, Indonesia, Nigeria and the Philippines.
6 In 2012, WHO produced a revised edition of the Guidance that updates clinical standards and retains the policy suggestions.
7 As a member of the US government delegation, I negotiated this outcome with delegates of Iran and Pakistan. The price was steep – dropping the term 'sexual rights' in return for their agreement to protect text on adolescents' SRHR from attack by other delegations.
8 The Center for Reproductive Rights and the International Campaign for Women's Rights to Safe Abortion are leading resources for abortion data and laws.

References

Anderson, I., Maliqi, B., Axelson, H. and Ostergren, M., 2016. How can health ministries present persuasive investment plans for women's, children's and adolescents' health? *Bulletin of the World Health Organization*, 94(6), pp.468–474. DOI: 10.2471/BLT.15. 168419.

Antrobus, P., Germain, A. and Nowrojee, S., 1994. *Challenging the Culture of Silence: Building Alliances to End Reproductive Tract Infections*. New York, NY: International Women's Health Coalition. Available at: https://iwhc.org/resources/challenging-culture-silence-building-alliances-end-reproductive-tract-infections [Accessed Oct. 10, 2016].

Asuagbor, L., 2016. *Press Release: Launch of the Campaign for the Decriminalization of Abortion in Africa: Women and Girls in Africa are Counting on Us to Save Their Lives!* [online] African Commission on Human and Peoples' Rights. Available at: www.achpr. org/press/2016/01/d287 [Accessed Jun. 19, 2016].

Chou, D., Tunçalp, Ö., Firoz, T., Barreix, M., Filippi, V., von Dadelszen, P., van den Broek, N., Cecatti, J.G. and Say, L., 2016. Constructing maternal morbidity – towards a standard tool to measure and monitor maternal health beyond mortality. *BMC Pregnancy and Childbirth*, 16, p.45. DOI: 10.1186/s12884-015-0789-4.

Committee on Economic, Social and Cultural Rights, 2016. *General Comment No. 22 (2016) on the Right to Sexual and Reproductive Health (Article 12 of the International Covenant on Economic, Social and Cultural Rights)*. [online] Available at: https:// documents-dds-ny.un.org/doc/UNDOC/GEN/G16/089/32/PDF/G1608932.pdf? OpenElement [Accessed Jul. 25, 2016].

Committee on the Rights of the Child, 2013. *General Comment No. 15 (2013) on the Right of the Child to the Enjoyment of the Highest Attainable Standard of Health (Art. 24)*. [online] Available at: http://tbinternet.ohchr.org/_layouts/treatybodyexternal/Download. aspx?symbolno=CRC%2fC%2fGC%2f15&Lang=en [Accessed Oct. 10, 2016].

Corrêa, S., Germain, A. and Sen, G., 2015. Feminist Mobilizing for Global Commitments to the Sexual and Reproductive Health and Rights of Women and Girls. In: E. Chesler and T. McGovern, eds., *Women and Girls Rising: Progress and Resistance Around the World*, Global Institutions. London; New York: Routledge, pp.51–68.

Cottingham, J., 2015. Historical note: How bringing women's health advocacy groups to WHO helped change the research agenda. *Reproductive Health Matters*, 23(45), pp.12– 20. DOI: 10.1016/j.rhm.2015.06.007.

Cottingham, J., Germain, A. and Hunt, P., 2012. Use of human rights to meet the unmet need for family planning. *The Lancet*, 380(9837), pp.172–180. DOI: 10.1016/S0140-6736 (12)60732-6.

Dixon-Mueller, R., 1993. The sexuality connection in reproductive health. *Studies in Family Planning*, 24(5), pp.269–282. DOI: 10.2307/2939221.

Dixon-Mueller, R., 2010. Review of international technical guidance on sexuality education: an evidence-informed approach for schools, teachers and health educators.

vol. I, vol. II, United Nations Educational, Scientific and Cultural Organization. *Studies in Family Planning*, 41(2), pp.159–162. Available at: www.jstor.org/stable/25681359 [Accessed May 14, 2016].

Dixon-Mueller, R. and Germain, A., 1992. Stalking the elusive 'unmet need' for family planning. *Studies in Family Planning*, 23(5), pp.330–335. DOI: 10.2307/1966531.

Dixon-Mueller, R. and Germain, A., 1994. Population Policy and Feminist Political Action in Three Developing Countries. In: J. Finkle and A. McIntosh, eds., *The New Politics of Population: Conflict and Consensus in Family Planning*. New York, NY: Population Council, pp. 197–219. (Also available on JSTOR: Population and Development Review. Vol. 20.)

Dixon-Mueller, R., and Germain, A., 2000. Reproductive Health and Demographic Imagination. In: H.B. Presser and G. Sen, eds., *Women's Empowerment and Demographic Processes: Moving Beyond Cairo*. New York, NY: Oxford University Press, pp.69–94.

Dixon-Mueller, R. and Germain, A., 2007a. Fertility regulation and reproductive health in the Millennium Development Goals: The search for a perfect Indicator. *American Journal of Public Health*, 97(1), pp.45–51. DOI: 10.2105/AJPH.2005.068056.

Dixon-Mueller, R. and Germain, A., 2007b. HIV testing: The mutual rights and responsibilities of partners. *The Lancet*, 370(9602), pp.1808–1809. DOI: 10.1016/S0140-6736 (07)61754-1.

Dixon-Mueller, R., Germain, A., Fredrick, B. and Bourne, K., 2009. Towards a sexual ethics of rights and responsibilities. *Reproductive Health Matters*, 17(33), pp.111–119. Available at: www.jstor.org/stable/40647616 [Accessed May 14, 2016].

Dunlop, J., Kyte, R. and Macdonald, M., 1996. Women redrawing the map: The world after the Beijing and Cairo conferences. *SAIS review (Paul H. Nitze School of Advanced International Studies)*, 16(1), pp.153–165. Available at: https://muse.jhu.edu/article/30292 [Accessed Jul. 25, 2016].

Every Woman Every Child, 2015. *Global Strategy for Women's, Children's and Adolescents Health 2016–2030*. [online] Available at: www.who.int/life-course/partners/global-strategy/globalstrategyreport2016-2030-lowres.pdf?ua=1 [Accessed Jul. 25, 2016].

Family Planning 2020, 2016. *Family Planning 2020*. [online] Available at: www. familyplanning2020.org [Accessed Jun. 19, 2016].

Germain, A., 2009. Review of integrating gender into HIV/AIDS programmes in the health sector: Tool to improve responsiveness to women's needs, by World Health Organization. *Bulletin of the World Health Organization*, 87(11), pp.883–884. DOI: 10.2471/BLT.09.071522.

Germain, A. and Dixon-Mueller, R., 2005. Reproductive health and the MDGs: Is the glass half full or half empty? *Studies in Family Planning*, 36(2), pp.137–140. DOI: 10.1111/j. 1728-4465.2005.00053.x.

Germain, A. and Dixon-Mueller, R., 2010. HIV is the biggest killer of women – but is it? *The Lancet*, 375(9726), pp.1592–1593. DOI: 10.1016/S0140-6736(10)60312-1.

Germain, A., Dixon-Mueller, R. and Sen, G., 2009. Back to basics: HIV/AIDS belongs with sexual and reproductive health. *Bulletin of the World Health Organization*, 87, pp.840–845. DOI: 10.2471/BLT.09.065425.

Germain, A. and Faundes, A., 1994. Women's Perspectives on Reproductive Health Research. In: P.F. Kanna, P.F.A. Van Look and P.D. Griffin, eds., *Challenges in Reproductive Health Research: Biennial Report 1992–1993*. [online] Geneva: World Health Organization, pp.58–65. Available at: www.who.int/iris/handle/10665/39653 [Accessed May 16, 2016].

Germain, A., Holmes, K.K., Piot, P. and Wasserheit, J.N. eds., 1992. *Reproductive Tract Infections: Global Impact and Priorities for Women's Reproductive Health*. Reproductive Biology. New York, NY: Plenum Press.

Germain, A. and Kim, T., 1998. *Expanding Access to Safe Abortion: Strategies for Action*. New York, NY: International Women's Health Coalition. Available at: https://iwhc.org/resources/expanding-access-safe-abortion-strategies-action [Accessed Oct. 10, 2016].

Germain, A. and Kyte, R., 1995. *The Cairo Consensus: The Right Agenda for the Right Time*. New York, NY: International Women's Health Coalition. Available at: https://iwhc.org/resources/the-cairo-consensus-the-right-agenda-for-the-right-time [Accessed Oct. 10, 2016].

Germain, A. and Liljestrand, J., 2009. Women's groups and professional organizations in advocacy for sexual and reproductive health and rights. *International Journal of Gynecology and Obstetrics*, 106(2), pp.185–187. DOI: 10.1016/j.ijgo.2009.03.038.

Germain, A., Sen, G., Garcia-Moreno, C. and Shankar, M., 2015. Advancing sexual and reproductive health and rights in low- and middle-income countries: Implications for the post-2015 global development agenda. *Global Public Health*, 10(2), pp.137–148. DOI: 10.1080/17441692.2014.986177.

Girard, Françoise (2009) Advocacy for Sexuality and Women's Rights: Continuities, Discontinuities, and Strategies Since ICPD. In: Laura Reichenbach and Mindy Jane Roseman, eds., *Reproductive Health and Human Rights The Way Forward*. Philadelphia: University of Pennsylvania Press.

Heise, L.L., McGrory, E. and Wood, S.Y., 1998. *Practical and Ethical Dilemmas in the Clinical Testing of Microbicides: A Report on a Symposium*. New York, NY: International Women's Health Coalition. Available at: https://iwhc.org/resources/practical-ethical-dilemmas-clinical-testing-microbicides-report-symposium [Accessed Oct. 10, 2016].

HERA Secretariat and International Women's Health Coalition, 1996. *Women's Sexual and Reproductive Rights and Health Action Sheets*. New York, NY: International Women's Health Coalition. Available at: https://iwhc.org/resources/hera-action-sheets [Accessed Oct. 10, 2016].

International Partnership For Microbicides, 2016. *International Partnership For Microbicides Home Page*. Available at: www.ipmglobal.org [Accessed Jun. 19, 2016].

International Planned Parenthood Federation and Sexual Rights Initiative, 2012. *Sexual Rights and the Universal Periodic Review: A Toolkit for Advocates*. [online] International Planned Parenthood Federation Arab World Region Press. Available at: https://issuu.com/ippfresources/docs/universalperiodicreview_toolkit_2012.

Irvin, A., 2004. *Positively Informed: Lesson Plans and Guidance for Sexuality Educators and Advocates*. New York, NY: International Women's Health Coalition. Available at: https://iwhc.org/resources/positively-informed-lesson-plans-guidance-sexuality-educators-advocates [Accessed Jul. 25, 2016].

Jahan, R., 2003. Restructuring the health system: experiences of advocates for gender equity in Bangladesh. *Reproductive Health Matters*, 11(21), pp.183–191. DOI: 10.1016/S0968-8080(03)02173-6.

Jahan, R., 2007. Securing maternal health through comprehensive reproductive health services: lessons from Bangladesh. *American Journal of Public Health*, 97(7), pp.1186–1190. DOI: 10.2105/AJPH.2005.081737.

Jahan, R. and Germain, A., 2004. Mobilising support to sustain political will is the key to progress in reproductive health. *The Lancet*, 364(9436), pp.742–744. DOI: 10.1016/S0140-6736(04)16954-7.

Joint United Nations Programme on HIV/AIDS, 2010. *Agenda for Accelerated Country Action for Women, Girls, Gender Equality and HIV – Operational Plan for the UNAIDS Action Framework – Addressing Women, Girls, Gender Equality and HIV.* [online] Geneva. Available at: www.unicef.org/aids/files/20100226_jc1794_agenda_for_accelerated_country_action_en.pdf [Accessed Jul. 25, 2016].

Marcelo, B. and Germain, A., 1994. Women's Perspectives on Fertility Regulation Methods and Services. In: P.F.A. Van Look and G. Pérez-Palacios, eds., *Contraceptive Research and Development 1984 to 1994: The Road from Mexico City to Cairo and Beyond.* Oxford: Oxford University Press, pp.325–342.

Office of the High Commissioner of Human Rights, 2016. *Joint Statement by UN Human Rights Experts* on the Occasion of the High-Level Meeting on ending AIDS by 2030.* [online] Available at: www.ohchr.org/EN/NewsEvents/Pages/DisplayNews.aspx?NewsID=20053&LangID=E [Accessed Jun. 19, 2016].

Presser, H.B., 1997. Demography, feminism, and the science-policy nexus. *Population and Development Review*, 23(2), pp.295–331. DOI: 10.2307/2137547.

Reproductive Health and Justice International Women's Health Conference for Cairo, 1994. The Rio Statement of 'Reproductive Health and Justice: International Women's Health Conference for Cairo 1994. In: *Reproductive Health and Justice: International Women's Health Conference for Cairo '94, January 24–28, 1994.* Rio de Janeiro: International Women's Health Coalition and Citizen, Studies, Information, Action. Available at: https://iwhc.org/resources/rio-statement-reproductive-health-justice [Accessed Oct. 10, 2016].

Rosenfield, A., Fathalla, M.F., Germain, A. and Indriso eds., 1989. Women's health in the Third World: the impact of unwanted pregnancy. *International Journal of Gynecology & Obstetrics*, 30(S3), pp.1–178. Available at: www.ijgo.org/issue/S0020-7292(00)X0149-X [Accessed Jul. 25, 2016].

Sedgh, G., Bearak, J., Singh, S., Bankole, A., Popinchalk, A., Ganatra, B., Rossier, C., Gerdts, C., Tunçalp, Ö., Johnson, B.R., Johnston, H.B. and Alkema, L., 2016. Abortion incidence between 1990 and 2014: global, regional, and subregional levels and trends. *The Lancet.* [online] Available at: http://linkinghub.elsevier.com/retrieve/pii/S0140673616303804 [Accessed Jun. 19, 2016].

Sen, G., Germain, A. and Chen, L.C. eds., 1994. *Population Policies Reconsidered: Health, Empowerment, and Rights.* Harvard Series on Population and International Health. Cambridge, MA: Harvard University Press.

Sen, G., Germain, A., Garcia-Moreno, C. and Shankar, M. eds., 2015. Sexual and reproductive health and rights for the next decades: What's been achieved? What lies ahead? *Special Issue, Global Public Health: An International Journal for Research, Policy and Practice*, 10(2), pp.135–272. Available at: http://www.tandfonline.com/toc/rgph20/10/2 [Accessed Jul. 25, 2016].

Singh, S., Darroch, J.E. and Ashford, L.S., 2014. *Adding it Up: The Costs and Benefits of Investing in Sexual and Reproductive Health 2014.* [online] New York, NY: Guttmacher. Available at: www.guttmacher.org/sites/default/files/report_pdf/addingitup2014.pdf [Accessed Jul. 25, 2016].

The World Bank Group, 2016. *Global Financing Facility.* [online] Available at: http://www.globalfinancingfacility.org [Accessed Jun. 19, 2016].

United Nations General Assembly, 1999. *Key Actions for the Further Implementation of the Programme of Action of the International Conference on Population and Development.* [online] Available at: www.un.org/documents/ga/res/21sp/a21spr02.htm [Accessed Jul. 25, 2016].

United Nations, 1995. *Report of the International Conference on Population and Development: Cairo, 5-13 September 1994.* [online] Available at: www.unfpa.org/sites/default/files/event-pdf/icpd_eng_2.pdf [Accessed Jul. 25, 2016].

United Nations, 1996. *Report of the Fourth World Conference on Women: Beijing, 4–15 September 1995.* [online] Available at: http://beijing20.unwomen.org/~/media/Field%20Office%20Beijing%20Plus/Attachments/BeijingDeclarationAndPlatformForAction-en.pdf [Accessed Jul. 25, 2016].

United Nations, 2015. *The Millennium Development Goals Report 2015.* [online] pp.38–43. Available at: www.un.org/millenniumgoals/2015_MDG_Report/pdf/MDG%202015%20rev%20(July%201).pdf [Accessed Jul. 25, 2016].

United Nations Educational, Scientific and Cultural Organization, 2015. *Emerging Evidence, Lessons, and Practice in Comprehensive Sexuality Education: A Global Review.* [online] France: UNESCO. Available at: http://unesdoc.unesco.org/images/0024/002431/243106e.pdf [Accessed Jul. 25, 2016].

Van Look, P.F.A. and Pérez-Palacios, G. eds., 1994. Appendix. In: *Contraceptive Research and Development 1984–1994: The Road from Mexico City to Cairo and Beyond.* Oxford: Oxford University Press, pp.543–546.

WHO Special Programme of Research, Development and Research Training in Human Reproduction and International Women's Health Coalition, 1991. *Creating Common Ground: Women's Perspectives on the Selection and Introduction of Fertility Regulation Technologies – Report of a Meeting Between Women's Health Advocates and Scientists.* [online] Geneva: World Health Organization. Available at: www.who.int/iris/handle/10665/62687 [Accessed May 16, 2016].

World Health Organization, 2003. *Safe Abortion: Technical and Policy Guidance for Health Systems (First Edition).* [online] Available at: http://apps.who.int/iris/bitstream/10665/42586/1/9241590343.pdf [Accessed Jul. 25, 2016].

World Health Organization, 2015a. *Health Worker Roles in Providing Safe Abortion Care and Post-Abortion Contraception.* [online] Geneva: World Health Organization. Available at: http://apps.who.int/iris/bitstream/10665/181041/1/9789241549264_eng.pdf?ua=1&ua=1 [Accessed Jul. 25, 2016].

World Health Organization, 2015b. *Sexual Health, Human Rights and the Law.* [online] Geneva: World Health Organization. Available at: www.who.int/reproductivehealth/publications/sexual_health/sexual-health-human-rights-law/en [Accessed May 16, 2016].

World Health Organization, 2016. *The World Health Assembly Endorses the Global Plan of Action on Violence Against Women and Girls, and also Against Children.* [online] WHO. Available at: www.who.int/reproductivehealth/topics/violence/action-plan-endorsement/en [Accessed Jun. 19, 2016].

7 Solving Nandi

The personal embodiment of structural injustice in South Africa's Child Support Grant

Tessa Hochfeld

Introduction

> *Nandi, I want you to solve Nandi for me. Nandi drinks alcohol, she doesn't come home and she doesn't know if the children eat. She doesn't even know if the children's clothes are washed . . . And when she gets paid the children's grant money, she uses it all at the tavern . . . [And this drinking], it started a long time ago, but she used to drink and come home . . . [Now] what I see is that she has given herself to alcohol.*

(Mother of research participant, in face-to-face
interview with author)

During research on the implications of cash transfers for women's lives in South Africa, I met Nandi and her family (all names used are pseudonyms). Nandi is a young mother with two children, both receiving state-funded Child Support Grants (CSGs). Her life story is one of hardship and lack of support. Here I argue that the end result, the misuse of state support as described by her mother in the above quote, is not just a result of her individual shortcomings, but a reflection too on a society that has neglected Nandi from early on. Nandi's story raises a dilemma about social justice in South Africa: what has failed Nandi in a developing country that has intentionally created a remarkably generous welfare regime?

South Africa's functional democracy, progressive pro-poor policies, and assumptions of equality are critical to social justice, as they provide the formal opportunity for all citizens to reach their life goals. However, the substantive freedom to achieve these goals is often missing, due to failures in their functioning, wider structural constraints, and problematic informal social institutions. The result is compromised security for individuals in the broad realm of the social, which has negative impacts on their health, especially mental health. The irony is that these insecurities are produced by the very structural, political and institutional systems that are also responsible for the progressive policies targeting these very individuals.

Nandi's story represents the multifaceted and complex experiences of social injustice. 'Solving Nandi' is solving the justice gap: the gap between the state's policy framework, which focuses largely on the delivery of material support as distributive justice, and the domain of the social. In this chapter I use a micro-level approach to draw out the issues of the social, as a way to raise questions about social justice, security and the health of those living hard lives in the context of a progressive developmental welfare state. The purpose of this close-up engagement with real lives, is to richly illustrate why a one-dimensional conception of justice, focusing only on resource distribution in the form of cash transfers, fails to deliver social justice for ordinary people struggling to live their lives in ways that they 'have reason to value' (Sen, 1999). This close-up view additionally offers up a meta-narrative of the gendered nature of care, and illustrates how structural and institutionally caused insecurities can have devastating impacts on women as caregivers. I use critical feminist scholarship as a lens to understand the context and consequences of care in the midst of institutional and structural insecurity.

The stories of two women living in a low-income urban community, and both receiving CSGs for their children, offer us insight into why cash transfers are an important but minimal response to injustice. I met with each of these two women multiple times using a feminist narrative framework for in-depth interviews for research investigating the social and gendered impacts of CSGs. The study as a whole included four other case studies, but here I will focus on just these two, as these women's stories clearly complicate the effects of cash transfers. The women, selected purposively via my knowledge of and involvement in the geographical community at the time, agreed to take part in this study voluntarily and without incentives, and were referred to various external support services when necessary. As a white, middle-class social worker, working predominantly with black, low-income women, navigating power issues and access to resources was complicated. Using a feminist ethic of care (Sevenhuijsen, 2003; Tronto, 2010) helped to manage and balance this process (this is discussed further in Hochfeld & Graham, 2012).

In their narratives, the two women interact with the state as provider, employer, administrator, and justice agent. They also experience and respond to societal norms and expectations around the relationships between the individual and the state. These stories expose the everyday insecurities that arise specifically from the formal and informal socio-economic, political, and cultural organisation of society. Their value, therefore, lies in the detail, as a focus on policy alone is not nuanced enough to raise these issues.

I turn now to a description of the current socio-economic conditions of South Africa, and the state responses to poverty, as a way to explain the current context. This is followed by a discussion of the notion of social justice, and then an application of these ideas to excerpts from the narratives of the two women under discussion to expose experiences of insecurity. Finally, I consider the implications of a comprehensive social justice framework in evaluating the outcomes of South Africa's developmental welfare regime, and how this relates to security.

Conditions of poverty and state responses

Current socio-economic conditions in South Africa are serious. Unemployment is at 36%, including discouraged work-seekers who have stopped looking for work (StatsSA, 2016). This has been a driver for poverty and high levels of inequality, with a Gini co-efficient of 6.5 in 2011 (StatsSA, 2014). The consequences are economic, political and social: 56% live below the 'upper bound' poverty line, which is calculated to include minimally adequate food and non-food items such as energy (StatsSA, 2017), with black, rural women and children the most vulnerable (Posel & Rogan, 2012; StatsSA, 2014). There are high levels of interpersonal violence (especially against women), substance use, and family disintegration (Abrahams, Martin, & Vetten, 2004; Budlender & Lund, 2011).

The South African state considers itself 'developmental', which is not analogous to the developmental states of the 'Asian Tigers', but is rather describing post-apartheid pro-poor policies with a commitment to spending on social, health, and welfare services (Patel, 2015). Indeed, the achievements in this regard are impressive. Relevant for our discussion are welfare services: social assistance spending is around R128 billion (USD9.2 billion) per year (SASSA, 2016a), and unconditional social grants reach 17.1 million South Africans monthly (SASSA, 2016b). This is one of the largest social protection programmes on the continent along with Ethiopia's (Patel, 2015). It has been extensively praised as a functional and well-managed programme (Devereux & Lund, 2010; DSD, SASSA, & UNICEF, 2012; Patel, Hochfeld, & Moodley, 2013; Woolard, Harttgen, & Klasen, 2011), with important positive outcomes in the reduction of poverty nationally (World Bank, 2014), and in improved household food security (DSD *et al.*, 2012). In the early months of 2017 this discourse began to shift, due to a serious crisis around the grant distribution system. In an unexpected series of events, the state's bungling of a contract with a private grant distribution service stripped assumptions of the security and solidity of the right to cash transfers for the poor. Far from being a shining example of the delivery of the promise of protection, the ability of the state to disburse grants in the short and long term was suddenly under question. Grants were, indeed, paid in this instance, but going forward there is heightened anxiety about the vulnerability of institutional structures to political interference.

The second arm of welfare provision, welfare services, has long been poorly funded, poorly managed, and attracted vehement criticism from civil society (Hochfeld, 2015; Patel, 2015; Vetten, 2016). The White Paper for Social Welfare of 1997 (Department of Welfare and Population Development, 1997), the primary welfare policy document, places a lot of emphasis on the integration and good articulation of different kinds of welfare services (Patel, 2015). The material in this chapter will convey some of the critical gaps severely limiting our ability to achieve this aim.

The Child Support Grant is the cash transfer with the furthest reach, and is thus the largest state-funded poverty alleviation strategy in South Africa. It supports 12 million children to the modest value of R380 (USD29) every month. This grant is means-tested but unconditional, meaning any child who lives in a household with an income below a set threshold will be eligible for a grant. In an innovative design, the CSG is given to the primary caregiver of the child, whoever that may be. In 98% of cases, this is a woman (Patel, 2015), illustrating the powerfully gendered nature of care in South Africa. These carers are biological mothers or grandmothers in the main, although other female relatives are also primary care-givers. For such a small monthly sum, the CSG has delivered some remarkable achievements, with clear benefits in relation to nutritional improvements for children (Agüero, Carter, & Woolard, 2006), improved household food security (DSD *et al.*, 2012; Neves *et al.*, 2009; Woolard *et al.*, 2011; Zembe-Mkabile, Surrender, Sanders, Jackson, & Doherty, 2015), increased numbers of years children complete at school (DSD *et al.*, 2012; Eyal & Woolard, 2014), lowered health and social risks (such as a decrease in risky sexual behaviour among adolescent girls) (Cluver *et al.*, 2013; DSD *et al.*, 2012), as well as labour promoting, savings and investment, and empowerment effects for caregiver recipients (Eyal & Woolard, 2014; Patel, Hochfeld, Moodley, & Mutwali, 2012). The impacts go beyond the targeted child as cash transfers in South Africa are pooled in households to a large extent (Duflo, 2003; Woolard *et al.*, 2011). It is for this reason I focus on female caregiver beneficiaries, as they receive the grant and make decisions on its use.

Social justice

The contributions of the CSG listed above are important, and definitely relieve the worst vagaries of poverty via dependable material support. This offers a basic level of material security for millions of households. The weaknesses of the workings of South Africa's developmental state rest not merely on the adequacy of the monetary value of the grant, which is acknowledged as limited, but on the narrow conception of social justice which implies that monetary support is sufficient for security (Hochfeld, 2015; Zembe-Mkabile *et al.*, 2015).

Nancy Fraser's (2007, 2009, 2013) work offers us a more holistic view of social justice, which helps to explain why a cash grant is insufficient. Her feminist theory of justice suggests that social justice is a balance of redistribution, recognition, and representation. South Africa's level of unemployment, and resulting poverty and material inequality, is an example of how a range of institutionalised economic mechanisms 'systematically deny some of its members the means and opportunities they need in order to participate on a par with others in social life' (Fraser, 2003, p. 49). While the cash transfer system cannot restructure the economy for a fairer deal for all, the publically funded nature of this massive programme does mean that money from the well-off are redistributed to the poor via progressive taxation. This substantial fiscal commitment of the CSG has real, material impacts and is certainly a form of redistribution and improves the security of millions.

The value of Fraser's approach is to show why this is important, but not enough for justice. She integrates the notion of the 'social' into a framework for justice, and show why justice in the sphere of what she calls recognition is critical to the real outcomes for real lives. The 'intersubjective condition' (Fraser, 2003, p. 36) is critical to the social valuing of individuals and groups of people, and has powerful social effects. Sexism, racism, classism, and other social inequalities are effective means of stratifying inter-subjectivity, and are key contributors to creating mis-recognition. Central to recognition, therefore, is the nature of social relationships;

not just between individuals, but also in the interaction between the state, society, groups, and individuals. Useful proxies for this dimension are the ideas of dignity and respect; a lack of these is prevalent in the narratives to come, and illustrate the power of misrecognition to undermine people's life choices.

Finally, Fraser's idea of representation is political voice, and the legitimacy of rights in a contract between the person and the state or society (Fraser, 2013). While her notion is focused more on the global stage, representation in this study can be understood as *who* is seen as *legitimate* for *which* claims.

It is in the dimensions of recognition and representation that significant injustices and resulting insecurities arise in the case of welfare needs of individuals, and it is ironic that these are felt so acutely by those benefiting from the redistributive rights delivered by the CSG. The stories that I draw from illustrate this potently in the next section.

Recognition

Institutional failures

A set of institutional injustices for a woman named Jabulile demonstrates serious misrecognition, or the destruction of dignity. Her story reveals the importance of differentiating actual and substantive rights vs symbolic or formal rights, something that Sen (1999, 2009) addresses extensively in his work on the capabilities approach. He makes the point that having formal rights to something does not mean you have the opportunity and freedom to fulfil those rights, and that assuming institutions based on just principles will, by definition, always deliver just outcomes is a major error (Sen, 2009). Jabulile's formal rights do not change in the course of this narrative, nor do the institutions of democracy, the state and its obligations, the context of labour regulations, and so on. It is rather that the functioning of these institutions fails in some fundamental ways, and in doing so they deny Jabulile her *substantive* rights to these institutions, undermine her dignity, and thus change Jabulile's life for the worse.

Jabulile is an articulate, confident, educated woman who has fallen on hard times. She lives with her boyfriend, Nathi, and with five of her six children, plus takes care of two young relatives, making the household nine people. The family lives in a small three-bedroom flat in a very run-down building. Jabulile, who has a vocational qualification and was working as a civil servant for government, was dismissed from her job while in hospital with severe depression. The depression was a result of extreme trauma after the abduction and murder of her late husband. Her boyfriend gets varying and unpredictable income from work as a freelance plumber. Their only other income is four Child Support Grants.

As Jabulile was dismissed from her position during the worst of her illness, she had none of those supports she was entitled to as an employed individual at a large state institution in the context of extensive regulatory protection of workers in South Africa. The services due to her should have been paid sick leave, the guarantee of her previous position when she was able to return to work, the continuation of her work-funded medical insurance, and the continuation of her work-linked accommodation without the threat of eviction. The way Jabulile describes the process of dismissal she underwent illustrates serious institutional injustice:

> *Jabulile: [Rebecca] works for [the state institution where Jabulile was employed] . . . she was here as a social worker to witness [the dismissal]. So when I was filing [my request for a review of the dismissal], she called me one day. She says: I was worried that we brought you the [dismissal letter that day]. Do you know, do you remember what happened? I told her I don't know what you are talking about. Then she said: I did see that, you didn't see what was happening, it was wrong for us to give you the letter of dismissal in that condition you were. You looked very sick and you looked confused. Then she said to me: the day they want witnesses at the court I want to be there [to speak on your behalf].*

Dismissal while severely ill is a direct contravention of law specifically designed to protect employees. But it is moreover a profound experience of misrecognition, as this event 'erased' Jabulile's status as an employed and economically independent member of society. It also precipitated her need for the CSG, a need she never had prior to this.

Further to this, Jabulile twice had the strange experience of being accused of grant fraud: routine state check-ups on the employment status of recipients led to the immediate cancellation of her grants as the state unit responsible for administration of cash transfers (The South African Social Security Agency, SASSA) still had her recorded as employed, as the unfair dismissal case was still pending. Just when she needed help the most, she was accused of fraudulently getting grants for personal enrichment, rendering her very real struggle for survival and for caring for her family invisible. The experience is captured in the following conversation:

> *Jabulile: I am, my heart [can't take the stress]. So now I have got a case whereby, they said I have done . . . fraud and corruption, yes, [they say] I am getting the grants illegally and they have [cancelled] them, oh . . . Anything I fix, the other one breaks. [If I was working] I would not even go to the Social Services to ask for the grant, why would I, and even if they can check, I applied for the grant last year and I was dismissed the year before. So with this now we didn't get the grant last month . . . Now we are suffering. I don't even have . . . the money to buy soap and to buy them bread tomorrow. There is nothing in the kitchen (she begins to cry).*

Being wrongly accused of fraud and having her grants withdrawn cancelled Jabulile's substantive political rights to social assistance. In addition, to get the grant reinstated was not just a case of presenting the right documents, but also a fight for political voice and entitlements. As Fraser comments, by having your rights denied, you are forced into a space of 'non-rights'. She says that the erasure of your rights erases your claim entitlements, your political voice, and your dignity (Fraser, 2013).

So one experience of institutional injustice forced Jabulile into a position of need, and therefore a grant claimant, and the other experience of institutional injustice erased even that status and stripped her of political legitimacy and dignity. These experiences are specific to this woman and her exact circumstances, but they offer us a window into how problems in institutions can have such a strong effect on the dignity and justice of a grant claimant. It is remarkable how insecure these failures left Jabulile in the context of such a strong set of formal rights.

Welfare services

I will now turn to the issue of welfare services failure. Just as the one arm of social development, social assistance, is an important demonstration of the state's commitment to assisting the poor, the other arm, welfare services, is a demonstration of the state's failure to do so. There is a glaring imbalance between the strong social assistance side of state welfare and the poorly funded, overloaded, poorly supported social services side (Patel, 2015). The state relies heavily on the NGO sector to deliver services on its behalf, but its funding models are woefully inadequate, pushing many NGOs into ongoing financial crisis which directly affects service delivery (Vetten, 2016). In addition, services are unintegrated and unconnected, and so just exactly when you are in need of support, you have to find out about and access a maze of services in different places in order to meet your need (Hochfeld, 2015). That is, if you are lucky enough to live in an urban area that has services – many are not.

Previous research has identified that the failures of welfare and other services have substantially eroded the benefits of the CSG. In these discussions the erosion has been identified as an *economic*, and thus *distributive*, concern, such as when grant money pays for healthcare or educational costs that should be freely available (Patel, 2012; Patel *et al.*, 2012). However, these narratives demonstrate that it can be misrecognition too, which comes from having to continually reassert your needs or continually fight to claim benefits, as described in Jabulile's story.

Jabulile is also a good example of the failings of *access* here because she is an educated, literate, confident woman living in a central urban area who was overwhelmed by the difficulties of sourcing, negotiating, and using the range of services her family needs: how much harder is it for those with fewer personal and other resources? During the process of the research, I referred Jabulile to six different welfare services, in both the public and the Non-Profit Organisation (NPO) sectors. The services ranged from health, welfare, education, housing and emotional and social support services. They were for herself, and various members of her immediate household.

None of these referrals is particularly complicated, nor are the services that difficult to find out about. But in the context of overwhelming care responsibilities, frequent bouts of depression, and severe financial concerns, she would not have managed to access any of these without my assistance. Jabulile's experience prompts me to rethink how we engage people in service delivery. The failure of delivery is not just the well-criticised 'silos' and 'sectorisation' of services (Patel, 2015), but that people are not understood as embedded in a life of complicated relationships and complex needs, rather than one-dimensional and narrow single needs. The authority to define needs lies with those in power, and is deeply politically loaded. The failure to 'problematise the social and institutional logic of processes of need interpretation' (Fraser, 2013, p. 56), which sees people in relation to a single need and cannot grapple with the complexity of real life, is, in effect a failure of formal rights.

The receipt of a CSG should automatically entitle the recipient to a range of benefits, and then open up avenues to necessary social services without the person in need having to fight for or negotiate the confusing landscape of state and NPO offerings available.

Instead, benefits often have to be fought for, and sometimes lost, individually. An illustration is Jabulile's experience when trying to get a school fee exemption for her sister's seven-year-old daughter, Thenjiwe, who lives with Jabulile's family and for whom Jabulile is receiving a CSG. All children in South Africa are constitutionally entitled to education, which means state education has to be free for those who are poor. The complicated system of public school fee charges means that if a poor child goes to a state, but fee-charging, school, then they are entitled to a fee-reduction or fee-exemption on application. This describes the case for Thenjiwe. However, Thenjiwe's mother is a drug addict and lives on the streets. Jabu described the frustrating and undignified experience of trying to apply for a fee-exemption:

> *Jabulile: So when I apply for an exemption, they tell me that I must have the full custody of the child from court. And I cannot, my sister is alive. I am just helping because I cannot just ignore the child. They said I must go to court for it and I can't do that. And then they make me walk around the streets to look for my sister to sign the forms, I found her in Joubert Park but she would not come with me so I made her sign there on the street. But the school, they said every year she had to come every time if she doesn't make her life better so it's up to her and then they won't give the child the exemption.*

These are failures of access and integration, and make claiming entitlements complicated and burdensome for those who need it most. This is partly explained by the simplification of people's need in order to suit institutional functioning and prevailing ideology, rather than recognising the inter-relationships of needs and thus designing services to suit this. The interpretation of needs is a political contest (Fraser, 2013), and by placing the burden of proof on individuals who have to consistently re-verify their right to claim, we stack the cards against those who are poor and without power. Their rights should be the basis of respect and a sense of security; instead they are the basis for political conflict between the individual and the state. Further, the consequences are strongly gendered as welfare and social services lie strongly in the domain of care, and care is overwhelmingly considered a women's responsibility in South Africa. Making caring onerous is significantly more damaging to women's material and symbolic well-being than men's; and it impacts negatively on distribution and recognition for women.

In addition, care burdens can also initiate or exacerbate mental or physical health vulnerabilities due to the physical and emotional strain involved, especially when caring in the context of a severe lack of resources. Jabulile's experience is illustrative here: the violent death of her husband precipitated a severe bout of clinical depression, the consequences of which were her dismissal, and subsequent range of challenges, including further periods of depression, poverty and lack of food security.

In addition to failures of access and integration, there are many examples of the actual failure of service *delivery*. An example comes from Nandi's story. I did a formal referral of the family to state social services, with a particular concern for Nandi's children, and followed up for over a year, but no social worker ever contacted the family to offer assistance. The referral indicated concerns for the safety of Nandi's children at particular time when she was not coping well, and by law a social worker should have contacted her and conducted a home assessment. This didn't happen, indicating a serious break in state statutory commitments to child protection in this case. This is a critical institutional failure, which has impacts on material and symbolic security for the specific children involved, but also for children generally, as it indicates an unresponsive and uncaring system.

The lack of service integration, the constant battle to assert your needs despite getting a CSG which is already means tested, and the delivery failures, all result in the undermining of individual dignity and detracts from the attainment of social justice. The next section focuses on representation justice.

Representation

Delving further into Nandi's story offers us a chance to consider the notion of representation as a dimension of social justice. Representation can be understood as the legitimacy of *who can claim for what and under what circumstances* (Fraser, 2013). Social security is a constitutional right, as long as you meet the eligibility criteria. Nandi's narrative reveals that this entitlement has social and political limits, and raises the question of how normative expectations can undermine entitlements.

Nandi is a young woman; 23 years old when I met her. Nandi grew up in a poor household with many social problems, including domestic violence and alcohol abuse, and herself suffered numerous experiences of violence, rape and trauma in her life. So she has a very difficult history.

At the time of the interviews, she and her two very young daughters, both getting a CSG, lived with her parents and others in a very crowded flat in a pleasant mixed-class suburb near the inner city. Her parents both worked in low-skilled part-time domestic work positions, and while Nandi occasionally did a bit of casual domestic work, she had no other income aside from the two grants. The father of Nandi's two children was murdered in a stabbing at work just prior to my meeting her.

In my research, I wanted to find the best in people with whom I worked. This is a reflection of my worldview as well as my research ethics. But Nandi tested this view. She was at times the responsible mother and dutiful daughter, caring for her young children attentively and looking after the household while her parents worked. But when Nandi was frustrated, angry, or fed up, she was the epitome of the irresponsible and wayward mother and rebellious teen. The consequences of Nandi acting out these different identities are real, and often contradictory, being both positive and negative at different times.

The mother that was proud of her children, that periodically gave her grant money to her mother or the crèche teacher for safekeeping to ensure that she herself didn't misuse it, or that spent it all immediately on nappies, milk and food in order for it to go to the correct expenses: this is the mother for whom the grant is a reliable, secure monthly protection for her and her children. These are the behaviours envisaged by the state when designing the grant, and the behaviours that research shows most mothers enact.

But Nandi's other enactment of motherhood is when she avoids looking for work, neglects her children, drinks with her friends, and disappears for days on end without notifying anyone of her whereabouts. She borrows money from microlenders who charge exorbitant rates of interest so that she and her friends can drink, and then uses CSG money to repay her debts. This is the Nandi who lies as a matter of course, can be violent and aggressive towards others, and has a long string of boyfriends. In this permutation, she is the perfect picture of the 'bad' young mother who 'eats' her children's money that South Africans love to hate.

The perception that some people are *undeserving* of support is an old and very persistent idea. The post-industrial ideal has become the independent, economically productive individual, in stark opposition to those who need help to manage the structural injustices of a socio-economic world pitted against the disadvantaged. Those who need help are assumed to be morally inferior, are accused of a lack of work ethic, and perceived as a serious drain on state resources (Fraser, 1989; Fraser & Gordon, 1994, p. 334). The remarkable power of this notion is evidenced by its insidious creep into the discourse of not only the politically conservative who use it to limit claims on the state, but also those who consider their politics to be left-leaning and socially responsible: numerous South African politicians have been heard using language implying those needing help were prone to dependence, laziness and 'bad' behaviour (Hassim, 2006; Marais, 2011). These are views that are often echoed by the public. This is despite research demonstrating no evidence of widespread perverse incentive effects of social grants (Makiwane, 2010; Rosenberg *et al.*, 2015; Steele, 2006) and research demonstrating, conversely, the poverty-alleviating and social investment effects of the CSG and other grants.

These politically shaped attitudes mean that when there are anecdotal cases of grant 'misuse', which of course exist, as Nandi's story shows, they are interpreted in the current conservative and punitive public space as both proof of extensive misuse as well as an indication of the value of distinguishing between deserving and undeserving recipients.

However, in South Africa there are some practices that are so common, even across socio-economic divides, that they are perceived as normative, for example, high levels of indebtedness, the consumption of alcohol as a form of leisure, the perception that airtime for mobile phones is a necessity not a luxury purchase, and motherhood at a young age. Despite the widespread nature of these practices, they are strongly disapproved of if the individual is a grant recipient (DSD, SASSA, & UNICEF, 2011; Makiwane, 2010). I argue that this moral surveillance is a powerful form of misrepresentation, as it implies that only certain people have the 'right' to claim entitlements, a classic case of political and social othering.

I am not condoning the use of cash transfers to buy alcohol rather than food for children, or any number of other uses that do not promote the well-being of households. Rather, Nandi's difficult history and destructive coping mechanisms have starkly demonstrated how society expects the receipt of a grant to magically change the behaviour and social challenges of ordinary members of our communities. This destructive behaviour is unfortunate, and not in the interests of her or her children. But this behaviour pre-dated receiving the CSG, and a grant on its own cannot substantively change Nandi's coping mechanisms, whether productive or dysfunctional. It is remarkable that the moment she claims the CSG, an entitlement, she moves into a new category as 'passive claimant' and social expectations of her behaviour shift too. In fact, the very idea of an entitlement is to eliminate judgements around how people use the entitlement. Hence the fact that a small group may misuse the money cannot be the basis for the removal of the entitlement for all.

Nevertheless, now she receives two grants, we believe we are at liberty to judge her behaviour. It is assumed that because the CSG money comes from the public purse, all of us have a right to judge the appropriateness of its use. However, this level of surveillance is accorded only to those who publically acknowledge their need, and the need is derived from structural, socially constructed, relations of deprivation and power.

This is rooted in the distinctions that are made in conservative societies between poor and non-poor, between deserving and non-deserving (Ulriksen & Plagerson, 2014). Those receiving state assistance are perceived to be social parasites as it is assumed that they make no contributions to society, despite, in reality, substantial contributions made in relation to tax (such as general sales tax or value added tax), community engagement, and substantial social care and social reproduction (Pateman & Murray, 2012; Ulriksen & Plagerson, 2014).

This raises the question of rights and duties, a classic conundrum amongst political philosophers, where arguments about which comes first traditionally marks your ideological stance from conservative to progressive. A restricted one-to-one contractual exchange of rights and duties is largely meaningless in the real world when contributions are made often at the same time as rights are being claimed, and structural inequalities exclude large portions of the society from traditional forms of income taxation (Sen, 2009; Ulriksen & Plagerson, 2014). In the case of Child Support Grants specifically in South Africa (discourses around the Old Age Pension are somewhat different), while we assume that the entitlement to the grant should obligate recipients to behave responsibly, we do not also recognise that we have *a responsibility* to support grant recipients, *if they need it*, beyond offering them income support.

However, it is a failure of our socio-political system that we expect a cash transfer to not only provide a means of economic survival, but also fill many other social, emotional and relationship needs. This is of course impossible, so those who were self-destructive before getting a grant will not be any less destructive after doing so. Expecting any different without other inputs is a form of injustice.

This raises the political philosophical question of the relationship between rights and duties as citizens. Nandi has a right to social assistance that precedes her duty to behave in particular ways. If we were to link the CSG to specific required behaviours we would be undermining the social right everyone, including Nandi, has to support for her children.

Ulriksen and Plagerson (2014, p. 755) argue that tensions between rights and duties are softened in a context of social solidarity; in other words, the notion of social solidarity 'provides a unifying premise for the promotion of social rights among citizens, to provide and care in times of ability in order to enjoy in times of vulnerability, thus avoiding a stark separation between rights-holders and duty-bearers'. A society guided by relations of social solidarity, by feelings of altruism to 'others', by understanding the delicate equilibrium between obligations and rights, and by ideas of reciprocity, is a society that can authentically deliver social care (Ulriksen & Plagerson, 2014; Yeates, 2011).

My argument does not, of course, nullify the need to ask questions in the case of a mother using the CSG on alcohol. But withdrawing rights in response to behaviour is punitive, and would erode the basis on which democratic South Africa is built. Her rights and her duties to her children should not be linked in a linear way. Rather, in a context of genuine social care, Nandi would be encouraged and supported to use more constructive coping mechanisms through functional social services, and not left to continue to fail.

Conclusions

It is of critical importance in that in receiving services, programmes, rights, cash transfers and other public goods, people's dignity and legitimacy to claim these public goods are not intentionally or unintentionally undermined. Unintended consequences of protective and progressive social policies cannot be dismissed just because they fall out of the scope or control of the state; symbolic, cultural, or representative injustice is surely as intolerable as material injustice (Sabates-Wheeler & Devereux, 2008; Ulriksen, Plagerson, & Hochfeld, 2015). Symbolic and representative injustices result in unacceptable insecurities, and often, as illustrated in these case studies, compromised mental health.

The pro-poor and progressive social policies such as social assistance in South Africa offer demonstrated material support and redistributive symbolism. However, this achievement does not mean the state has dispensed with its social, welfare, and health obligations to recipients. Institutional, service delivery, and political failures, as well as the negative views of recipients and social judgements about who is worthy of the support and who is not, are all strong forms of misrecognition and misrepresentation. Understanding these issues in the context of a social justice framework allows us to move beyond the assumption that justice and security are inevitably being accomplished because such a large amount of money is being spent by the state for so many poor individuals in the form of social assistance.

The events of early 2017 forcefully underlined the potential for institutional insecurity in times of peace and, consequently, the undermining of recognition and representation justice. A looming expiration of the contract between the state and the private service provider which distributes the grants exposed deep problems in the system. Suddenly, the most secure form of institutional protection was shown to be vulnerable to inefficiency, mismanagement, profit-seeking, and political interference. The surprising dependence of the state on an outsourced and privately run distribution system lays bare the insidious dominance of the market-driven 'growth economy' ideology even within a self-styled develop-mental state. The fragility of a seemingly solid state service resulted in a wave of structural insecurity for both the millions of grant beneficiaries (*Will my grant be paid? If not, what will I do next month to feed my family?*), and for the general public, who, for the first time, were united in their support of grants as a foundation of the state's responsibility to the poor.

As the above illustrates, social justice is partly a condition of the formal state machinery and how it is organised. Laws and policies frame the expectations citizens can have about their lives, and prompt their definition of a 'life they have reason to value', Amartya Sen's (2009) description of 'the good life'. To question institutional functioning and enquire how it can be improved 'is a constant and inescapable part of the pursuit of justice' (Sen, 2009: 86). The everyday needs and struggles that are experienced at an individual level are linked to the public and the political via social vulnerabilities created by structural, institutional and sym-bolic insecurities. They create multifaceted experiences of injustice that cannot be addressed through policy 'fixes' and state expenditure alone. By not vigorously and resolutely protecting securities, improving institutions and recognising the power of symbolic harms, the state is suggesting that income support is sufficient to deliver social justice. The lived experiences of women receiving the CSG dem-onstrate that economic solutions, essentially the tools of capitalism, cannot resolve fundamental social problems alone. The notion of the developmental state as a caring state is diluted by its lack of questioning the market-driven global economic system in which it functions.

Recognition and representation failings detract from the material and non-material benefits of the CSG, and thus undermine justice and security outcomes. The delivery of a minimal set of good quality social services is a vital start to a pathway of state commitment to the notion of care. This would contribute substan-tively to the justice, health, and security outcomes of people like Jabulile. 'Solving Nandi' is probably more complex; but certainly the delivery of social supports and care would make a major difference to her and her children's well-being. Beyond actual service delivery, both women's experiences would be fundamentally different if the state assumed that it has a leading role to play in facilitating recognition and representation justice, and took responsibility for eliminating gaps in services, remedying institutional failures, addressing unintended consequences, and responding strongly to negative views on state support.

Thus despite an impressive set of laws and regulations protecting the rights of individuals and communities in South Africa, and significant state expenditure directed at addressing economic inequality, these narrative accounts expose the irony that the actual functioning of formal and informal democracy in times of peace may serve to deny substantive rights, with tangible implications for justice and security.

References

Abrahams, N., Martin, L. J., & Vetten, L. (2004). An Overview of Gender-Based Violence in South Africa and South African Responses. In S. Suffla, A. van Niekerk, & N. Duncan (Eds), *Crime, Violence and Injury Prevention in South Africa: Developments and Challenges* (pp. 40–64). Pretoria: Medical Research Council.

Agüero, J. M., Carter, M. R., & Woolard, I. (2006). *The Impact of Unconditional Cash Transfers on Nutrition: The South African Child Support Grant*. Retrieved from Cape Town: www.opensaldru.uct.ac.za/bitstream/handle/11090/46/06_08.pdf?sequence=1 7 March 2013

Budlender, D., & Lund, F. (2011). South Africa: A Legacy of Family Disruption. *Development and Change, 42*(4), 925–46.

Cluver, L., Boyes, M., Orkin, M., Pantelic, M., Molwena, T., & Sherr, L. (2013). Child-Focused State Cash Transfers and Adolescent Risk of HIV Infection in South Africa: A Propensity-Score Matched Case-Control Study. *Lancet Global Health, 1*(e), 362–70.

Department of Welfare and Population Development, D. (1997). *White Paper for Social Welfare, Government Gazette (1108 of 1997)*. Retrieved from Pretoria: www.gov.za/sites/www.gov.za/files/White_Paper_on_Social_Welfare_0.pdf 2 February 2009.

Devereux, S., & Lund, F. (2010). Democratising Social Welfare in Africa. In V. Padayachee (Ed.), *The Political Economy of Africa* (pp. 152–171). London: Routledge.

DSD, SASSA, & UNICEF. (2011). *Child Support Grant Evaluation 2010: Qualitative Research Report*. Retrieved from Pretoria: www.unicef.org/southafrica/resources_10734. html 5 November 2013

DSD, SASSA, & UNICEF. (2012). *The South African Child Support Grant Impact Assessment: Evidence From a Survey of Children, Adolescents and their Households*. Retrieved from Pretoria: www.unicef.org/southafrica/resources_10737.html 5 November 2013

Duflo, E. (2003). Grandmothers and Granddaughters: Old-Age Pensions and Intrahousehold Allocation in South Africa. *The World Bank Economic Review, 17*(1), 1–25.

Eyal, K., & Woolard, I. (2014). *Cash Transfers and Teen Education: Evidence from South Africa*. Retrieved from Cape Town: https://editorialexpress.com/cgi-bin/conference/download.cgi?db_name=CSAE2015&paper_id=234 31 October 2014

Fraser, N. (1989). *Unruly Practices: Power, Discourse, and Gender in Contemporary Social Theory*. Minneapolis: University of Minnesota Press.

Fraser, N. (2003). Social Justice in the Age of Identity Politics: Redistribution, Recognition, and Participation. In N. Fraser & A. Honneth (Eds), *Redistribution or Recognition? A Political-Philosophical Exchange* (pp. 7–109). London: Verso.

Fraser, N. (2007). Re-framing justice in a globalising world. In T. Lovell (Ed.), *(Mis) recognition, Social Inequality and Social Justice* (pp. 17–35). London: Routledge.

Fraser, N. (2009). *Scales of Justice: Reimagining Political Space in a Globalizing World*. New York: Columbia University Press.

Fraser, N. (2013). *Fortunes of Feminism: From State-Managed Capitalism to Neoliberal Crisis*. London: Verso.

Fraser, N., & Gordon, L. (1994). A Genealogy of Dependency: Tracing a Key Word of the U.S. Welfare State. *Signs: Journal of Women in Culture and Society, 19*(2), 309–36.

Hassim, S. (2006). Gender Equality and Developmental Social Welfare in South Africa. In S. Razavi & S. Hassim (Eds), *Gender and Social Policy in a Global Context: Uncovering the Gendered Structure of the 'Social'* (pp. 109–29). Basingstoke: Palgrave.

Hochfeld, T. (2015). *Cash, Care and Social Justice: A Study of the Child Support Grant*. Johannesburg: Thesis submitted for Doctoral Degree, University of the Witwatersrand.

Hochfeld, T., & Graham, L. (2012). A Feminist Reflection on the Ethics of Social Work Research. *The Social Work Practitioner-Researcher, 24*(1), 31–47.

Makiwane, M. (2010). The Child Support Grant and Teenage Childbearing in South Africa. *Development Southern Africa, 27*(2), 193–204.

Marais, H. (2011). *South Africa Pushed to the Limit: The Political Economy of Change*. Cape Town: University of Cape Town Press.

Neves, D., Samson, M., van Niekerk, I., Hlatshwayo, S., & du Toit, A. (2009). *The Use and Effectiveness of Social Grants in South Africa*. Retrieved from Cape Town: www.finmark.org.za/sites/?publication_type=the-use-and-effectiveness-of-social-grants-in-south-africa-case-studies 17 July 2010

Patel, L. (2012). Poverty, Gender and Social Protection: Child Support Grants in Soweto, South Africa. *Journal of Policy Practice, 11*(1–2), 106–20.

Patel, L. (2015). *Social Welfare and Social Development in South Africa* (Second ed.). Cape Town: Oxford University Press, South Africa.

Patel, L., Hochfeld, T., & Moodley, J. (2013). Gender and Child Centred Social Protection in South Africa. *Development Southern Africa, 30*(1), 69–83.

Patel, L., Hochfeld, T., Moodley, J., & Mutwali, R. (2012). *The Gender Dynamics and Impact of the Child Support Grant in Doornkop, Soweto*. Retrieved from Johannesburg: https://ujcontent.uj.ac.za/vital/access/manager/Repository/uj:6605 3 March 2012.

Pateman, C., & Murray, M. C. (2012). Introduction. In M. C. Murray & C. Pateman (Eds), *Basic Income Worldwide: Horizon of Reform* (pp. 1–8). Basingstoke: Palgrave Macmillan.

Posel, D., & Rogan, M. (2012). Gendered Trends in Poverty in the Post-Apartheid Period, 1997–2006. *Development Southern Africa, 29*(1), 96–113.

Rosenberg, M., Pettifor, A., Nguyen, N., Westreich, D., Bor, J., Bärnighausen, T., Mee, P., Twine, R., Tollman, S. and Kahn, K. (2015). Relationship between Receipt of a Social Protection Grant for a Child and Second Pregnancy Rates among South African Women: A Cohort Study. *PLoS ONE, 10*(9). doi:e0137352. doi:10.1371/journal.pone.0137352

Sabates-Wheeler, R., & Devereux, S. (2008). Transformative Social Protection: The Currency of Social Justice. In A. Barrientos & D. Hulme (Eds), *Social Protection for the Poor and Poorest: Concepts, Policies and Politics* (pp. 64–84). London: Palgrave MacMillan.

SASSA. (2016a). *SASSA Annual Report 2015/2016*. Retrieved from Pretoria: www.sassa.gov.za/index.php/knowledge-centre/annual-reports 3 July 2016

SASSA. (2016b). *A Statistical Summary of Social Grants in South Africa: Fact Sheet: Issue no 9 of 2016 – 30 September 2016*. Retrieved from Pretoria: www.sassa.gov.za/index.php/statistical-reports 25 October 2016

Sen, A. (1999). *Development as Freedom*. Oxford: Oxford University Press.

Sen, A. (2009). *The Idea of Justice*. London: Penguin.

Sevenhuijsen, S. (2003). Principle Ethics and the Ethic of Care: Can They Go Together? *Social Work / Maatskaplike Werk, 39*, 393–399.

StatsSA. (2014). *Poverty Trends in South Africa: An examination of absolute poverty between 2006 and 2011*. Pretoria: Statistics South Africa. Accessed on 18 February 2017: http://beta2.statssa.gov.za/publications/Report-03-10-06/Report-03-10-06March 2014.pdf.

StatsSA. (2016). *Quarterly Labour Force Survey Quarter 2: 2016, Statistical release P0211*. Retrieved from Pretoria: www.statssa.gov.za/publications/P0211/P02112nd Quarter2016.pdf 6 November 2016

StatsSA. (2017). *Poverty Trends in South Africa: An Examination of Absolute Poverty Between 2006 and 2015, Statistician-General Report No. 03-10-06*. Retrieved from Pretoria: www.statssa.gov.za/publications/Report-03-10-06/Report-03-10-062015.pdf 28 August 2017.

Steele, M. (2006). *Report on Incentive Structures of Social Assistance Grants in South Africa*. Retrieved from Pretoria: www.socdev.gov.za/documents/2006/gps.pdf 18 May 2008

Tronto, J. (2010). Creating Caring Institutions: Politics, Plurality, and Purpose. *Ethics and Social Welfare, 4*(2), 158–171.

Ulriksen, M. S., & Plagerson, S. (2014). Social Protection: Rethinking Rights and Duties. *World Development, 64*, 755–65.

Ulriksen, M. S., Plagerson, S., & Hochfeld, T. (2015). Social Protection & Justice: Poverty, Redistribution, Dignity. In C. Boisen & M. C. Murray (Eds), *Distributive Justice Debates in Social and Political Thought: Perspectives on Finding a Fair Share* (pp. 191–211). London: Routledge.

Vetten, L. (2016). Unintended complicities: preventing violence against women in South Africa. *Gender & Development, 24*(2), 291–306. doi:10.1080/13552074.2016.1194560

Woolard, I., Harttgen, K., & Klasen, S. (2011). The History and Impact of Social Security in South Africa: Expereinces and Lessons. *Canadian Journal of Development Studies, 32*(4), 357–80.

World Bank, W. (2014). *South Africa Economic Update: Fiscal Policy and Redistribution in an Unequal Society*. Retrieved from Washington: http://documents.worldbank.org/curated/en/933231468101334970/South-Africa-economic-update-fiscal-policy-and-redistribution-in-an-unequal-society 5 November 2016

Yeates, N. (2011). Going Global: The Transnationalization of Care. *Development and Change, 42*(4), 1109–1130. doi:10.1111/j.1467-7660.2011.01718.x

Zembe-Mkabile, W., Surrender, R., Sanders, D., Jackson, D., & Doherty, T. (2015). The Experience of Cash Transfers in Alleviating Childhood Poverty in South Africa: Mothers' Experiences of the Child Support Grant. *Glob Public Health, 10*(7), 834–51. doi:10.1080/17441692.2015.1007471

8 Responses to recent infectious disease emergencies

A critical gender analysis

Colleen O'Manique

Introduction

One of the consequences of the systemic environmental disruption of expanded globalization has been the intensification of human–animal pathogen relations, hastening the rise of novel epidemics and pandemics. The drivers of novel disease outbreaks are varied: they include the interrelated processes of increased human mobility and migration, rapid urbanization, and the growth and consolidation of our increasingly globalized agro-industrial food system. The subtle and not so subtle impacts of climate change in tandem with the erosion of biodiversity and habitat loss can transform the life cycles and habitats of animal vectors, intensifying zoonotic spread, while large industrial farms can provide ideal breeding grounds for viral mutation (Bennett and McMichael, 2012; Bardosh, 2016; Davis, 2005). Given declining biodiversity and intensifying global warming, it is likely that our planet will experience new and more virulent viral epidemics. But as Bardosh explains, we are far from an understanding what drives novel viruses – from the molecular level to global circuits of capital (Bardosh, 2016: 6). What is becoming clear is that novel pathogens and their emergency responses can reinforce and intensify existing structural inequalities and invisibilities that underlie our more virulent present.

A common incantation is that all humans on our crowded planet are under increasing threat from novel pathogens that cross national borders; that viruses don't discriminate. But in fact, we are not all equally vulnerable. While recent global patterns of production and consumption have deepened insecurities and polarized life chances, a particular narrative of health security has emerged that privileges some interests, while erasing others. One's geographic location, class, ethnicity, gender, and sexuality can potentially shape vulnerability to novel disease outbreaks, the capacity to seek emergency treatment, and the longer-term impacts. In what places are robust public health systems and disease surveillance intact? Whose bodies are more prone to infectious disease? Who has access to healthcare and medicines, and who bears the social, economic, and cultural burdens of disease? What *don't* we see in the evolving knowledge production on 'health security' discussed in national and global policy responses to novel infectious disease? And whose bodies are left out altogether in contemporary health security narratives?

This chapter casts a critical feminist lens on global health security, the dominant policy approach to global health that has been strengthened to respond to viruses that have been constructed as global public health emergencies. The chapter begins by briefly introducing how global health agendas have changed over time in health bilateral and multilateral governance, and the place of novel pathogens in that evolution. It then exposes the gender blindness contained in the emergency policy responses to contemporary infectious disease outbreaks, drawing examples from HIV/AIDS, Avian Influenza, Ebola, and Zika. The focus is on two key areas of concern that are largely invisible in policy responses to, and impacts of public health emergencies. The first is how novel viruses come up against the exercise of sexual and reproductive health and rights (SRHR) in contexts in which disease is spread through sex or impacts biological reproduction; in essence, the ways in which one's gender and sexuality shape one's experience of infectious disease and its aftermath. The second concern is the impacts of novel epidemics on livelihoods, labour, and social reproduction. These two interrelated exclusions, linked to everyday insecurities and identities, challenge the meaning and practices of the current regime of global health security. The conclusion suggests how a critical gender lens might offer pathways toward a more expansive understanding and practice of health security.

Securing health

There are a variety of meanings of health security, but the frame that has come to dominate has its roots in the early days of European conquest and colonization, in practices to control infectious diseases such as the quarantining of people and goods suspected of harbouring infectious disease (King, 2002: 64). The foundations of today's International Health Regulations date to back to 1851, when representatives of European states met in Paris to negotiate a treaty to control the international spread of infectious disease, their objective, to protect growing commercial interests in the colonies (Markel, 2014: 124). Health security was essential to the expansion of commercial trade and colonial networks of the eighteenth-century Atlantic political economy, with approaches to disease control built on multilateral cooperation that standardized systems of knowledge and health practice (Arner, 2013: 773–5). A series of international conferences to address containment strategies for cholera, plague, and yellow fever eventually culminated in the International Sanitary Regulations of 1903, the precursor to today's recently revised International Health Regulations (IHR), the legal instrument that is binding on all member states of the World Health Organization (WHO).

While public health measures of the nineteenth century helped to bring major epidemic illnesses under control through better living and working conditions, water and sanitation, and nutrition, these changes did little to undermine the dominance of a regime of global health that focused on disease containment and biomedical technologies to control infectious disease (Birn, 2012). The WHO rhetorically embraced the social determinants of health, first in its expansive definition of health encoded in its 1948 constitution as 'a state of complete physical, mental, and social well-being and not merely the absence of disease or infirmity' (WHO, 2003) and later in the Alma Ata Declaration of 1978, where the world's nation-states signed on to the WHO campaign: Health Care for All by the Year 2000. One of a number of UN new world order declarations, Alma Ata had as its constitutional objective 'the attainment by all citizens of the world by the year 2000 of a level of health which will permit them to lead a socially and economically productive life' and the means to achieving this, primary health care (PHC) (WHO, 1987). There was a clear recognition that disease and poverty were deeply inter-twined and that health policies should be community-driven, support local health priorities and health's determinants, and use appropriate technologies (WHO, 1987). Corresponding to the advent of the oil and debt crises in the early 1980s, Alma Ata was eclipsed by cost-recovery, privatization, and 'selective primary health care', an approach focused on the few diseases responsible for the greatest mortality, to the detriment of strengthening health care systems and health's social determinants (Werner, 1994: 11). Still, as late as 2008 the report of WHO's High Level Commission on the Social Determinants of Health contained in its overarching recommendations to 'improve daily living conditions; tackle the inequitable distribution of power, money and resources; measure and understand the problem and assess the impact of action' (WHO 2008). The commission's work was undertaken during the time that the power of the WHO to steer to global health agenda was on the decline. The World Bank (WB), pharmaceutical and other corporations, and philanthropists began to play a larger role in global health policy within and outside of UN bodies. Donor interests increasingly shaped the global health agenda while huge profits were to be gained from private sector involvement in providing 'public goods'. Vertical, single disease campaigns that focused on technological quick-fixes crowded out prevention and health systems strengthening.

Global health security at the intra-state level evolved to become more closely aligned with the specific interests of corporate capital, disguised as "national" or "global" interests. The WHO aspirational definition of health remains, but as little more than rhetoric; a 2009 editorial in *The Lancet* re-defined health in rather apolitical terms as 'the ability to adapt' given that the obstacles to health 'seem so huge and complex' that it makes sense to offer a more modest view of what health means (Lancet, 2009: 781). Under the rubric of development and humani-tarianism, global health policy is driven through a specific neoliberal rationality that leans toward market-based and technocratic solutions to address complex and intransigent health problems, constructing individuals as responsible for their own health. The emergency rationalities that dominate the institutional landscape are often described through the language of rights, development, and humanitarian-ism, which serves to mask corporate political influence in state and multilateral processes (Biehl and Petryna, 2013). Lakoff (2010) views 'humanitarian biomedi-cine', which addresses the individual suffering of people afflicted by the neglected diseases of poverty as '. . . a philanthropic palliative to nation-states lacking public health infrastructure in exchange for the right of international health organizations to monitor their populations for outbreaks that might threaten wealthy nations'

(p. 75). Delivered through organizations such as Médecins Sans Frontières, the Bill and Melinda Gates Foundation, and the Global Fund to HIV/AIDS, Tuberculosis and Malaria, non-government actors avoid 'political entanglement' (Lakoff, 2010) through the provision of goods such as drugs, vaccines, and bed-nets, and we can add to the list, emergency food aid and hospitals in zones of war, famine, or natural disaster.

The tensions amongst competing conceptions of health are reflected in the contemporary "securitization" of new, emerging, and re-emerging diseases (EID) that '. . . mainly acts to prevent the diseases of the poor in the South from spreading to the North and laterally to other areas in the South' (Weir, 2015: 27). The practices constituting global health security have come to exclusively *mean* global infectious disease security, and have been codified in the development through the WHO of more robust International Health Regulations and interventions to enhance the capacity and compliance of nation-states, to follow the new regulations (Davies, Kamradt-Scott, and Rushton, 2015). Significant investments have been made to shore up international networks for epidemic alert and response and strengthen disease surveillance, laboratory systems, risk communication, and public education. These investments as well as the development and stockpiling of vaccines and drugs will continue to be highly uneven and influenced by vested interests, with Western countries focusing on their own preparedness while the beleaguered UN system copes with assisting poor countries (Weir, 2015). As Lakoff (2010) has suggested, both projects are ostensibly 'apolitical'; both are socio-technical projects; both can be seen essentially as responses to the erosion of the basic constituents of health and bare life. These include clean water and sanitation, nutritious food, shelter, security, health knowledge, and access to preventative and comprehensive health care. Competing and overlapping conceptions of health security remain, and are reflected in the tension between the conception of health as a human security issue linked to a broader analysis of the ideological and structural forces that shape human health, and the hegemonic view of health as a national and global security concern in which new pathogens that pose threats to particular (and largely northern) interests need to be contained. Indeed, the threat of the spread of a communicable disease such as Avian Influenza or Zika can cause very real economic and political disruption and human suffering within and well beyond the afflicted communities. The prospect of a novel influenza strain mutating and setting off a chain of human-to-human transmission in the future could have quite significant global impacts. The dominant narratives, however, pay scant attention to the conditions incubating those novel viruses, nor do they address in any meaningful way the social suffering of those who fall ill or experience most intensely the multiple impacts of epidemics.

Gender, health, and security

Feminist approaches to security are engaged in a project of transforming the field of Security Studies into one that takes gender relations seriously, whether the focus is security in the military sense, or the broader view of human security that transcends the pragmatic orthodoxy of the narrow, state-centric definition of national and global security. The traditional concerns of Security Studies obscure how the tight alliance between corporate and state interests and the structural privileging of men and masculinity operates to shape what are commonly understood as "gender neutral" policies. Deeply entrenched gendered power relations, intersecting with other hierarchical axes of differentiation such as class, race, ethnicity, and sexuality, operate to produce discourses and practices that render invisible, or normalize the gendered structural violence of the current global order. Feminist scholars have illuminated the pathways between contemporary neoliberal governance at both supra-national and state levels and the local conditions that underpin poverty and deepen gendered insecurities that are experienced differently by different racialized, classed, and gendered bodies. A central theoretical contribution of critical International Relations has been to expose the essential contradiction between the public sphere of politics and economics and the "private" sphere of the household and its (feminized) labours, where the activities of social reproduction – the unpaid and invisible care labours that keep bodies alive are undertaken. Capital accumulation depends upon the intensification of this contradiction, this invisible care labour largely the responsibility of girls and women, given the intransigence of socially constructed gendered and racialized divisions of labour (Cohen and Brodie, 2007; Peterson, 2012; Gill and Roberts, 2011; Marchand and Runyan, 2011). The labours of social reproduction continue to intensify as nation-states and global governance institutions increasingly guarantee the security of capital at the expense of human security (Bakker and Gill, 2003).

A critical feminist perspective can illuminate what remains invisible in the current regime of global health security: the ideologies and practices of the governance of health that shape the underlying determinants of health at the level of the body, the household, community, and beyond, and the impacts of health security practices on differently classed, racialized, and gendered bodies. Systemic intersectional inequalities can magnify the structural violence of specific policies and practices that are designed to respond to viral emergencies, resulting in the undermining of the livelihoods, and the sexual and reproductive health rights (SRHR) of women and girls. The understanding of the right to health for women has evolved to encompass a broad range of protections and entitlements that include freedom from coerced contraception and forced sterilization, unwanted sexual relations, sexual and gender-based violence, and involuntary maternity, including access to safe abortion. It also includes rights to comprehensive health services including, but not limited to, maternal and child health care, as well as access to health's social determinants including proper nutrition, water and sanitation, and shelter/security (Petchesky, 2003; Sen and Ostlin, 2008; Nowicka, 2011; Kabeer, 2015). This framing of SRHR is consistent with the concept of human security that gained prominence in the 1990s, based on the idea that the individual (although embedded in community) is the only reducible focus of security, and that the claims of other referents (states, economies, the globe) emerge from the person's inherent right to dignity and to what is necessary to survive and flourish. Yet feminist perspectives have not figured in any prominent way in either the "human" or "health security" debates, despite the central role of gendered power relations in shaping the security of girls and women.

The four examples that follow, while far from exhaustive, serve to illuminate the gendered structural violence emerging from recent responses to pandemic disease "threats". The accounts are based on a combination of primary sources from UN and government organizations, feminist and civil society advocacy organizations, and academic publications.

Responses to health threats

HIV and AIDS

The Human Immunodeficiency Virus is spread from human to human through sexual contact, blood, and from mother to foetus or infant. In the early 1980s when the disease made its first appearance in urban gay communities in North America, initial research was driven by the hypothesis that the new syndrome resulted from "promiscuity" and "drug abuse", confining the health threat to stigmatized risk groups – initially gay males and injecting drug users. At its outset, gender non-conforming identities were subject to coercive practices and homophobic/trans-phobic violence. By 1986 the view that a virus (HIV) was the cause of AIDS (the virus having been isolated in 1984) shifted policy responses toward a seemingly simple solution: avoid sharing bodily fluids. The development of anti-retroviral therapy (ART) (the first drug in 1987) and the widespread availability by the mid-1990s of Highly Active Antiretroviral Therapy (HAART) – a potent combination of antiretroviral drugs – transformed HIV into a chronic treatable condition, at least for those who could afford them or who lived in places in the world where the patent-protected drugs were made publically available. In countries on the African continent there was no such widespread availability of ART until years later, when prices dropped. In East and Southern African countries with serious epidemics, the provision of even the most basic palliative care was lacking. Estimates of annual health spending on the African continent for the year 2000 amounted to as little as 31 cents per person, and $8.16 for person living with HIV, '. . . spending so miniscule as to leave millions without care and support' according to a report of the AIDS Economics Network (McGreevey *et al.*, 2002: 3).

The casting of HIV/AIDS as a health emergency of global proportions is dated to January 2000 with the UN Security Council's designation of the pandemic as a security threat, marking the first time in their history that their interpretation of a threat fell outside the domain of armed security. The looming "threat" was ostensibly unfolding on the African continent, where the prevalence and incidence of HIV were highest. Given that mortality was concentrated amongst the most productive members of society – workers in private and public sector institutions, the military, and labourers contributing to GDP – the security concern was that high HIV-related mortality could lead to instability across the continent. HIV spread could potentially undermine military and state capacity and economic growth, threatening Western geopolitical interests in the region (ICG, 2001). But as coinciding epidemics unfolded there was '. . . no significant co-variation between HIV/AIDS prevalence and military security, social uprising, macroeconomic instability, or democratic consolidation' (Fourie, 2015: 114). The reality on the ground was that communities adapted, but not without costs. Those modelling various epidemics likely did not take into account that the evolution of coping strategies, of familial and communities of care, would keep the "security crisis" at bay.

Women were constructed as the "victims" of HIV, as epidemics became more feminized with steady rises in the proportion of young women living with HIV and AIDS. Within mainstream accounts of risk and vulnerability, gender relations were largely understood through a focus on individual sexual behaviour, perceived to be amenable to change through women's empowerment campaigns; the individual 'the bearer of risk and the locus of action' (Das, 2011: 32). Development projects were rolled out to provide income generation and microcredit to women to make up for the loss of labour attributed to HIV related mortality, along with strategies to keep girls in school, given the strong correlation between girls' education and sexual debut (O'Manique, 2004). Invisible was the fact that complex gendered power relations and non-consensual sex were rooted in relations of production and social reproduction, supported by state-mandated distortions in structures of production, physical mobility, and familial relations (Das, 2011: 30).

Vertical programs were initially put in place to prevent and contain viral spread (first targeted at 'high risk' groups, which included soldiers in the military and sex workers), while the provision of comprehensive health care, the protection of human rights, and addressing the foundations of HIV spread and its impacts were largely neglected. But the securitization frame was seen as a positive development because it did in fact mobilize an increase in global spending for HIV/AIDS, by constructing it as exceptional. The AIDS industry flourished, with investments in ART scaling up at a remarkable speed. The re-medicalization of AIDS – a growing emphasis on treatment alone, as well as 'treatment as prevention' in 2010 raised concerns that the progress that had been made with regard to understanding the deeper contexts and drivers of HIV spread would be reversed (Nguyen *et al.*, 2010) thus pushing aside the gender question.

The securitizing rationality of AIDS skewed responses away from the human security "crisis" of HIV/AIDS, a significant one, the feminized crisis of social reproduction at the household level (O'Manique and Fourie, 2010: 250). Women's central roles in formal, informal, and in household care economies were neglected in analyses of gender relationships, and their implications for the links between poverty, insecurity and HIV and AIDS. Female care-givers were the invisible health workers whose adult children were coming home to die, their informal and subsistence labours intensified in efforts to provide the care that was needed in the absence of health care systems and other social supports. Research carried out in Uganda (O'Manique, 2004), in Zimbabwe (Tiessen, Parpart and Grant, 2010), and in Malawi (Anderson, 2015) tell a similar story: time from home-based care and trips to hospital, time away from cultivating and wage labour, difficulties providing food and medicines for patients and other family members, and taking on debt to pay for funerals and other necessities. The burden of care was invisible in the understanding of "crisis", and predictably the poorest households shouldered the most difficult burdens.

In the framing of HIV/AIDS in conflict situations, women were also invisible, apart from the recognition of their increased risk of infection through sexual violence or prostitution, but without consideration of their underlying drivers (Sekinelgin, Birirumwami, and Morris, 2010). The single-minded focus on rape and prostitution obscured the complex nature of girls' and women's insecurities in zones of conflict and post-conflict situations and had the effect of removing women's agency to define their own vulnerabilities. Feminist security scholars have drawn attention to the ubiquity of sexual violence in conflict and post-conflict situations, but call for gender sensitive analyses of the communities in which the conflict is unfolding, including the power relations that shape individual and collective gendered and ethnic/racialized identities, alliances, and behaviours. After protracted low intensity war, the physical and psychological trauma of violence, malnutrition, and disease in the absence of basic health services and livelihood options does not disappear, and sexual violence can remain as part of the everyday fabric of daily life (see Liebing, this volume, Chapter 3).

The long-wave nature of the HIV/AIDS pandemic has resulted in its normalization, and its move largely outside of the health emergency paradigm. But the structural violence that shapes individual risk and resilience and the social suffering of those without access to adequate care and support continues. In 2015, HIV took over one million lives. HIV/AIDS remains exceptional to the extent that treatment has been made widely available through international development assistance and subsidies to public health systems. The situation remains that the invisible gendered care labour of women underpins the health care economies in regions of high HIV prevalence, to the point that, in South Africa, grandmothers are still, today, celebrated as the indispensable "backbone" of care for AIDS orphans.

Avian Influenza

Prior to the 2003 global outbreak of Highly Pathogenic Avian Influenza (HPAI) (H5N1) that spread throughout China and Southeast Asia, wild birds, small-scale poultry farming, and live markets for poultry had coexisted, relatively unproblematically, for centuries (GRAIN, 2006). The emergence of this more virulent strain included rare human infections with severe mortality rates, the vast majority of victims having had prolonged and close contact with infected birds. Risk of H5N1 was that a viral mutation that would make possible human-to-human spread could lead to a global catastrophe (Davis, 2005). In the end, human infections remained very low with the cumulative number of human cases reported to the WHO as of 2016 at 856, with 452 deaths and only a handful the result of human-to-human contact (WHO, 2016a). Still, reports in the media during the height of the HPAI pandemic constructed the virus as a threat to human health with devastating consequences for the global economy. A worst-case scenario modelled for the Food and Agricultural Organization (FAO) predicted extensive shocks to global poultry markets, higher meat prices, and lower global meat consumption should the virus reach the European Union (EU). While the most apocalyptic predictions did not play out, the cost to the global economy was estimated to be in the billions of dollars (Velasco *et al.*, 2008).

The emergency response to HPAI was not uniform but was shaped by the severity of regional outbreaks and the varying capacities of different states to report and address animal disease. Davies, Kamradt-Scott, and Rushton found that in Asia, the WHO's 2006 resolution calling on states to respond to H5N1 as an IHR Emergency, was generally accepted at a normative level, but was significantly hindered by the ability of some states to meet their IHR core capacities, such as virus strain detection, veterinary services, and compensation to poultry farmers for culled birds (2015: 88–92). Thailand and Indonesia were regularly criticized for substantial lags in their reporting of poultry and human cases, the presence of large poultry producers who stood to suffer major economic losses a possible reason (Davies, Kamradt-Scott, and Rushton, 2015: 85). Chuensatiansup's (2008) analysis of the response in Thailand documented the deliberate complicity of the government to protect the largest agribusiness exporters by waiting months before declaring an epidemic, giving them time to process their inventory, and disinfect their plants. In the next year, 60 million free-range chickens and ducks were ordered slaughtered, undermining the livelihoods of those dependent upon them (p. 55).

The emergency "rapid response" elides the complex drivers that give rise to novel infectious disease events, in this case, an infection with very different consequences for different people's lives and livelihoods. In the case of HPAI, the few studies of the gendered consequences that emerged from the "rapid response" suggest the undermining of poor, rural women's subsistence through a focus on biosecurity measures that favoured large-scale industrial poultry producers while undermining the already vulnerable positions of female backyard poultry farmers. Backyard farming is one of the foundations of food security and a source of income for hundreds of millions of rural poor in Asia, with chicken production providing up to one third of the protein intake for the average rural household, and often the only livestock that poor families can afford (GRAIN, 2006: 3).

A 2008 report focusing on the gendered aspects of the HPAI crisis in Laos, Thailand, and Vietnam based on interviews and consultations with planners, project implementers, and government authorities uncovered a general lack understanding and acknowledgment in HPAI responses across the board of potential gendered impacts in terms of loss of livelihoods and incomes, health risks, and household and community roles and responsibilities (Velasco *et al.*, 2008). The few analyses of the gendered impacts of the response exposed the preference for bio-secured and predominantly male-managed market-oriented poultry production resulting in income displacements for many poor rural women. A common understanding was that backyard and village free-range poultry was the main vector of disease spread, a hypothesis that was challenged by research that located the emergence of the pandemic in the self-regulated, mammoth, transnational poultry industry (GRAIN 2006). Poultry production in South-East Asian countries had skyrocketed in the previous decades, most of it concentrated in large factory farms that were integrated into transnational production systems, which are overwhelmingly the beneficiaries of the demand for more meat. According to the transnational NGO Genetic Resources Action International, HPAI provided a rationale to consolidate the commercial industry and do away with small-scale production (GRAIN, 2006). Fertile conditions for the spread of HPAI in the region were provided by huge industrial poultry factories that operated in close proximity to densely populated human settlements where chickens and ducks freely co-mingled with humans (Davis, 2005: 153–55). These industries provide ideal breeding grounds for viral mutation given that a large number of genetically uniform birds confined to a small area can generate enough virus for a mutation to occur, while, historically, the low density and genetic diversity of much smallholder production served as checks on viral load (GRAIN, 2006; Alders *et al.*, 2014).

Field studies in various hard-hit communities found that when compensating backyard producers for culling chickens it was common practice to use commercial poultry prices as the benchmark for backyard chickens, which undervalued women's contributions to household food security (Alders *et al.*, 2014; Bagnol, 2009). It was also a common practice to pay male "household heads" instead of women, making them suspicious of, and reluctant to engage with, official HPAI control programs (Bagnol, 2009). Bagnol's field research uncovered that the overwhelmingly male veterinary and extension staff were unaware of women's needs, and left them out of information campaigns. Top-down biosecurity measures were mandated such as the housing of birds to segregate flocks altered the production system from one in which birds freely scavenged, to a more labour and capital intensive enterprise in which women in poor households were required to build pens, purchase feed, provide water and clean out the flock (Bagnol, 2009: 235). Initiatives to control H5N1 in village poultry has shown to work, but has meant the active involvement of the local community, working together in line with local conditions (Alders *et al.*, 2014). In sum, strategies of containing the epidemic undermined the economic security of women poultry producers, their roles in social reproduction, and left out their potential contributions to improving responses.

Ebola

Ebola is a deadly haemorrhagic fever transmitted through infected fruit bats or primates to humans, as well as through direct human-to-human contact with body fluids. Small outbreaks of Ebola have occurred in a handful of Central African countries since the mid-1970s and tended to be quickly contained. But the most recent epidemic, which began in a remote village in Guinea located in the Mano River region, went undetected for months, allowing it to quickly spread from Guinea across borders to Liberia and Sierra Leone and to escalate into a global health emergency (WHO, 2014). The slate upon which the epidemic was written was the legacy of colonialism and the protracted violent conflicts that brutalized Sierra Leone and Liberia from the late 1980s and spread to Guinea in 2001, ending in a fragile post-conflict peace in 2003. During the civil unrest, mining and timber companies disrupted the densely forested region, the habitat of Ebola's natural reservoir, the fruit bat (Bardosh, Leach, and Wilkinson 2016). The conflicts in the sub-region fostered highly militarized societies and the '. . . absence of strong local institutions that might diagnose and stop such outbreaks and care for the afflicted' (Farmer, 2015: 25). Structural violence took the form of a lack of durable government functions, socio-economic infrastructure and services, particularly in the rural areas (Ogbonnaya, 2015: 30). The vast wealth of the small political elite classes tied to resource extraction and the aid industries was in stark contrast to the insecurity of the majority of the population who experience multidimensional poverty (Anderson and Beresford, 2016; Bardosh, Leach, and Wilkinson, 2016).

Local clinics were overwhelmed as the virus spread through Sierra Leone, Guinea, and Liberia. The WHO declared the outbreak a Public Health Emergency of International Concern (PHEIC) in August 2014. In Liberia it took months for medical outreach and infrastructure to reach hard hit areas, and the epidemic curve had largely passed by the time Ebola Treatment Centres and Community Care Centres were on the ground (Bardosh, Leach and Wilkinson, 2016: 78). Nokov (2015) observed that the crisis framing of the Ebola epidemic intensified once a case showed up in the United States (on 23 October 2014) at which point it was overtly framed in the media as an "African" disease with potential "global" consequences (p. 9). Media reporting in North America focused on the potential risk to American citizens and the legitimacy of strategies of containment – of border controls, suspension of airline travel, contact tracing and quarantine of people from the region. Xenophobia was reflected in ongoing calls for travel bans from the Ebola zone, despite any evidence that they would have an effect (Dionne and Seay, 2015: 7). A more rapid response would indeed have made a difference. But as Bardosh, Leach, and Wilkinson (2016) explain, 'the interlocking socio-political, economic and historical processes that have effectively perpetuated deep-seated inequalities in income, health and political inclusion' is where the source of the epidemic was located (p. 76). The authors describe several patterns as the crisis unfolded: fragmented, confusing and top-down messages that bred suspicion of strangers; severely under-equipped health systems that were rapidly overwhelmed; a dramatic collapse of civil society and local economies; personal tragedy as loved ones died; the normalization of road checkpoints, curfews, and massive quarantine (pp. 77–78).

Sophie Harman's (2016) literature survey of gender narratives in Ebola strategies and in the WB and WHO health system strengthening plans in the epidemic's aftermath uncovered a number of "conspicuous invisibilities" at every point in the international response. While some attention was paid to the different biological impact on men and women, such as the maternal health crisis that unfolded as health systems were overwhelmed by Ebola patients, Harman exposes the invisibility of gender, which in turn 'ignores and subsequently reinforces gendered norms of care and social reproduction' (p. 524). When "women" were mentioned in broader reports, it was often in a few scant sentences, and there was little evidence that specific concerns were addressed in the wider response (pp. 528–30). Others observed that women were reduced to a 'vulnerable group' of mothers, with no acknowledgement of their role as caregivers in both formal and informal health care systems, in caring for orphaned children, and as traders and income providers. Acknowledgement of women's particular vulnerabilities to personal and economic losses, despite their critical roles in food production and cross-border trade, was also absent (Diggins and Mills, 2015; IASC, 2015).

That healthcare centres were so under-resourced and unable to provide essential care implicitly meant that women were already taking on the care burden that the state and other actors were not providing, while the closure of schools presented additional care burdens for women and an increased risk for girls. The tendency to emphasize "non-modern" or "culturalist" explanations for women's specific vulnerabilities such as maternal mortality as located in patriarchal practices masked the extent to which they were driven by broader structures of impoverishment and inequality. State Diggins and Mills (2015: 2):

> Given the utterly shattered state of [its] post-war health system, we might question how logical it was to view poor reproductive health as evidence of gender discrimination; or how possible it could ever be to address Ebola or maternal mortality as stand-alone problems, in isolation from each other or more comprehensive structural investment, building the basic capacity of health care systems.

Although the virus has been contained, the gendered consequences of the epidemic in West Africa will remain for years to come. The 'emergency within the emergency' (Vetter *et al.*, 2016) is the thousands of Ebola survivors with a range of sequelae, some very serious, including neurological complications, vision problems, severe fatigue, and muscle weakness. Mental health challenges of survivors are magnified by increased food insecurity, the scarcity of access to medical services, the closing of schools and businesses, and local people's distrust of the health care system (pp. 85–89). Caring for survivors may well intensify women's unpaid care labours for years to come. The CDC reported in August 2006 that fragments of Ebola virus were found in semen of 9 per cent of 429 men after recovering from the disease: of 429 tested, and 63 per cent of those still tested positive one year later (CDC, 2016). Whether this will put women at risk of Ebola infection through sex remains unknown. Calls from the Inter-Agency Standing Committee Reference Group on Humanitarian Action highlight the most pressing issues for gender justice in the epidemic's aftermath, calling on the need for an explicit gender-integrated response and the participation of women and girls in all communities in the recovery process across the board, including livelihood support, the protection needs of women and girls in the context of the curtailment of security including family planning and access to contraception, social and justice services, girls' education, and entitlements for caregivers (IASC, 2015).

But now that the virus has been contained and the emergency is over, attention has moved elsewhere. US$510 million that had been allocated to the post-crisis reconstruction by the American government through the Department of Health and

Human Services and Department of State/USAID was re-directed toward containing the Zika virus:

> . . . on immediate, time-critical activities such as mosquito control, lab capacity, development of diagnostics and vaccines, supporting affected expectant mothers and babies, tracking and mapping the spread and effects of Zika infections in humans, and other prevention and response efforts in the continental United States, Puerto Rico, other U.S. Territories, and abroad, especially within the Americas.
>
> (Donovan, 2016)

Zika

Zika is a virus first discovered in 1947 in Uganda and transmitted through the bite of the *Aedes aegypyi* species of mosquito. It can also be transmitted through the blood, semen, and vaginal fluids of an infected person. Zika was declared a PHEIC by the Director-General of the WHO in February 2016 on the basis of an extraordinary cluster of microcephaly in infants born to mothers with the virus in Brazil. In October 2015 the Brazil Ministry of Health reported a 20-fold increase in cases of congenital syndrome in foetuses and infants that corresponded to a high prevalence of suspected Zika cases in the northeast of the country. The virus subsequently spread throughout South and Central America and into the Caribbean and the United States, but the overwhelming number of babies born with microcephaly were concentrated in Brazil, particularly the northeast of the country: 2,366 of the global 2,726 cases, as of 23 February 2017 (PAHO/WHO, 2017). The mosquito population in the poor favelas of Brazil has proliferated due to inadequate municipal sewage management, extremely dense urban development and reliance on open-reservoir stagnant drinking water (Truong *et al.*, 2015: 1,089). There is no vaccine for the virus. About 80 per cent of people with Zika are asymptomatic, and when symptoms do occur, they are typically mild.

While Zika's emergency status was the result of virus' link to microcephaly, the response offered little to women of childbearing age or pregnant. The mainstay of prevention messages from institutions such as the CDC and WHO was to minimize exposure to mosquito bites though eliminating mosquito vectors, and encouraging through public health campaigns, personal protective measures such as wearing long sleeves, pants and hats, using insect repellent and bed nets, and staying indoors with screened or closed windows, or air-conditioning. Women were specifically instructed to put off pregnancy through the use of family planning and contraception, and screening and monitoring for congenital birth defects was recommended for pregnant women. There was silence on the very different realities of girls and women with regard to the extent to which they could follow such directives. The great majority of women who gave birth to babies with Zika lived in dense zones of poverty where access to such protections was not readily available. In the city of Recife, considered "ground zero" of the epidemic, volunteers and soldiers went door to door to provide information to people on how to protect themselves, but as journalist Sarah Bosley reported, many women in the favelas could not even afford insect repellent, or a new set of window screens, and given the absence of piped water and sanitation, vector control was difficult and also accounts for the endemic status of Dengue in the region.

But the directive to "avoid pregnancy" was the most problematic. Although research on the sexual transmission of the virus is ongoing, the current science demonstrates that it can remain in semen longer than in other bodily fluids, and that the majority of cases of sexual transmission have been male-to-female (CDC, 2017). The HIV/AIDS pandemic exposed the complexities addressing "high risk" sexual behaviour; of how poor health care systems, gender based-violence, and inequalities across gender, race/ethnicity and class undermined the impacts of particular policy responses (O'Manique, 2004). It became clear that sexual behaviour takes place within a broader context of power relations, which include gendered power relations. For the impoverished women living in "ground zero" of the Zika health emergency, 56 per cent of pregnancies were unintended (Roa, 2016: 843). According to Roa, shaping the 'tragic failures of reproductive health and rights' was the poor quality of sex education, poor access to contraception, a high prevalence of gender-based violence and gendered power relations that made the negotiation of safe sex less than straightforward (p. 843).

Laws that govern girls' and women's sexual reproductive rights in South America are amongst the most draconian in the world. Brazil has amongst the strictest anti-abortion laws in the region, and the recent conservative backlash fuelled in the region called for even stricter laws, and in some countries, a total ban. In Brazil it is a crime punishable for up to three years in jail, with exceptions for rape, or where the woman's life is at risk. While wealthy women can find discreet and safe access to abortion services, poor women must seek out clandestine and dangerous ways to terminate pregnancies (Yamin, 2016). Donald Trump's recent re-instatement of the "global gag rule", which withholds USAID funding from any organization overseas that so much as offers information on abortion, or reproductive health services, has produced a chilling effect in the region while emboldening evangelical legislators to further curtail women's exercise of sexual and reproductive health rights. The response has also been remarkably silent on the impact of those who face the long-term burden of caring for a children with microcephaly whose needs would continue throughout their lives, and women were having to stop work, and girls were leaving school (Bosley, 2016).

On 18 November 2016 the status of Zika was changed from a PHEIC '. . . into a sustained programme of work with dedicated resources to address the long-term nature of the disease and its associated consequences' (WHO, 2016b). According to the WHO, it would remain a 'significant enduring public health challenge requiring intense action' (WHO, 2016b). The epidemic has, however, mobilized feminist activists throughout the Americas against the antipathy toward women's SRHR in global health governance as well as in state laws, and has cast a light on the systemic inequality experienced by racialized women living in critical poverty.

Conclusion

Gary Finnegan makes the case that Zika has pushed other major health challenges out of the spotlight, and has distracted the world from other "medical emergencies." He contrasts the 2015 incidence of Zika in the Americas at just under half a million with the 390 million global incidence of Dengue, spread through the same mosquito, and Malaria, at 214 million (Finnegan, 2016). Finnegan is right in observing that the narratives and practices of public health emergencies deflect attention away from other critical global health concerns. But the argument that they focus on specific diseases at the expense of others promotes the faulty idea that diseases exist in isolation from each other. What is lost from view is that unequal global disease burden and its impacts are a consequence of deep structures of inequality and structural violence, regardless of specific origin. The chronic, endemic diseases of poverty and inequality do not have the potential to dramatically disrupt the state and material interests of Northern countries, nor do they pose a threat to the lives of the rich. But new pathogens will likely continue to develop with increasing frequency and speed, given that the conditions of their emergence are advancing rather than abating. The institutionalization of both global health security and humanitarian biomedicine invite technocratic and market-based solutions and entrench neo-liberal systems of political and economic management that pose no threat to capital's hegemony, and in fact support its expansion into "development." Hence the urgency of developing a deeper understanding of the gendered and racialized structural violence that shape both the conditions that incubate health emergencies, and their responses, not just for girls and women, but for humanity as a whole.

Where does this leave us? The individual cases point to the need for a broader-based shift away from emergency epistemologies that focus on containment, and that leave the foundations of health emergencies intact, and their deep impacts imprinted on the bodies and lives of people who already pay the largest price for a world order that is anything but human rights- and life-sustaining. Without denying the need for rapid responses for infectious diseases, it is becoming clear that the two regimes of global health that dominate are palliative, at best. Conventional thinking on global health emergencies maintains a system that does not call into question the political order and vested interests that shape the epidemiology of novel infections and the problematic nature of emergency responses. The serious global economic and ecological crises that we now face are also gendered and sexualized. A starting point in terms of emergency responses might involve paying attention to the material conditions that nurture viral contagion and the impacts of pandemics on the most vulnerable. The larger political project involves a deeper challenge to the legitimacy of a global health governance system that is accountable not to flesh-and-blood bodies, but to capital.

References

Alders, Robyn, Awuni, Joseph Adongo, Bagnol, Brigitte, Farrell, Penny and de Hann, Nicolene (2014) 'Impact of Avian Influenza on Village Poultry Production', *EcoHealth* 11: 63–72.

Anderson, E-L. (2015) *Gender, HIV and Risk: Navigating Structural Violence.* Basingstoke: Palgrave Macmillan.

Anderson, E-L., Beresford, A. (2016) 'Infectious Injustice: The Political Foundations of the Ebola Crisis in Sierra Leone', *Third World Quarterly* 37(3):468–486.

Arner, K. (2013) 'Making Global Commerce into International Health Diplomacy: Consuls and Disease Control in the Age of Revolutions', *Journal of World History* 24(4): 771–96.

Bakker, I. and Gill. S., (2003) 'Ontology, Method and Hypotheses', in I Bakker, S. Gill (Eds) *Power, Production, and Social Reproduction.* Basingstoke: Palgrave Macmillan.

Bagnol, B. (2009) 'Gender Issues with Small-scale Family Poultry Production: Experiences from Newcastle Disease and Highly Pathogenic Avian Influenza Control', *World's Poultry Science Journal* 65: 231–241.

Bardosh, K. (2016) 'Unpacking the Politics of Zoonosis Research and Policy', in K. Bardosh (Ed.) *One Health: Science, politics, and Zoonotic Disease in Africa.* Oxon: Routledge.

Bardosh, K., Leach, M., and Wilkinson, A. (2016) 'The Limits of Rapid Response: Ebola and Structural Violence in West Africa', in K. Bardosh (Ed.) *One Health: Science, Politics, and Zoonotic Disease in Africa.* Routledge Oxon: Routledge.

Bennett, C. and McMichael, A. (2012) 'Global Environmental Change and Human Health', in T. Schrecker (Ed.) *The Ashgate Research Companion to the Globalization of Health.* Farnman: Ashgate.

Biehl, J. and Petryna, A. (2013) *When People Come First: Critical Studies in Global Health.* Princeton: Princeton University Press.

Birn, A.E. (2012) 'From Plagues to Peoples: Health in the Global/International Agenda', in T. Schrecker (Ed.) *The Ashgate Research Companion to the Globalization of Health.* Farnham: Ashgate.

Bosley, S. (2016) 'Heartbreak and Hardship for Women in Brazil as Zika Crisis Casts Deep Shadow', *The Guardian International* Thurs. 5 May 2016. Available: https://www.theguardian.com/global-development/2016/may/05/zika-crisis-brazil-women-heartbreak-hardship (accessed 24 February 2017).

CDC (2016) 'Traces of Ebola Virus Linger Longer than Expected in Semen'. Available: https://www.cdc.gov/media/releases/2016/p0830-ebola-virus-semen.html (accessed 22 February 2017).

CDC (2017) 'Centres for Disease Control: Zika and Sexual Transmission'. Available: https://www.google.ca/search?q=Zika+chances+of+spread+through+sex&ie=utf-8&oe=utf-8&gws_rd=cr&ei=ZbCxWJeNMKu3jwTK0bHYBQ (accessed 29 January 2017).

Chuensatiansup, K. (2008) 'Ethnography of Epidemiologic Transition: Avian Flu, Global Health Politics and Agro-industrial Capitalism in Thailand', *Anthropology and Medicine* 15(1): 53–9.

Cohen, M.G. and Brodie, J. (2007) 'Remapping Gender in the New Global Order', in M. Griffin Cohen and J. Brodie (Eds.) *Remapping Gender in the New Global Order*, London and New York: Routledge.

Das, V. (2011) 'The New Geography of HIV: Introductory Essay', in J. Klot, V-K Nguyen (Eds.) *The Fourth Wave: Violence, Gender, Culture and HIV in the 21st Century.* Paris: UNESCO.

Davies, S., Karmadt-Scott, A., and Rushton, S. (2015) *Disease Diplomacy: International Norms and Global Health Security.* Baltimore, MD: John Hopkins University Press.

Davis, M. (2005) *Monster at Our Door: The Global Threat of Avian Influenza.* New York: New Press.

Diggins, J. and Mills, E. (2015) 'The Pathology of Inequality: Ebola in West Africa', *IDS Practice Paper in Brief* 25 February Institute of Development Studies/UK Aid.

Dionne, K.Y. and Seay, L. (2015) 'Perceptions about Ebola in America: Othering and the Role of Knowledge About Africa', *Political Science and Politics* 48(1): 6–7.

Donovan, S. (2016) 'Taking Every Step, as Quickly as Possible, to Protect the Amerian People from Zika,' *White House Blog, Washington D.C.* Online. Available: https://www.whitehouse.gov/blog/2016/04/06/taking-every-step-necessary-quickly-possible-protect-american-people-zika (accessed 10 September 2016).

Farmer, P. (2015) 'The Caregivers' Disease', *London Review of Books*, 21 May pp. 25–28.

Finnegan, G. (2016) 'Outbreaks like Zika Distract Us from other Medical Emergencies', *Guardian UK*, Wednesday 28 December. Available https://www.theguardian.com/global-development-professionals-network/2016/dec/28/outbreaks-like-zika-distract-us-from-other-medical-emergencies (accessed 12 January 2017).

Fourie, P. (2015) 'AIDS as a Security Threat: The Emergence and Decline of an Idea', in S. Rushton and J. Youde (Eds.) *Routledge Handbook of Global Health Security.* London: Routledge.

Gill, S. and Roberts, A. (2011) 'Macroeconomic Governance, Gendered Inequality, and Global Crises', in B. Young, I. Bakker and D. Elson (Eds.) *Questioning Financial Governance from a Feminist Perspective.* New York: Routledge.

GRAIN (2006) 'Foul Play: The Poultry Industry's Central Role in the Bird Flu Crisis.' Available: https://www.grain.org/article/entries/22-fowl-play-the-poultry-industry-s-central-role-in-the-bird-flu-crisis (accessed 10 December 2016).

Harman, S. (2016) 'Ebola, Gender, and the Conspicuously Invisible Wwomen in Global Health Governance', *Third World Quarterly* 37(3): 524–541.

(IASC) Inter-Agency Standing Committee Reference Group for Humanitarian Action (2015) 'Humanitarian Crisis in West Africa (Ebola) Gender Alert'. Available: www.unwomen.org/~/media/headquarters/attachments/sections/library/publications/2015/iasc%20gender%20reference%20group%20-%20gender%20alert%20west%20africa%20ebola%202%20-%20february%202015.pdf (accessed 20 October 2016).

International Crisis Group (2001) 'AIDS as a Security Issue'. Available: https://www.crisisgroup.org/africa/hivaids-security-issue (accessed 23 August 2016).

Kabeer, N. (2015) 'Tracking the Gender Politics of the MDGs: Struggles for Interpretive Power in the New International Development Agenda', *Third World Quarterly* 36(2): 377–95.

King, N.B. (2002) 'Security, Disease, Commerce: Ideologies of Post-colonial Global Health', *Social Studies of Science* 32(5–6): 763–89.

Lakoff, A. (2010) 'Two Regimes of Global Health', *Humanity: An International Journal of Human Rights, Humanitarianism, and Development* 1(1): 59–79.

Lancet (2009) 'What is Health? The Ability to Adapt', *Lancet* 373(9666); 781–781.

Markel, H. (2014) 'Worldly Approaches to Public Health: 1851 to the Present,' *Public Health* 128(2): 124–28.

Marchand, M. and Runyan, A.S. (2011) 'Introduction: Feminist Sightings of Global Restructuring: New and Old Conceptualizations', in M. Marchand and A. Runyan (Eds.) *Gender and Global Restructuring: Sightings, Sites and Resistances.* New York: Routledge.

McGreevey, S., Bertozzi, S., Gutierrez, J., Opuni, M. and Izazola, J.A. (2002) 'Current and Future Resources for HIV/ AIDS', in S. Forsythe (Ed.) *State of the Art: AIDS and Economics*. International AIDS and Economics Network. Online. Available: www. policyproject.com/pubs/other/SOTAecon.pdf (accessed 23 August 2016).

Nguyen, V-K., Bajos, N., Dubois-Arber, F., O'Malley, J. and Pirkle, C.M. (2010) 'Remedicalizing an Epidemic: From HIV Treatment as Prevention to HIV Treatment is Prevention', *AIDS* 24. Online. Available: http://chiasm.hypotheses.org/files/2012/10/ remedicalizing.pdf (accessed 11 November 2016).

Nokov, J. (2015) 'Infecting the Constitution', *Political Science and Politics* 48(1): 9–10.

Nowicka, W. (2011) 'Sexual and Reproductive Rights and the Human Rights Agenda: Controversial and Contested', *Reproductive Health Matters* 19(38): 119–128.

Ogbonnaya, U. (2015) 'Political Conflicts, State Collapse and Ebola Virus Disease', *Africa Insight* 45(1): 30–51.

O'Manique, C. (2004) *Neoliberalism and AIDS Crisis in Sub-Saharan Africa: Globalization's Pandemic*. Basingstoke: Palgrave Macmillan.

O'Manique, C., Fourie, P.P. (2010) 'Security and Health in the 21st Century', in M. Dunn Cavelty and V. Mauer (Eds) *The Routledge Handbook of Security Studies*. London: Routledge.

PAHO/WHO. Zika Cumulative Cases, 23 February 2017. Available: www.paho.org/hq/ index.php?option=com_content&view=article&id=12390&Itemid=42090 (accessed 24 February 2017).

Petchesky, R. (2003) *Global Prescriptions: Gendering Health and Human Rights*. London: Zed Books.

Peterson, V. S. (2012) 'Rethinking Theory', *International Feminist Journal of Politics* 14 (1): 5–3.

Roa, M (2016) 'Zika Virus Outbreak: Reproductive Health and Rights in Latin America', *The Lancet* 387: 843.

Sekinelgin, H., Birirumwami, J., and Morris, J., (2010) 'Securitization of HIV/AIDS in Context: Gendered Vulnerability in Burundi', *Security Dialogue* 41(5): 515–535.

Sen, G. and Östlin, P. (2008) 'Gender Inequity in Health: Why it Exists and How We Can Change It', *Global Public Health* 3(S1): 1–12.

Tiessen, R., Parpart, J., and Grant, M. (2010) 'Gender, HIV/AIDS and Human Security in Africa', *Canadian Journal of African Studies* 44(3): 503–523.

Truong, Lisa, Gonnerman, Greg, Simonich, Michael T. and Tanguay, Robert L. (2016) 'Assessment of the Developmental and Neurotoxicity of the Mosquito Control Larvicide, Pyriproxyfen, Using Embryonic Zebrafish', *Environmental Pollution* 218 (2016): 1089–1093.

Velasco, E., Dieleman, E., Supakankunti, S., and Phong, T.T.M. (2008) 'Gender Aspects of the Avian Influenza Crisis in Southeast Asia: Laos, Thailand and Vietnam: Final Report for the D. G. External Relations, Avian Influenza External Response Coordination, European Commission'. Available: http://ec.europa.eu/world/avian_influenza/docs/gender_study_ 0608_en.pdf (accessed 10 September 2016).

Vetter, P., Kaiser, L., Schibler, M., Cigenecki, I, and Bauch, D.G. (2016) 'Sequelae of Ebola Virus Disease: The Emergency within the Emergency', *Lancet Infectious Diseases* 16(6): e82–91.

Weir, L. (2015) 'Inventing Global Health Security: 1994–2005', in S. Rushton and J Youde (Eds.) *Routledge Handbook of Global Health Security*. London: Routledge.

Werner, David (1994) 'The Life and Death of PHC' *Third World Resurgence* 42/43: 10–15.

WHO (1987) 'Declaration of Alma Ata'. Online. Available: www.euro.who.int/__data/assets/pdf_file/0009/113877/E93944.pdf (accessed 17 June 2016).

WHO (2003) 'WHO Definition of Health'. Online. Available: www.who.int/about/definition/en/print.html (accessed 17 June 2016).

WHO (2008) 'Social Determinants of Health'. Online. Available: www.who.int/social_determinants/en (accessed 17 June 2016).

WHO (2014) 'Six Months after the Ebola Outbreak was Declared, What Happens When a Deadly Virus Hits the Destitute?' Available: www.who.int/csr/disease/ebola/ebola-6-months/en/ (accessed 10 September 2016).

WHO (2016a) 'Cumulative Number of Confirmed Human Cases for Avian Influenza (H5N1) Reported to WHO 2003–2016'. Available: www.who.int/influenza/human_animal_interface/2016_12_19_tableH5N1.pdf?ua=1 (accessed 10 September 2016).

WHO (2016b) 'Fifth Meeting of the Emergency Committee under the International Health Regulations (2005) Regarding Microcephaly, other Neurological Disorders and Zika Virus WHO Statement 18 November 2016'. Available: www.who.int/mediacentre/news/statements/2016/zika-fifth-ec/en/ (accessed 12 December 2016).

Yamin, A.E. (2016) 'To Fight Zika, We Must Fight Poverty and Powerlessness and Ensure that Women Enjoy their Rights', FXB Center for Health and Human Rights, Harvard University. Available: //fxb.harvard.edu/4941-2/ (accessed 21 December 2016).

9 The invisible men
HIV, security, and men who have sex with women

Simon Rushton

Introduction

Over the past 30 years, AIDS has come to be widely seen as a security threat, both in terms of human security, through its impacts on individuals and communities, and of national and international security, through the potential effects that high levels of HIV and AIDS could have on social, political and economic stability. One of the fears that has been raised by critics of the 'securitization' of AIDS is that People Living with HIV (PLWHIV) could come to be viewed as a source of 'security threat', leading to further stigma and discrimination and 'pitting the interests of those living without HIV/AIDS against those affected by the illness through implying, however erroneously, that the healthy ones would be better off without the latter' (Elbe, 2005: 410–11).

At different times and in different places there have been countless cases where PLWHIV, or people suspected of being infected with the virus, have been viewed and treated as threats to the security of the wider community. Many examples have been documented over the years by AIDS and human rights activists, medical professionals, and academic commentators including notorious national policy responses such as the United States' quarantining of Haitian refugees at Guantanamo Bay in the early 1990s (Johnson, 1994; Farmer, 2003: Chapter 2) and the Russian Federation's repressive response that led to a failure to provide protection from infection for Intravenous Drug Users (Csete, 2004).

During the same period that AIDS has come to be seen as a threat to human, national and international security, the gendered dimensions of HIV epidemics around the world have come to be better comprehended – with significant progress being made in understanding the particular vulnerabilities of women and girls to infection, as well as the challenges they frequently face in accessing treatment and care. Whilst the nature of HIV epidemics varies significantly by region, in Eastern and Southern Africa – the region home to over half of all of PLWHA – the epidemics are overwhelmingly heterosexual and generalized: 2% of the total number of PLHWA being people who inject drugs; 4% sex workers; 6% men who have sex with men; 9% clients of sex workers and other sexual partners of key populations; and 79% the rest of the population (UNAIDS, 2016: 9). This places heterosexual men (or, perhaps more accurately, men who have sex with women – MSW) in

Eastern and Southern Africa as the predominant vector for the spread of the virus and potentially, if a security-based lens is adopted, as a threat to wider society.

The ways in which heterosexual men have been viewed in the global AIDS response has been criticized on a number of grounds, with echoes of threat–defence logics that are characteristic of security discourse being detectable in the dominant narratives. Some have argued that the focus on addressing gender inequalities that impact upon women's ability to access prevention, treatment and care has brought a concomitant assumption that men *are* able to access these things, and that their failure to do so makes them a source of the 'AIDS problem'. Others have pointed to a racial dimension in how this has been applied, most obviously in Africa, but also in other parts of the world. Authors such as Eileen Stillwaggon and Simon Watney, for example, have examined a range of sources including the media, academic research and policy statements and found a pervasive tendency to attribute the serious epidemics in sub-Saharan Africa to a hyper-sexualized and primitive culture, frequently (sometimes not even implicitly) constructing Africa as an undifferentiated 'deviant continent'. The types of interventions that have been targeted at men have also been critiqued for their focus on changing individual behaviours or implementing medico-technological 'fixes' for those behaviours rather than grappling with the thornier structural issues that impact on men just as they do on women. Each of these criticisms touches on the ways in which men and (what are assumed to be) male behaviours represent a threat, in particular to women and girls.

In this chapter, I examine whether these critiques apply to the declared strategies of four of the leading global AIDS institutions: the Joint United Nations Programme on HIV/AIDS (UNAIDS); the United States' President's Emergency Plan for AIDS Relief (PEPFAR); the World Health Organization (WHO); and the Global Fund to Fight AIDS, TB and Malaria (Global Fund). Through an analysis of the ways in which MSW are represented in the HIV strategies of those organizations, and the types of interventions that are promoted, I argue that there is no explicit evidence of the kinds of racialized assumptions about African sexuality that have been seen in previous eras, but that there continues to be a focus on men as part of the AIDS problem rather than part of the solution, and a continued failure to address the various ways in which MSW as well as women and MSM can be subject to structural violence resulting from a range of different sectionalities (for example of class, ethnicity, or social status).[1]

Before forwarding this argument, it is important to clarify two points. First, this chapter is not aimed at 'playing men off against women', still less at arguing that policy responses in respect of women have been adequate. Rather the point is to recognize that both women and men have been subject to discourses that simplify and caricature the realities of HIV epidemics around the world, and that these discourses have had negative effects on policy responses towards both genders, including a tendency to focus on behavioural at the expense of structural interventions. Second, it is of course the case that structural issues impact differently on different people – and that overwhelmingly those structures have tended to benefit men. Recognizing that structures are gendered in this way, however, does not mean that they cannot also impact negatively on (some) men – not least due to a variety of other sectionalities. Rather it behoves us to investigate the ways in which different men are affected by different structures – in other words, to avoid treating 'men' as a homogenous group. An essentializing discourse that constructs men as 'the problem' ignores the historical and social roots of hegemonic masculinities that are present at both the global and the local levels. Women are overwhelmingly the losers from these hegemonic masculinities. The point here is that men also pay a price.

Men who have sex with women as a 'health security' threat

That HIV represents a threat to human security has been discussed since the concept of human security first came into being (UNDP, 1994: 24), but it was in the late 1990s and early 2000s that HIV, in particular the large-scale generalized epidemics then taking hold in sub-Saharan Africa, first came to be widely discussed as a national and international security threat. The UN Security Council's discussion of the issue in January 2000, and its passing of Resolution 1308 later the same year, has generally come to be seen as a defining moment in the 'securitization' of AIDS. The Security Council spoke of its deep concern over 'the extent of the HIV/AIDS pandemic worldwide, and [. . .] the severity of the crisis in Africa in particular' and stressed that 'the HIV/AIDS pandemic, if unchecked, may pose a risk to stability and security' (UN Security Council, 2000: 1–2). Whilst the Security Council discussing a disease as an international security threat was new, the logics that underpinned that move have a far longer history, anchored as they are in longstanding fears about the ability of infectious diseases to undermine the stability of societies and to determine the outcomes of war (Price-Smith, 2009: Chapter 2).

Inseparable from those fears over disease's impact on social, political and economic stability has been the identification of particular individuals or communities as a source of threat to the wider population. In some cases (as can be seen through the implementation of quarantine regulations for the best part of 1,000 years (Gensini, Yacouba & Contia, 2004)), those threats have been perceived as coming from outside. In other cases, however, the threats have been internal. As Susan Sontag (1988: 27) argued in the late 1980s,

> Every feared epidemic disease, but especially those associated with sexual license, generates a preoccupying distinction between the disease's putative carriers (which usually means the poor and in this part of the world [Sontag is referring to the US], people with darker skins) and those defined – health professionals and other bureaucrats do the defining – as 'the general population'.

The stigma and discrimination that has resulted from such distinctions in the case of HIV has been well documented, and AIDS advocates within the US and around the world have made huge efforts (and significant progress) in addressing those problems. But just as the patterns and dynamics of HIV epidemics have varied around the world, so have the perceived sources of threat. In the US in the early 1980s it became common to talk of the '4 Hs': haemophiliacs, heroin addicts, homosexuals and Haitians (Gallo, 2006). In the discourse around African HIV epidemics, meanwhile, ideas of race and gender – either explicitly or implicitly – have frequently been at the heart of diagnoses of the AIDS problem. In particular, assertions about 'typical' male behaviours and supposed 'African cultural norms' have been put forward as explanations for the scale of the epidemics in sub-Saharan African countries, implicating ideas of gender and race in ways that are highly troubling.

For example, in 1989 Simon Watney published an article examining Western media reporting of 'African AIDS'. He sought to show the ways in which the media discourse consistently constructed Africa as a "deviant' continent'; an 'undifferentiated apocalyptic Africa', which condensed 'ancient fears concerning contagious disease, together with vengeful fantasies concerning 'excessive' sexuality, understood in essentially pre-modern terms as both the *source* and the *cause* of AIDS' (Watney, 1989: 59). In this discourse, Watney argued, differences between the epidemics in different places in Africa were obscured, with the source of threat being simplified in ways analogous to the American '4 Hs', equating 'black Africans and Western gay men as wilful "perverts" who are equally threatening to "family values"' (Watney, 1989: 52).

Such constructions of African (particularly African male) sexuality as lying at the heart of the continent's AIDS crisis have not been confined to the media. Eileen Stilwaggon, writing in 2003, examined some of the key works that had been 'cited repeatedly in the social science and policy literature' to explain the high prevalence of HIV in sub-Saharan Africa. This research, Stillwaggon argued, was plagued by sweeping generalizations about 'a hypersexualised pan-African culture' ('culture' being a word that effectively stood in for 'race') in which assumptions were made about higher levels of promiscuity in 'African culture' despite empirical evidence to the contrary. Whereas epidemiologists point to a wide range of factors underlying HIV/AIDS epidemics, not least poverty, Stillwaggon identifies the discursive dominance of a 'behavioural paradigm' grounded in an assumption of 'epic rates of sexual partner change in Africa for which empirical support is lacking' (Stillwaggon, 2003: 811). Although Stillwaggon points to research by WHO and UNAIDS in the mid-1990s that undermined the notion that promiscuity is responsible for high levels of HIV transmission in Africa (Stillwaggon, 2003: 811), she nevertheless finds subsequent evidence of these assumptions in the publications of some of the key global organizations seeking to address HIV/AIDS, including the United Nations Population Fund (UNFPA) and the World Bank. Importantly, she also argues for the existence of a policy paradigm that focuses primarily on behavioural solutions such as improving condom use, rather than grappling with structural factors such as socio-economic conditions, concluding that

> The behavioural paradigm and its assumption of Africa exceptionalism largely determine the questions that can be asked and the solutions that can be proposed

in AIDS research and AIDS-prevention policy for Africa and other profoundly poor populations.

(Stillwaggon, 2003: 830)

When taken together, Sontag's identification of a distinction between 'putative carriers' and 'general populations', and the insights about the ways in which Africa men have been depicted, leads us inevitably towards questions of blame: whose behaviour is seen as threatening to human security and/or social, political and economic stability? In turn, whose behaviour needs to be altered to address that threat?

The politics of blame

As already noted, stigma, discrimination, injustice and other harms have been pervasive throughout of the history of AIDS. Men who have sex with men (MSM), for example, have been blamed from a wide range of standpoints; from religious and moral discourses portraying HIV/AIDS as a consequence of 'unnatural' behaviours, to scientific discourses that rest on many of the same assumptions of promiscuity as Watney and Stillwaggon identified around 'African' sexuality. Women have suffered at the hands of the AIDS discourse too, on the one hand being blamed for the spread of the virus (as in the case of sex workers), on the other framed as disempowered victims unable to negotiate safer sex or to protect themselves from domestic violence. The point here is not to suggest that these things are never true: rather that they simplify a far more complex set of realities and lived experiences.

Over time, and through the sustained efforts of advocates, such narratives have been subject to critique, and a greater awareness has developed of the need to counteract them in policy discourse and approach. Simplistic interventions that focus narrowly on changing individuals' behaviours (an approach that seems to be very closely aligned with implicit apportionments of blame for infection) have been widely problematized by scholars, and this has begun to seep into the policy discourse. It is now widely appreciated, for example, that women are disproportionately affected by the HIV epidemic as a result not only of individual risk factors but also socio-economic conditions and cultural norms (Mane & Aggleton, 2001). It remains true that many policies directed at women have continued to have a behavioural bent – for example, interventions designed to empower women to negotiate safer sex, which approach structural issues through changing individual behaviours. But there has nevertheless been a growing policy rhetoric on the need to grapple with structural challenges, reflected in good practice guidelines from all of the major global AIDS institutions, even if national-level policymaking has in practice often lagged behind. The same is true of MSM, where the need to actively work to address structural violence such as discrimination is present in all international AIDS guidelines – even if these men continue to face huge challenges in achieving equality in many (indeed most) countries around the world.

The ways in which MSW are subjects of blame in the AIDS discourse (and the ways in which they are viewed as targets of policy) have been far more rarely examined. Mane and Aggleton make a convincing case for why this is regrettable, arguing for a need 'to focus on men if the course of the epidemic is to be influenced', but noting that instead 'the general approach is still one that sees men as adversaries and posing obstacles to women's advancement' (Mane & Aggleton, 2001: 27). Such approaches, they go on to argue,

> fail to acknowledge that gender, class, race, sexuality and age (among other factors) oppress men as well as women (albeit not with the same or necessarily equal consequences), and that it is the interaction between *different* systems of oppression that causes the most serious forms of disadvantage.
>
> (Mane & Aggleton, 2001: 28)

In the remainder of this chapter I examine four policy strategies produced by the most significant global AIDS institutions to see whether there is evidence of three tendencies that have been critiqued in the broader AIDS discourse: first, that MSW are viewed as a source of 'the AIDS problem' in sub-Saharan Africa but written out as part of the 'solution' to those problems; second, that underpinning such an understanding are (perhaps unstated) assumptions about 'African sexuality'; and thirdly, that the policy responses to this threat focus on changing individual problematic male behaviours rather than engaging with the structural issues that affect not only women, but also men (albeit in different ways and to different extents).

The place of MSW in four global AIDS strategies

In this section and the next I examine four strategy documents produced in the same time period by what are generally seen as being four of the foremost global AIDS institutions: UNAIDS, PEPFAR, WHO and the Global Fund. These four documents have been selected because they represent high-profile examples of the contemporary 'global AIDS discourse', each of which seeks to set out a comprehensive approach to addressing the AIDS pandemic, including the gender aspects of epidemics around the world. The documents examined here are,

- UNAIDS' *2011–2015 Strategy: Getting to Zero* (UNAIDS, 2010)
- PEPFAR's *PEPFAR Blueprint – Creating an AIDS Free Generation* (U.S. Department of State, 2012)
- WHO's *Global Health Sector Strategy on HIV/AIDS, 2011–2015* (WHO, 2011)
- The Global Fund's *Gender Equality Strategy Action Plan 2014–16* (Global Fund 2014).[2]

To begin quantitatively, the first striking commonality between the four documents is that men and boys appear much less frequently than women and girls. For the

Table 9.1 Word frequencies in the four documents

	UNAIDS	PEPFAR	WHO	Global Fund
Women	74	77	28	45
Men	64	34	22	3
Girls	27	40	7	17
Boys	1	2	2	1

Table 9.2 Word frequencies in the four documents, excluding specific references to MSM

	UNAIDS	PEPFAR	WHO	Global Fund
Women	74	77	28	45
Men (excl. MSM)	8	23	4	1
Girls	27	40	7	17
Boys	1	2	2	1

purposes of comparison, Table 9.1 provides the word frequencies of four gender terms – women, men, girls, and boys – in the four documents.

On these counts it is clear that in each case men appear less frequently than women, and boys less frequently than girls, in the four documents. However, when those word frequencies are examined in greater detail and the references specifically to MSM are removed, the differences become far more stark (see Table 9.2).

Whilst these figures are not claimed to accurately reflect the relative degree of policy attention, nor the allocation of funding, between females and males, they do provide an insight into the limited extent to which MSW are discussed in the four documents examined here. The visibility of such men is extremely low – in some cases they are almost entirely invisible – despite their clear centrality to both the AIDS problem and to AIDS solutions. Indeed the UNAIDS report recognizes this, specifically pointing to the need to engage both men and women in AIDS programmes:

> Heterosexual exposure is the primary mode of transmission in sub-Saharan Africa. As epidemics have matured, the number of people in 'low-risk' partnerships who are newly infected is often high. Nevertheless, programmes rarely focus on adults, married couples or people in long-term relationships or provide prevention services for serodiscordant couples.
>
> (UNAIDS, 2010: 32)

The Global Fund's Gender Equality strategy also establishes as one of its objectives the need to

> Develop a robust communications and advocacy strategy that promotes the Gender equality strategy and encourages programming for women and girls and men and boys.
>
> (Global Fund, 2014: 12)

Far more revealing than mere word frequencies in terms of the three critiques I examine in this chapter is analysis of what *is* said about MSW, and the contexts in which they *do* appear in the four reports. In the remainder of this section I show the contexts in which MSW are represented as part of 'the problem' in the reports, and the ways in which solutions are shown as involving MSW. In the next section I return to discuss these findings in the light of the three critiques outlined above. It is important to again stress that the purpose of the analysis is not to deny the truth of any of these issues, nor to claim that they should not be addressed, but rather to illustrate the limited range of different ways in which MSW are represented within these organizational strategies.

First, men are commonly depicted in the strategies as behaving in ways that both reinforce problematic gender norms and undermine the ability of women and girls to protect themselves. In some cases the risk they pose may be unwitting:

> because males are less likely to access medical services, men living with HIV are less likely to know their status and be on antiretroviral treatment, putting themselves and the women and girls they expose to *their disease* at greater risk.
>
> (U.S. Department of State, 2012: 33. Emphasis added)

In others, meanwhile, assumed male conformity with established gender norms means that

> Too often, the mutual responsibilities of both men and women in reducing the risks of HIV transmission cannot be realized, in part because women are excluded from sexual decision-making, have not had access to comprehensive sexuality education and have unequal access to prevention methods.
>
> (UNAIDS, 2010: 16)

The solution to such problems are seen as lying in a range of interventions that seek to change problematic male behaviours (as well as those of their female counterparts), challenge their presumed conformity with regressive gender norms, and promote the empowerment and protection of women and girls. In the case of PEPFAR, for example:

> PEPFAR programmes are focused on supporting countries to implement evidence-based, multisectoral activities that improve the health and well-being of women and girls and promote gender equality through:
>
> 1. Increasing gender equity in HIV/AIDS programmes and services, including access to reproductive health services.
> 2. Reducing violence and coercion.
> 3. Engaging men and boys to address norms and behaviors.
> 4. Increasing women and girls' legal protection.

5.   Increasing women and girls' access to income and productive resources, including education.

(U.S. Department of State, 2012: 31)

The importance of engaging men in behavioural change is echoed in the UNAIDS strategy, which notes that

> Recent research and experience in programme implementation emphasizes the importance of actively engaging men in addressing negative male behaviour and changing harmful gender norms such as early marriage, male domination of decision-making, intergenerational sex and widow inheritance. Scaling up effective gender-sensitive and gender-transformative interventions that engage men is needed just as much as efforts to ensure that women have roles in decision- making from the household level to the parliament.

(UNAIDS, 2010: 44)

Second, MSW are frequently identified within the four strategies as perpetrators of gender-based violence (GBV), which is closely associated with an increased risk of male-to-female HIV transmission and with barriers to women accessing prevention and treatment (Dunkle & Decker, 2013; Jewkes *et al.*, 2010). The Global Fund strategy points to the prevention of GBV as one of three areas part of 'a renewed focus on women and girls' (Global Fund, 2014: 6). WHO (2011: 15) identifies the need to address 'structural barriers to service access, such as stigmatization, discrimination and intimate partner violence', and also points to a positive role for national HIV responses which 'can significantly reduce gender-based vulnerability to HIV infection in their communities (such as intimate partner violence) and gender-based inequities in access to health services' (WHO, 2011: 27). The PEPFAR strategy features GBV similarly prominently, making the case for the 'importance of putting GBV at the centre of an effective HIV response' (U.S. Department of State, 2012: 34) and highlighting the particular vulnerabilities of 'adolescent girls and young women who often cannot negotiate condom use and experience high levels of GBV and are therefore at increased risk of acquiring HIV' (U.S. Department of State, 2012: 39). 'Zero tolerance for gender based violence' is identified as one of UNAIDS's 'Goals for 2015' (UNAIDS, 2010: 42).

Third, MSW appear in the strategies (at least implicitly, if not always explicitly identified) as clients of sex workers – a 'key population at higher risk'. In most cases, sex workers appear as part of a 'roll call' of key populations to be addressed alongside MSM, transgender people, drug users and (sometimes) prisoners. The only strategy that explicitly addresses the *clients* of sex workers (many, although not all, of whom will be MSW) is the UNAIDS strategy which highlights the fact that

> Prevention programming also remains unacceptably low for people at higher risk of infection, such as people who inject drugs, men who have sex with men,

transgender people and female, male and transgender sex workers and their clients.

(UNAIDS, 2010: 33)

It is primarily in these three ways that MSW are represented in the four strategies examined here. They are important parts of 'the AIDS problem', through: i) their conformity with problematic gender norms; ii) their perpetration of GBV; and iii) their use of sex workers. The only other places in which we may occasionally glimpse their presence are as part of more general groups – as youth/young people, as drug users, or as prisoners.

Notwithstanding the statements above about the need to engage men in challenging gender norms, in terms of interventions targeted at MSW the four strategies examined here reveal a strong concentration on medical and behavioural, as opposed to structural, interventions (which, as noted above, has also often been the case with interventions targeted at females). The most frequently discussed is encouraging voluntary male circumcision – a policy response that was gaining significant traction during the period that these reports were being written, primarily as a consequence of new scientific evidence on its effectiveness as a method of HIV prevention (Doyle *et al.*, 2010). UNAIDS (2010: 35) calls scaling up voluntary male circumcision 'critical to reshaping the response'; it is identified as a key 'Action Step' in the PEPFAR blueprint (U.S. Department of State, 2012: 21–3); and the WHO (2011: 11) designates it a 'Recommended Country Action'. As the PEPFAR blueprint notes, such programmes are expected to significantly reduce the risk of infection for both men and women:

> Mathematical modeling studies suggest that if eight of 10 adult men become circumcised, approximately 3.5 million new HIV infections may be prevented within 15 years, averting as much as $16.5 billion in HIV care and treatment costs. Almost half of these are among women, because women's probabilities of encountering HIV-infected sex partners decrease as HIV-prevalence in men decreases due to circumcision.

(U.S. Department of State, 2012: 21)

Elsewhere, UNAIDS recognizes the need for 'men and women [to] have access to and choose to use condoms' (UNAIDS, 2010: 32), one of the foremost HIV prevention strategies since the earliest days of the epidemic.

There is one place in which structural issues impacting on men (rather than on women via men) are mentioned. The PEPFAR strategy promises to

> a) Support countries in identifying the social, legal, economic and cultural barriers that prevent women and girls, as well as men and boys, from accessing essential health services, and tailor HIV prevention, treatment and care programmes to address these barriers and meet their needs.

(U.S. Department of State, 2012: 34)

Assessing the place of MSW within the strategies

To return to the three critiques set out above, the evidence of the four global strategies examined here provides some support to the idea that MSW are identified as a source of the 'AIDS problem' (although not, in these documents at least, in a way that explicitly draws on security language). This does not, however (at least explicitly), seem to rest upon assumptions about African sexuality, although there are certainly claims made about the negative impact of cultural gender norms. With some limited exceptions it does seem to be the case that the proposed interventions targeted at MSW do focus primarily on behavioural and medical interventions rather than on addressing structural issues.

On the first critique, it is immediately notable that MSW appear most prominently in the strategies as perpetrators of GBV, clients of sex workers, and conformers to (and reproducers of) unequal gender norms. Some MSW are, of course, all of these things. Furthermore, these do represent genuine challenges for HIV prevention, and in each case are supported by significant bodies of empirical evidence. Yet such depictions at the very least represent a simplistic portrayal of MSW's role – in the same way as critics of the international AIDS discourse have long pointed to simplistic portrayals of women as mothers or whores (Booth, 1998; Sacks, 1996), repositories of infection for either their babies or their clients, or to disempowering narratives of women as victims (Rao Gupta, 2000). The point, then, is not that the AIDS discourse is any 'kinder' to women than to men, but that it is problematic in its relationship to both.

Here we find echoes of longstanding discussion in the masculinity studies literature (or, some authors prefer, 'critical studies on men'), in particular work on hegemonic masculinities that has identified the generally negative assumptions about male characteristics (such as aggressiveness, competitiveness, a tendency to take risks and emotional illiteracy) and how these behaviours have come to be taken as explanations for the statistical fact that men commit more (and more violent) crimes (Collier 1998). As Connell and Messerschmidt (2005: 838) have argued, such hegemonic masculinities can be constructed despite the fact that they 'do not correspond closely to the lives of any actual men' – and certainly not all actual men. Also important in the masculinity literature, however, have been the discussions of the relationship between individual 'masculine' behaviours and broader social structures – including the ways in which male identities articulate with other sectionalities. In terms of health, there has been a call for focusing research on the diverse ways in which masculinity and health interrelate and relating this diversity "to the broader social and economic milieu" (Lohan 2007: 498). In the strategies examined here there is little recognition in the strategies that structural issues also impact negatively upon men, nor that the identities and behaviours of men can be impacted by a range of other sectionalities: of race, social class, nationality and so on. In other words, the different effects that structural issues can have on different men become obscured. Nor is there any significant discussion in the strategies examined here of the positive roles that some men play. In relation to caregiving, for example, the UNAIDS strategy (2010: 40) notes that

'The bulk of care and support is provided by families – specifically women'. This may be true in the majority of families, but it is certainly not true of all men in all places – not to mention the roles played by male doctors, nurses and other professional caregivers.

As Peacock *et al.* argue, such homogenizing depictions can have their own negative consequences as

> Messages that only target men as holders of power and privilege miss the many men who do not to identify as such and who may in fact be committed to challenging rigid gender roles that negatively impact men and women. Simplistic portrayal of men as 'advantaged' may not resonate those who are disadvantaged by intersecting forms of discrimination (race, ethnicity, nationality, class, sexuality, disability, and so on), and excessive stereotyping about men as violent oppressors may only reinforce regressive norms.
>
> (Peacock *et al.*, 2009)

The impact of structural violence on HIV risk-facing women is beginning to be recognized, although even in that case policy responses continue to be ineffective. Emma-Louise Anderson, for example, points to the claims of development actors to be pursuing the 'empowerment' of women without effectively grappling with the deeper-rooted issues of inequality and structural violence (Anderson, 2015: Chapter 5). That being true for women does not mean that it cannot also be true for (at least some) men. Just as it has been argued Western AIDS policies have positioned 'Western professionals as superior to some homogenous "Third World Woman"' (Booth, 1998: 118), so it can be the case that global AIDS strategies fail to get beyond a homogenous 'Third World Man' (with the notable, and welcome, exception of its focus on the particular issues facing MSM in many countries of the Global South).

It would be unfair, however, to go so far as to say that there is evidence in the strategies examined here to support the second critique, of explicitly racialized depictions of 'African sexuality'. There is not – a fact that illustrates both the progress that has been made in understanding HIV epidemics and the dominance of a liberal Western orthodoxy in these documents (and, more generally, in the statements of these organizations) that conforms to notions of non-discrimination and the centrality of human rights to the global AIDS response. What we do find, however, is an absence of discussion of the structural issues facing MSW (at least those MSW who do not fall into the category of a 'key population' such as drug users, prisoners, or sex workers).

This leads to the third critique: that interventions targeting MSW are likely to be behavioural and/or medical in character rather than structural in the sense of promoting health through 'altering the structural context within which health is produced and reproduced' (Blankenship *et al.*, 2006). As is already noted above, that is overwhelmingly borne out in these four strategies. Voluntary male circumcision is highlighted – an individualized medical intervention that, whilst it may indeed reduce the risk of HIV transmission, does not engage with the broader social context in which those men's identities are constructed and their behaviours shaped. Here, and even more clearly in the depictions of men as perpetrators of GBV, clients of sex workers, and conformers to unequal gender norms, we get a clear (if implicit) depiction of what Mane and Aggleton call 'The "Problem" of Men', but also of their claim that the 'inability to differentiate between the individual and the social misses the very core of how gender is constructed and influences vulnerability in the context of prevalent gender constructions' (Mane & Aggleton, 2001: 28) – something that is true of both men and women. As Mane and Aggleton go on to argue,

> Analyses that condemn men also paint an abstract and, simultaneously, an individualizing picture of men. Such a picture is abstract in the sense that 'men' are all too frequently constructed as a monolithic whole that requires to be changed. It is individualizing in that it is largely individual men who are to be blamed for their actions, and for contributing to women's disadvantage, rather than larger social structures. Within such a scenario, differences between men – for example between caring and abusive husbands, between listening and controlling fathers, and between elders and younger men – simply disappear. The existence of dominant and subordinate masculinities, or of alternative and even oppositional ways of being a man, remains unacknowledged. Masculinity comes across in such analysis as much the same (broadly speaking), and as needing to be changed.
>
> (Mane & Aggleton, 2001: 28–9)

The strategies examined here pay little or no attention to the historical and cultural embeddedness of hegemonic masculinities, which are evident at both local and global levels and which affect everything from individual behavioural choices to the likelihood of particular policies being adopted (or not). Changing such deeply rooted social norms is notoriously difficult – especially when, as in this case, those who tend to hold the preponderance of power (again, both locally and globally) are those who tend to benefit most from them. However, a recognition that not all men benefit from structural gender inequalities in the same ways or to the same extent seems to be a prerequisite for building momentum for change. For this reason if for no other, simplistic homogenizing discourses should be seen as deeply problematic.

Conclusion

It would be absurd to even attempt to argue that heterosexual men are in some way an oppressed minority. But it would be naïve to assume that those men are a homogenous whole, that they exercise uninhibited agency, or that they are immune to the impacts of structural violence of various forms. MSW can be victims of (health) insecurity as well as posing a threat to the health security of their sexual partners. Men are not all the same, and it has been argued here that in failing to explicitly recognize this, the effectiveness of the strategies examined here is likely to be undermined – failing to protect the health of both men and women, and failing to provide a nuanced critique of the interlocking structural inequalities that pose risks to both women and men. The challenge that is raised by such a critique lies in specifying what a 'better' policy approach would look like, and how a more nuanced approach could simultaneously engage both with the very real problems caused by men (and in many cases inflicted on women) but also the potential of (at least some) men to be positive agents of change. Such an approach would, undoubtedly, bring some risks of its own.

In the broadest sense, there would be a danger in jettisoning the clear and specific focus on 'key populations' that permeates all four of the strategies examined here. These populations have come to be understood as 'key' for valid epidemiological and historical reasons. They do face disproportionate risk of infection. They are frequently subjected to stigma and discrimination – and to legal structures that make it more difficult for them to access prevention, treatment and care services. Losing the clarity of the 'key populations' communication strategy could raise the problem of a message targeted at everyone in practice reaching no one.[3] It would also be a retrograde step if the focus that has been put on the risks faced by women were undermined. However inadequate current policy responses may be in addressing the structural roots of those risks, major progress has been made in including and 'mainstreaming' considerations of gender (at least as it relates to women) in HIV/AIDS policies. Indeed, the shift from 'blaming women' in the early days of the epidemic to 'blaming men' in the contemporary era represents progress of a sort in the light of globally pervasive gender inequalities. Yet blaming men risks disengaging men, and missing out on opportunities to involve them in positive response efforts.

A range of approaches to achieving this have been proposed in the literature, some of which are specific interventions (for example, addressing gender norms through educational programmes for boys and helping men to play a greater roles in caring for the sick and for orphans (Mane & Aggleton, 2001: 30)), whilst others – of direct relevance to the discussion in this chapter – point to the power of discourse, in particular the need to avoid simplistic stereotypes that homogenize male behaviours and to recognize men as holders of rights (which they are not always able to realize) and not just of responsibilities (Peacock *et al.*, 2009). The instrumental ways in which men tend to be included in HIV interventions have been seen as problematic, engaging men only for the protection of women's health, not for the benefit of both men *and* women.

Such initiatives are not entirely absent in the global AIDS response – and there have been good examples of interventions designed to address the structural issues MSW face, for example to involve them in efforts aimed at gender transformation. Peacock *et al.* (2009) highlight the existence of programmes that have sought to engage men in changing gender attitudes and in behaviours, and in playing roles in improving women's health as well as men's. Outside Africa, Bowleg and Raj (2012) have examined a range of approaches to engaging black heterosexual men in HIV prevention the US. The UN's Division for the Advancement of Women has also recognized the important roles that men and boys have to play in advancing gender equality, and documented successful policy initiatives in this regard (United Nations, 2008).

Whether or not we align ourselves with the view that HIV/AIDS represents a threat to the stability of countries in sub-Saharan Africa or elsewhere, it clearly represents a significant threat to the human security of women, men and children around the world. Yet simplistic notions of threat and blame can lead not only to stigma and discrimination, but also to a narrowing of the types of interventions that come to be seen as valid, and in particular an occlusion of the structural factors that shape individual identities and condition individual behaviours. This can be threatening to the human security of all people, regardless of their gender.

Acknowledgements

I am grateful to the participants in the workshop on 'Global Health, International Relations & Gender: How to Govern Global Challenges' held at the University of Heidelberg in September 2014, and also to Jeremy Youde, Pieter Fourie and Colleen O'Manique for helpful comments on earlier versions of this chapter.

Notes

1 In this chapter I use the terminology 'sectionalities' rather than 'identities' in order to highlight the ways in which particular identities (e.g. that of a heterosexual man) interact with other identities (for example, of social class, religion or race). For a useful recent discussion of intersectionality research see Collins (2015).
2 I analyse the Global Fund's gender equality strategy because its more general strategy document (Global Fund, 2012) focuses on the Fund's investment strategies and funding models rather than on the types of policies addressed in the other three strategies.
3 This, indeed, was a criticism that was raised of the early AIDS response, e.g. Kolata, (1993).

References

Anderson, E-L. (2015) *Gender, HIV and Risk: Navigating Structural Violence*, Basingstoke: Palgrave Macmillan.
Blankenship, K.M., Friedman, S.R., Dworkin, S. and Mantell, J.E. (2006) 'Structural Interventions: Concepts, Challenges and Opportunities for Research', *Journal of Urban Health*, 83(1): 59–72.
Booth, K.M. (1998) 'National Mother, Global Whore, and Transnational Femocrats: The Politics of AIDS and the Construction of Women at the World Health Organization', *Feminist Studies*, 24(1): 115–139.
Bowleg, L. and Raj, A. (2012) 'Shared Communities, Structural Contexts, and HIV Risk: Prioritizing the HIV Risk and Prevention Needs of Black Heterosexual Men', *American Journal of Public Health*, 102(S2): S173–7.
Collier, R. (1998) *Masculinities, Crime and Criminology: Men, Heterosexuality and the Criminal(ised) Other*. London: Sage.
Collins, P.H. (2015) 'Intersectionality's Definitional Dilemmas', *Annual Review of Sociology*, 41:1–20.

Connell, R.W. and Messerschmidt, J.W. (2005) 'Hegemonic Masculinity: Rethinking the Concept', *Gender & Society*, 19(6): 829–859.

Csete, J. (2004). 'Lessons Not Learned: Human Rights Abuses and HIV/AIDS in the Russian Federation', *Human Rights Watch*, 16(5): 1–62. Available: www.hrw.org/reports/2004/russia0404/russia0404.pdf (accessed 24 June 2016).

Doyle, S.M., Kahn, James G., Hosang, Nap and Carroll, Peter R. (2010) 'The Impact of Male circumcision on HIV Transmission', *Journal of Urology*, 183: 21–26.

Dunkle, K.L. and Decker, M.R. (2013) 'Gender-Based Violence and HIV: Reviewing the Evidence for Links and Causal Pathways in the General Population and High-risk Groups', *American Journal of Reproductive Immunology*, 69(S1): 20–6.

Elbe, S. (2005) 'AIDS, Security, Biopolitics', *International Relations*, 19(4): 403–419.

Farmer, P. (2003) *Pathologies of Power: Health, Human Rights and the New War on the Poor*, Berkeley: University of California Press.

Gallo, R.C. (2006) 'A Reflection on HIV/AIDS Research after 25 Years', *Retrovirology* 3:72. DOI: 10.1186/1742-4690-3-72.

Gensini, G.F, Yacouba, M.H. and Contia, A.A. (2004) 'The Concept of Quarantine in History: From Plague to SARS', *Journal of Infection*, 49(4): 257–261.

Global Fund (Global Fund to Fight AIDS, TB and Malaria) (2012) *The Global Fund Strategy 2012–2016: Investing for Impact*. Geneva: Global Fund.

Global Fund (Global Fund to Fight AIDS, TB and Malaria) (2014) *Gender Equality Strategy Action Plan 2014–16*. Geneva: Global Fund. Available: www.globalfundadvocatesnetwork.org/wp-content/uploads/2014/10/Publication_GenderEqualityStrategy_ActionPlan_en.pdf (accessed 27 July 2016).

Jewkes, R.K., Dunkle, K., Nduna, M. and Shai, N. (2010). 'Intimate Partner Violence, Relationship Power Inequity, and Incidence of HIV Infection in Young Women in South Africa: A Cohort Study', *The Lancet* 376/9734: 41–8.

Johnson, C. (1994) 'Quarantining HIV-infected Haitians: United States' Violation of International Law at Guantanamo Bay', *Howard Law Journal*, 37(2): 305–331.

Kolata, G. (1993) 'Targeting Urged in Attack on AIDS', *New York Times*, 8 March: 1.

Lohan, M. (2007) 'How Might We Understand Men's Health Better? Integrating Explanations from Critical Studies on Men and Inequalities in Health', *Social Science & Medicine*, 65: 493–504.

Mane, P. and Aggleton, P. (2001) 'Gender and HIV/AIDS: What Do Men Have to Do with It?', *Current Sociology*, 49(6): 23–37.

Peacock, D., Stemple, L., Sawires, S. and Coates, T.J. (2009) 'Men, HIV/AIDS, and Human Rights', *Journal of Acquired Immune Deficiency Syndrome*, 51(S3): S119–S125.

Price-Smith, A. (2009) *Contagion and Chaos: Disease, Ecology, and National Security in the Era of Globalization*. Cambridge, MA: MIT Press.

Rao Gupta, G. (2000) 'Gender, Sexuality, and HIV/AIDS: The What, the Why, and the How', Plenary Address, XIIIth International AIDS Conference, Durban, South Africa. Available: www.med.uottawa.ca/sim/data/assets/documents/DurbanSpeech.pdf (accessed 28 June 2016).

Sacks, V. (1996) 'Women and AIDS: An Analysis of Media Misrepresentations', *Social Science Medicine*, 42(1): 59–73.

Sontag, S. (1988) *AIDS and its Metaphors*. London: Penguin.

Stillwaggon, E. (2003) 'Racial Metaphors: Interpreting Sex and AIDS in Africa', *Development and Change*, 34(5): 809–832.

UN Security Council (2000) S/RES/1308.

UNAIDS (2010) *2011–2015 Strategy: Getting to Zero,* Geneva: UNAIDS. Available: www.unaids.org/sites/default/files/sub_landing/files/JC2034_UNAIDS_Strategy_ en.pdf (accessed 27 July 2016).

UNAIDS (2016) *Global AIDS Update 2016.* Available: www.unaids.org/sites/default/files/ media_asset/global-AIDS-update-2016_en.pdf (accessed 23 June 2016).

UNDP (1994) *Human Development Report 1994.* New York: UNDP.

United Nations (2008) *The Role of Men and Boys in Achieving Gender Equality.* New York: UN Division for the Advancement of Women. Available: www.un.org/womenwatch/daw/ public/w2000/W2000%20Men%20and%20Boys%20E%20web.pdf (accessed 30 June 2016).

U.S. Department of State (2012) *PEPFAR Blueprint – Creating an AIDS Free Generation.* Washington DC: Department of State. Available: www.pepfar.gov/documents/organization/ 201386.pdf (accessed 27 July 2016).

Watney, S. (1989) 'Missionary Positions: AIDS, "Africa", and Race', *Critical Quarterly,* 31(3): 45–62.

WHO (2011) *Global Health Sector Strategy on HIV/AIDS, 2011–2015,* Geneva: WHO. Available: http://apps.who.int/iris/bitstream/10665/44606/1/9789241501651_eng.pdf (accessed 27 July 2016).

10 Labouring bodies in the global economy

Structural violence and occupational health

Teresa Healy

Introduction

What defines the terrain of 'security' in global affairs has long been the subject of fierce debate, with different epistemic communities constructing arguments in favour or against the view that the security of the state is the ultimate guarantor of human security (Walker, 1990; Fierke, 2007; Baylis *et al.*, 2014). When it comes to public health issues on a global scale, the premise of this volume is that, in the field of International Relations, health is placed 'between the discourse of state securitization and the discourse of biomedical safety and the need to control the physical body and order of the Other' (Kadetz, 2016: 27). Critical feminism asks us to re-think the gendering of politics within and between states; that kind of gendering that silences the voices of diverse populations in favour of a singular, competitive and national interest. This chapter takes on the challenge by considering the health insecurities of workers whose bodies bear the impact of transnational production processes and privatized social reproduction under conditions of neoliberal, capitalist social relations. Because the research on occupational health and safety is empirically grounded in workers' experiences of particular households, workplaces, economic sectors and national social formations, I ask what can we learn about structural violence from this rich literature on workers' health? By means of a literature review, this chapter presents a framework for understanding similarities and differences, as well as absences and promising avenues for research agenda alive to the embodied, the intersectional, and the diverse impacts of globalized power relations where security is not seen from the perspective of the nation-state, but from that of the embodied worker and (their) collectivities.

Methodology

In this chapter, I work from the understanding based in critical social theory that knowledge is produced within a social context built on discourses of domination and exclusion, making it difficult to bring workers' experiences into the study of international relations. Many of the authors considered here carry similar concerns, and have chosen from among different methods that bring a social constructivist's appreciation for the subjective meanings and views of injured workers themselves

(Cresswell, 2013). Thus, it is my intention to work with the concept of structural violence in a nuanced way throughout this paper. In Johan Galtung's (1975) idea of structural violence, the activities of specific institutions are not of particular interest. Rather, an abstracted understanding of indirect violence explains how individuals' rights to self-realization are left unrealized (Quesada *et al.*, 2011; Badami, 2014). Farmer *et al.* (2006) draw heavily on Galtung (1969) to bring the concept to medical research where they define structural violence as a complex of socially embedded and inequitable economic, political, legal, religious and cultural social practices that cause physical and psychological harm to people (Flynn *et al.*, 2015; Bitton *et al.*, 2011). In other words, structural violence turns large historical and social dynamics into systemic and everyday practices that injure the most marginalized:

> The concept covers structural forms such as the deeply rooted racism and social inequality that have their origins in colonialism, the everyday forms that are evidenced in ongoing power relationships, humiliations, discriminations, recriminations and injustices between people and institutions, and the symbolic forms, which are the embodiment and naturalisation of everyday and structural forms, as the marginalised themselves accept their position in a social hierarchy expressing it as shame, timidity and inferiority and embody this as ill health and illness.
>
> (Gamlin and Hawkes, 2015: 80)

A structural understanding moves ill health out of the frame of individual circumstance, and supports claims to health care as a universal human right (Bourgois and Hart, 2011). It can also help us understand occupational health inequities in light of their provenance in broader social practices and processes (Flynn *et al.*, 2015; Rodriguez *et al.*, 2016).

For this review of previous research, I first turned to the Scholars Portal Journals database of articles covering 19,808 full-text journals. For the first search, my keywords were 'health and safety'. I chose the most recent 460 results covering the period January 2013 to November 2016 and recorded the names of the 178 journals from which these articles came, without downloading or reading the articles. These became the basis for Figure 10.1 below. From the same database, I conducted a second search of the years 2000–2016 using the keyword search terms 'occupational' and 'health and safety' to select and then download 50 of the 628 articles for further study. I chose the most relevant from the most recent articles and stopped arbitrarily after deciding that 50 was an adequate number. Since I had not identified sufficient references to diverse women's experiences, I conducted a third search covering the same years, using the keyword search 'health and safety' and 'gender' and received 11 results. After scrubbing industry articles, and snowballing for 'cited by' and 'related articles', I imported 66 articles into NVivo and coded for 'gender' and 'security'. I then ran a fourth search using the words 'structural violence' and 'health' from 2004 to 2016 and collected 23 articles for review and imported these to NVivo and coded for 'structural violence'. These 89 articles became the basis for this literature review.

The chapter begins with a discussion of the globalized social structure of employment that has resulted in a return to precarious work with specific gendered health implications for workers. The discussion then moves to an analysis of the role of neoliberalism and the welfare state in which I discuss individualization and the intersectional implications for women's health. This is then followed by a presentation of literature in the area of gender and migration in which I focus on hegemonic masculinity and the health inequities faced by workers with new or disputed citizenship status. Finally, I discuss structural violence and contestation and end with a call for engagement by students of world order.

The globalized social structure of employment

For almost 40 years, working people have experienced a series of recessions and ongoing economic restructuring that has fundamentally altered the post-1945 era of Fordist *Pax Americana* (Rupert, 1990). Where workers' organizations once sought inspiration in the social compromise of the post-war period, weakened labour movements have been unable to prevent the impoverishment of whole communities when owners shift production to low-wage and more flexible 'greenfield' sites (Carter *et al.*, 2013). Part of the restructuring of production has been enacted through the extension of globalized supply chains, but it is also characterized by firms' decisions to outsource production to smaller firms creating an even more 'flexible' work force as a core component of their competitiveness strategy (Benach *et al.*, 2014). Unions have had few successes in mitigating the intensification of work in old or new industries, and the influence of employers' interests within the state has meant that public sector unions have been able to keep privatization at bay only with great difficulty and to a limited extent. Otherwise, 'accumulation by dispossession' (Harvey, 2004) and de-regulation in the wider economy prevail.

In this changing context, researchers look beyond specific workplace hazards to the broader social structure of employment to better understand the health risks of precarious work (Clarke *et al.*, 2007). From Benach *et al.* we learn that occupational health research rooted in psychosocial perspectives restricts our understanding of the work environment, but by including employment conditions as a determinant of health, one can bring sociological understandings to the study of work and health (2014). Workers' health and safety is increasingly seen by occupational health and safety researchers to expand beyond the physical and psychosocial aspects of workplaces previously structured by Fordism to the broader dynamics of economic restructuring and the return to instability in employment practices (Premji *et al.*, 2010). These are among the most useful approaches bringing the concerns of occupational psychology and biomedical approaches together with sociological approaches to the study of work organization and ill-health (Carter *et al.*, 2013).

The return to non-standard or 'precarious' work is certainly a sociological phenomenon, but it is also a premise of economic globalization. Apart from the health impacts of outright unemployment, which most certainly does cause significant negative health outcomes for workers, intensely stressful workplaces provoke physiological, psychological and behavioural responses (Landsbergis *et al.*, 2014). Clarke *et al.* offer the metric of 'employment strain' as an indicator of poor health in jobs where workers experience i) uncertainty over the future of their work and working conditions; ii) effort in finding and keeping employment; and iii) lack of support from family, co-workers, a union, or welfare state benefits such as health insurance, rent-control and public child care (Clarke *et al.*, 2007). Similarly, Rodriguez *et al.* consider the combination of i) job demands; ii) job control, and iii) job support, as a measure of 'job strain' associated with physical and mental health problems for workers and work-family conflict for women (2016). Benach *et al.* define precarity as involving 'employment insecurity, individualized bargaining relations between workers and employers, low wages and economic deprivation, limited workplace rights and social protection, and powerlessness to exercise workplace rights' (2014: 230). Vosko (2015) includes i) degree of certainty; ii) regulatory protection; iii) control over the labour process; and iv) income level in her influential work on precarious employment (Daly and Armstrong, 2016). Rather than seeing psychosocial stress as arising in the workplace only, here we see a number of approaches taking broader approaches that consider employment conditions, work organization and the extent of 'precarity' as objective measures of the insecurity facing workers (Landsbergis *et al.*, 2014). These processes are not characteristic of particular economic sectors or workplaces bounded by specific geographic regions, but widely found and are matters for empirical comparative and transnational research. If we are to understand the underpinnings of global power, then it would be fruitful to examine the specific ways in which embodied workers are subjected to production patterns extending beyond workplaces and national borders.

Embodied workers are located within production relations that are themselves constituted by unequal and gendered power relations. Beginning from such an assumption, Carter *et al.* identified the gendered hazards facing women clerical workers in a 'lean' public sector workplace, after management had introduced standardization, labour process efficiencies and individual productivity goals. They found that women clerical workers with low levels of authority faced overwork and job insecurity and were most susceptible to mental fatigue, stress, headaches and musculoskeletal conditions (Carter *et al.*, 2013). Carter *et al.* offer us a way to examine the embodied gendered worker in terms of their 'proximate environment' (workstation), 'ambient environment' (building), and 'social environment' (organization of work) (2013). An international political economy perspective might usefully add 'global environment' (organization of production) to this model so as to locate the individual worker in transnational, gendered processes where flesh and blood are rarely seen.

Neither are they easily heard. One of the difficulties facing workers who experience negative psychosocial effects at work is that it is difficult to present objective measures of their complaint. Unlike an acute injury, psychosocial hazards create conditions that have a delayed onset and are experienced in different ways by different individuals. Studies have found that if a worker perceives job insecurity, it will be as a 'chronic rather than an acute experience' (Benach *et al.*, 2014). Researchers show that both job instability and job insecurity are associated with psychological ill health, but not necessarily with physical ill health, although some studies show an increase of occupational injury (Landsbergis *et al.*, 2014). For example, one study found that male workers in the EU faced mental health problems as a result of high demands and low levels of autonomy at work (Cottini, 2012). As workers are moved into nonstandard arrangements such as contract work, research shows their level of insecurity might be such that they would not object to more hazardous work. If they lack training or access to protective equipment, or if they have no social networks in the workplace that might protect them from hazards, or if the lines of responsibility are confused by the nature of their contract in the 'gig economy', they could be at higher risk of injury or illness (Howard, 2017). After conducting a review of the literature on the rise of non-standard work arrangements, Menendez *et al.* concluded that women's health is negatively affected by new forms of employment more than is the case for men (2007). Together, these results ask us to consider how these deeper effects of economic change may become part of what we think of when we analyse globalisation. It also raises the methodological question of who it is that 'speaks for' workers who face the chronic, ill-effects of global power inequalities and the extent to which international relations scholars will permit workers to articulate their most intimate health insecurities in an effort to *revitalize* and *enliven* not just the study of global power, but the very conditions under which we earn our daily bread.

That daily bread is very likely to have been prepared in a household. The globalized social structure of employment also includes the relationship between workplaces and household labour. In their recent call for a robust research agenda on the health effects of precarity, Benach *et al.* call for a more complex understanding of the intersections of gendered workplaces and women's household responsibilities (2016). In industrialized countries, musculoskeletal and repetitive strain injuries are reported more frequently among women facing gender-segregated work, but also because of the caring work they do in addition to their paid employment (Breslin *et al.*, 2013). Women find different strategies to cope with the competing demands of household labour. Research with elderly women in Sweden revealed the health-promoting strategy which included women seeking solitude or autonomy, in order to find a 'room of one's own' away from household labour. Without it, they reported 'never being left in peace and not getting enough sleep, as well as feelings of insufficiency, worry, guilt and loneliness. Several had sustained injuries from the physically and mentally strenuous work of caring for their families' (Forssén and Carlstedt, 2001: 155). Just as we must look beyond the workplace to the extra-local dynamics of globalized production patterns, so too must we look to the gendered dynamics of the household in order to analyse the multiple sites where workers' health insecurities are constructed.

Part of the difficulty in re-defining security to include the concerns of political economy lies in the engagement of disciplines with very different foundations. From an initial distance, the field of occupational health and safety (OHS) evokes an image of regulatory norms and procedures meant to protect the male, white body, regularly employed in an industrial workplace in a northern climate. These are the concerns of chemicals and toxics; physical injury; slips, trips and falls; occupational diseases and other sources of workplace-related injuries and illness (Safety, 2016). Psychosocial and musculoskeletal concerns are also addressed, but these do not seem to be as well considered. OHS calls to mind structures of governance including joint labour-management health and safety committees governed by collective agreements. Some of this is accurate. Even if he is not unionized, the potentially injured worker works in a sector where unions have worked with or fought with employers and with government agencies to undertake research, create technical standards, and ensure that management bears its responsibility to ensure a safe and healthy workplace in which workers have the right to health and safety education, protective equipment, and to refuse unsafe work (Confederation, 2016). These issues lie far from the traditional concerns of interstate relations but the field of international relations and occupational health and safety do share a similar recourse to an ideal hegemonic masculinity characterized as autonomous, able-bodied and rational. This shared androcentric preoccupation must be overcome.

A beginning point is to recognize that work hazards are not restricted to the 'standard' work relationship, resource-extraction or industrial work-sites. Women in non-standard employment relations, working in the service sector are also affected by serious occupational health and safety issues, but there has been a 'gendered blind spot' preventing regulatory frameworks from seeing and understanding the causes of illness and injury in gender-segregated workplaces where women predominate (Carter *et al.*, 2013). Jamieson found that although the state of New South Wales in Australia enacted gender-neutral health and safety legislation, the health and safety authority only brought the winnable cases of traumatic injuries to court. These had occurred overwhelmingly in construction and manufacturing which meant that the government did not prosecute cases of disease or injury with delayed onset. As a result, women's injuries and illness were ignored (Jamieson, 2005). Feminist research has shown that in dismissing psychosocial and musculoskeletal hazards, women's injuries are less visible than the traditional concerns of occupational health and safety practitioners (Messing, 1998; Carter *et al.*, 2013).

An intersectional approach, however, requires that we dig even more deeply to interrogate the concept of 'women' to ask about the social hierarchies that racialized women experience in addition to that of class. One study found epidemic levels of depression among African American women working in a poultry processing plant in the southern United States. Not only did they experience low wages, but ongoing racism as well. These were women facing low levels of support at work, workplace hazards, job insecurity and fast-paced and repetitive assembly work (Lipscomb *et al.*, 2007). As Thurston and Vissandjée. describe it, 'gender interacts with other Symbolic Institutions—in particular race, class and sexuality—to form hierarchies of inclusion and exclusion, is never seen alone and is essential to understanding the organization of society' (2005: 235). Consider the scenario presented by Thurston *et al.*: a woman fleeing war and racial conflict, who is defined in her country of refuge according to her ethnicity and first language, who then encounters a health care provider from the very group with whom she is at war (2013). What health insecurity is she now presented with? Racialized women workers carry deeply intersecting identities that do not conform to the prevailing hegemonic masculinity neither in the field of occupational health and safety, nor international political economy.

Under conditions of post-Fordist restructuring, workers bear the costs of processes arising beyond the boundaries of their particular workplaces. Work-related injuries and ill-health occur because of social and global processes that are fundamental to the global economy. Gender is a central element, interwoven with neo-colonial hierarchies. The structural violence experienced by injured workers is constituted in unequal gender relations lying behind white, able-bodied, masculine ideals. The reason we know this ideal is hegemonic, is because everything else is considered to be 'non-standard'. This is the challenge of transdisciplinary work in which researchers must examine the accepted boundaries of their field. Without giving voice to workers, then these deeper processes remain obscured.

Neoliberalism and the welfare state

Coming to terms with the role of gendered bodies in the global economy means thinking about diverse workers engaged in social reproduction, as well as produc-tion, which leads to a consideration of the role of the state as well as the organization of work in the public sector. The non-profit sector, as part of the broader public sector, relies upon high-stress social environment, the unpaid labour of women and low-wages to keep agencies running in times of austerity and cutbacks to public funding (Charlesworth and Baines, 2015). In their cross-national study, Charlesworth and Baines found that gendered assumptions governed work practices and shaped expectations by management and workers themselves that women would engage in remarkable levels of self-sacrifice (2015). Following on Baines (2006), Choiniere *et al.* argue that just as there are gendered assumptions in the provision of health care services portraying 'women's caring labor as endlessly elastic, natural, reliable and altruistic' so too do these managerial practices extend the competitive efficiencies of the market economy into public sector workplaces, and offer nurses little support in confronting the racist behaviours of patients, families or co-workers. This further embeds the social practices of institutional racism in the neoliberal workplace (Choiniere *et al.*, 2014: 40). According to the researchers, structural violence:

> further situates those on the frontlines of care in a persistently precarious position in which the health and safety, of both nurses and patients may be compromised, undermined or ignored and where new hazards and risks may be introduced.
>
> (Choiniere *et al.*, 2014: 46)

In line with managerial strategies that individualize workers' responsibilities to protect their own health and safety, Choiniere *et al.* see nurses' experiences of workplace assault within the broader dynamics of neoliberalism, gender and racialization. Mental health nurses who experience violence at work are enmeshed within power structures that put them at risk (Choiniere *et al.*, 2014)

The post-Fordist return to such high levels of workplace insecurity did not happen automatically. Over the past four decades, powerful governments and international economic institutions have actively sought to increase workers' insecurity by reducing the protections offered by the welfare state and weakening the regulations governing collective bargaining (Benach *et al.*, 2014). What this meant was that governments in the north and in the south imposed structural adjustment on their populations in ways that significantly undermined twentieth-century reform liberal and social democratic laws and regulations providing workers in the 'standard' employer-employee relationship with basic protections. The United States welfare state was never as inclusive as was European standards of social provision but still, a significant institutional framework provided for (i) old-age assistance and disability benefits; (ii) collective bargaining rights; (iii) minimum wage, overtime, and child labour protections; (iv) employment discrimination protections; (v) safety and health protections; (vi) pension, health, and other employee benefits; and (vii) unemployment insurance and workers compensation benefits (Howard, 2017). In contrast to this role for the state, it is one of the central tenets of neoliberalism that individual freedoms are guaranteed by free markets and state protection of private property rights (Harvey, 2005). This assumption takes shape in policies:

> . . . such as privatization and deregulation, capital mobility and free trade, anti-inflation rather than full employment, and a limited and fiscally constrained state. Applied to social policy, it is defined by measures such as promotion of individual responsibility, including user-pay mechanisms, private delivery of services, attachment of strict conditions and obligations to receipt of benefits (e.g., workfare), and tougher qualification requirements and lower benefit levels for recipients of social programs.
>
> (McBride *et al.*, 2015: 6)

The level of social protection has declined significantly in the neoliberal era and inequality has increased exponentially (Milanovic, 2016).

After the economic crisis of 2008, the governments of the most hard-hit economies chose to face their fiscal dilemmas by choosing austerity over redistributive tax policies. This transnational alignment of government policies led to either unemployment or a rapid decrease in the quality of jobs for millions of workers. The most marginalized in the economy, including migrant workers, have been thrown into very precarious circumstances indeed (Benach *et al.*, 2014). Benach *et al.*'s extensive review of the literature concluded that the character of the welfare regime has a bearing on employment-related health. Precarious workers in Scandinavian welfare states reported better or equal health outcomes in comparison with their permanent counterparts. This was not the case for precarious workers in other welfare regimes who reported adverse health outcomes (Benach *et al.*, 2014).

Workers engaged in project-based work fare much better in societies with a social security net (Ekstedt, 1999).

When applied to social policy, neoliberal discourse moves away from the guarantee of individual freedoms and towards the assumption of individual responsibilities. There is an unmistakable class division constructed in the process. While individual freedoms may be guaranteed to property owners within neoliberal capitalism, individual responsibility falls on the shoulders of those who work for wages. If they cannot bring themselves safely home at the end of the day, then their responsibility for their own health care causes them to navigate alone the neoliberal health care maze of public or private economies, or the workers' compensation health system which also runs according to neoliberal principles. This process of individualization extends to workers who are made to shoulder the risk of becoming injured at work or worse. It is a double bind for workers inside and outside of the formal health care system who must care for patients under conditions of precarious working conditions and ongoing austerity (Daly and Armstrong, 2016). What appears at the outset as an instance of unequal, class-based power relations is carried in the gendered and racialized bodies of workers' experiences. One study looked to the social practices causing indigenous women to experience shame and exclusion from health services. Once recognized as structural violence, these barriers must be met with policy responses that:

> shift the focus away from the level of the individual (e.g., individual risk behaviours or lack of health care seeking) and towards the political, legal and social context in which behaviours occur . . . and would take into account the educational, linguistic and cultural barriers that hinder equitable health care access.
>
> (Gamlin and Hawkes, 2015: 87)

For Gamlin and Hawkes, a structural policy response is 'inter-sectoral' in its linking of health outcomes to better education and welfare-state reforms. Thus, while neoliberal policy frameworks give priority to individualized solutions to health inequalities, structural approaches embed individual experiences in longer-term social processes (2015).

When we turn our attention to social reproduction, we see that governments have increasingly introduced market-dynamics into the public sector. As a result of work intensification and individualised responsibilities, workers increasingly assume the burden of austerity budgets and the secular decline in social spending. This burden is manifested in physical and psychological injuries. If they are not organized into unions, workers will face racialization and gender discrimination alone.

Gender and migration

Globalized production processes become rooted in society by shifting material power upwards and away from the local contexts. This market dynamic is not a narrowly defined economic process, but one that has been built upon various

gendered arrangements that become hegemonic in different national social formations. We can identify hegemonic masculinities that subordinate other devalued
masculinities and all femininities (Connell and Messerschmidt, 2005) to neo-
colonial forms of social reproduction. Hegemonic masculinity takes shape in the
economic dynamics of sex work established alongside trade routes, underpins
the migration of female nurses across borders, and conditions the development of
northern markets for domestic workers that the International Labour Organization
(2003) has identified as exposing women to the 'double hazards of precarious work
and the insecurities of migration' (Menendez *et al.*, 2007: 777). Hegemonic masculinity in the service sector extends into the transnational hotel industry where room
attendants' sense of security and well-being depends upon their individual abilities
to safely manage their interactions with male guests. As Kensbock *et al.* argue,
'(b)y rationalizing sexual harassment as normal for men, room attendants internalize the view that these interactions are part of the broader sociocultural behaviour,
thus sustaining a hegemonic gendered culture rather than an urgently needed change
to their workplace culture' (2015: 46). Without a strong union, the most vulnerable
workers are exposed to workplace hazards (Landsbergis *et al.* 2014). According to
Scott-Samuel *et al.*:

> The linkages between hegemonic masculinity and structural violence are
> clear. Both refer to institutionalised forms of social, cultural and political domi-
> nance which work to systematically oppress those groups who find themselves
> powerless in the face of patriarchal and economic domination.
>
> (2009: 291)

Not only women, but immigrant men find themselves having to navigate the
dangers of a new environment where they are subject to the hegemonic masculinity of that social space. Gendered assumptions are often challenged in the new
environment and men might be required to change their ways of expressing their
masculinity, or they might hold fast to their pre-migratory expectations (Thurston
et al., 2013; O'Daniel, 2008). For example, as honourable men, undocumented
Latino day-labourers meet their family responsibilities by working in the United
States but their gendered identities are under constant assault within a context that
demands both strength and docility (Walter *et al.*, 2004). When workers are injured
on the job, leaving them unable to support their family at home, their identity is
profoundly threatened.

Along with production patterns that move across borders, so do the producers
themselves. There are 12 million undocumented immigrants in the United States
who find themselves disproportionately subject to dangerous working conditions resulting in higher rates of injury and death than native-born workers. Flynn
et al. (2015) propose that undocumented status may be seen as one of the social
determinants of health, in particular of occupational health.

Undocumented workers work in agriculture, construction, services and manufacturing doing dangerous and low-paid work that result in disproportionately high
levels of accidents and fatalities each year (Smith, 2012). As Mora *et al.* found for

example, the undocumented status of Latino workers in the chicken processing industry in the southern United States robs them of labour law protections. Unprotected, workers must contend with physical hazards in jobs considered by the wider society to be 3-D 'dirty, dangerous, and demanding' (2016). Even when jobs offer workers a certain amount of stability, set hours, relatively good wages and benefits, structural violence can still prevent workers from having access to training, job advancement or the mobility they need to find less dangerous work (Mora *et al.*, 2016).

Some cultural explanations suggest that migrant workers are disadvantaged because of poor language and communications skills in the host-country environment (Wasilkiewicz *et al.*, 2016), but the idea that migrant workers' vulnerability to accidents is somehow related to their cultures of origin and the safety values of that nation was debunked by a European study in which it was found that language barriers, lack of health and safety training, the pressure to be compliant given the limited time they have to make money, and whether or not they had official status were the reasons migrant workers experienced high rates of injury due to accidents (Guldenmund *et al.*, 2013). Instead of reproducing assumptions about marginalization that focusses on the presumed deficits of individuals, Thurston and Vissandjée call for further research into the intersection of gender and migration in health promotion (2005). Lacking alternative ways to meet their families' needs, undocumented workers are further marginalized by governments' failure to enforce regulations, as well as their lack of interest in new regulations that would establish ergonomic standards protecting the long-term health of workers in poultry processing (Arcury *et al.*, 2014). The psychological costs that come from having an undocumented status arise from fear of deportation, economic insecurity and limited mobility, but they also include the difficulty of working in a hostile environment, or prolonged separation from one's family (Flynn *et al.*, 2015). For Flynn *et al.*, it is essential to bring a structural analysis of occupational health and safety inequities in order to explore 'the additional, often pervasive structural barriers associated with immigration status, poverty, race, and gender and how they may be overcome or at least mitigated' (2015: 1135). A structural approach can identify the various inequalities presenting barriers to positive health outcomes.

Just as the broader context of employment relations should be considered when thinking about work-related health inequities, so too should we understand immigrant workers' health not by seeing only the individual worker, but in perceiving the person who is also affected by the stress of finding employment, setting up a home, losing social status and a support system and experiencing loneliness and social isolation, often in the context of significant language barriers (Thurston *et al.*, 2013). As Thurston *et al.* have found, lack of credential recognition and work experience; poverty, prejudice and discrimination; barriers to health care services; cultural shock, and ongoing uncertainty must be seen alongside the impact of working in hazardous workplaces (2013). That said, it is still the case that in Canada, immigrant men are at twice the risk of being injured at work in their first five years in the country, than their Canadian-born counterparts (Breslin *et al.*, 2013).

Immigrants face unfavourable working conditions and a higher incidence of injury, disease or work-related health problems than the Czech population (Brabcová *et al.*, 2014). In Canada, Chinese women were more likely than white women to have a low household income, to face discrimination, to not be a union member and to believe that making a worker's compensation claim would negatively affect their employment (Premji and Lewchuk, 2014). Although Chinese workers were more highly educated than whites, this afforded them no protection from health and safety risks. Premji and Lewchuk conclude that the prevalence of discrimination faced by Chinese workers may explain their disproportionate exposure to other hazards (2014). Researchers also found that in Canada, immigrants face a high risk of injury due to a combination of factors. They are less likely to be unionized, are under great economic pressure to accept available employment, and if they are without credential recognition, they take on jobs with which they are unfamiliar (Smith and Mustard, 2009).

By taking seriously the physical insecurities borne by workers in their injured bodies, we are presented with expressions of global power which, far from floating above and between the boundaries of the nation state, are experienced with immediacy and intimacy in the very centre of capitalist social relations. Variable structures of hegemonic masculinity subordinate migrant and immigrant workers who face unequal risks of ill-health and injury as they cross-borders seeking work and opportunity, or an escape from intolerable oppression only to find structural violence at their journey's end. Yet workers also analyse and organize and engage in the contestation of that which has hurt them.

Structural violence and contestation

Just as has occurred in other fields of inquiry, the structure-agency debate arose within health care studies and took shape among researchers seeking to understand individual and local responses to social and historical dynamics. Badami for example, examines high rates of suicide by the landless Paniya people and concludes they may be an expression of 'partial politicisation' in response to extreme social and economic marginalization (Badami, 2014). The Paniya community experiences these losses as they would any other 'bad' or premature death resulting from oppressive circumstances, and mourns the death through similar spiritual practices and funeral rites. By examining such systems of meaning held collectively, Badami argues that we may come to deeper understandings of the local impact of globalising forces (Badami, 2014). Like Badami, Bourgois and Hart situate an individual's psychological and social life in broader world views. They propose an approach that 'links political economic, material and cultural forces to psychodynamics and socially charged intimate ways-of being in the world ...' (2011: 1975). They critique the methodological individualism of public health discourse which is meant to shape decision-making by rational actors. Instead, they propose an alternative lens of 'structural vulnerability' which is 'a product of an individual's interface with 'class-based economic exploitation and cultural, gender/sexual, and racialized discrimination'(Bourgois and Hart, 2011: 1975).

In these approaches we find ways of situating the individual within their collective capacities to give meaning to their experiences of structural violence in the workplace.

As workers give meaning to their injuries in the context of their collective world views, so too will they organize collectively to resist and transform these conditions. Bitton *et al.* (2011) draw upon Friedrich's (2010) definition of corporate violence as well as Saussy (2010) to propose a mode of analysis that examines the local and the global dimension of corporate practices and to suggest a role for workers' organizations in confronting those practices. Research on the Ghanaian mining industry has shown that when workers in hazardous workplaces felt their employers did not care about their health and safety, workers did not show a great deal of commitment to the organization and manifested their discontent in high rates of absenteeism, and high turnover (Amponsah-Tawiah and Mensah, 2016). Other studies suggest that managers who do not sufficiently consider the value of providing safe and healthy workplaces, find that workers' commitment to the firm weakens and performance levels diminish (Beck-Krala and Klimkiewicz, 2016). In a study of HIV/AIDS service providers, O'Daniel posits 'a dynamic interaction between macro-level policy and the micro-politics of daily life' in which providers, patients and advocates struggle with the allocation of public funds in meeting the health care needs of African-American women (O'Daniel, 2008: 112). Workers' resistance to dangerous circumstances and physical insecurity will also appear in the work of immigrant settlement agencies and ethno-cultural organizations through which immigrants will self-organize to provide health care services for the community (Thurston *et al.*, 2013). While acknowledging structural barriers, it is also possible for researchers to observe more immediate strategies to prevent workplace illness and injury (Flynn *et al.*, 2015). There is a role for social scientists to conduct research with agencies to learn about migrant workers, and to learn from migrant workers by engaging them directly (Cottini, 2012).

Workers are not only damaged by the demands of global capitalism, they also capable of analysing their oppression within collective systems of meaning and may organise collectively to resist by withdrawing their support for the employment relationship, seeking public funds for health services, self-organising in ethno-cultural institutions, or by working with researchers in the shared hope that their individual experience of oppression might contribute to social change, in addition to efforts to combine their energies into unions and other forms of working-class organisations.

Conclusion

At the outset, I asked what can we learn about structural violence from the rich literature on occupational health and safety and suggested that I would present a critical feminist framework for understanding global power beginning with the embodied worker rather than the nation-state. From a research agenda framed by the concerns of work and labour, first of all, the organization of work continues to be structured by the inequalities of colonialism and racism. These historical processes are gendered in the sense that they depend upon multiple forms of exclusionary practices wresting surplus from women and men on the basis of their social identities with the result that structural violence, intimately felt and socially constructed, relegates workers' interests to the margins of capital accumulation in the twenty-first century. Second, it is useful to examine with care the various hegemonic masculinities arising out of particular national social formations and cultural hierarchies and the ways in which these are used to justify divisions between protected and unprotected workers. Third, I would argue that critical feminist work can be advanced as researchers consider both production and social reproduction and the role of the state in expanding market-based insecurities for public sector workers who face physical and psychological damage, and the injured workers who are the recipients of their services. Fourth, even a brief review of the experiences of immigrant workers shows us how significant is their risk of injury, occupational illness and disability. Finally, students of global (in)security can usefully bring their research and analyses into conversation with workers and their organizations seeking to resist the inequalities of global power and re-order the conditions under which structural violence is carried in the bodies of working-class people around the world.

A final note: I conducted my first literature search with the intention of better understanding the breadth of occupational health and safety as a field of inquiry. As described above, I identified 460 articles with keywords 'health and safety' published between January 2013 and November 2016. These articles were published in 178 different journals and, using an excel table, I logged these into 13 broad categories. With these parameters, the field of occupational health and safety (OHS) is primarily an area of concern to medical researchers. The broad categories of medicine, occupational medicine, disease and public health predominate and 73 journals were grouped here. Another 28 journals were primarily concerned with environmental issues, or production and technology, and 28 journals were generally dedicated to the study of chemicals, ergonomics, accident and injury, as well as disability and compensation. However, there were 49 journals

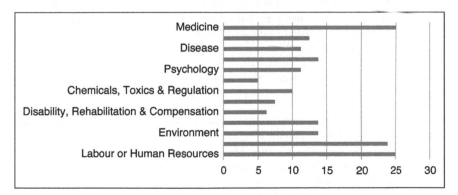

Figure 10.1 Categories of journals publishing articles with keywords 'health and safety'

Source: Scholars Portal Journals, January 2013–November 2016.

in the humanities and social sciences, as well as those covering labour and human resources research that also published occupational health and safety articles. It is notable that only three journals that regularly consider international affairs including *Journal of Development Economics*; *China: An International Journal*, and *International Labour Review* had published articles on topics where occupational health and safety were named in the keywords. I conclude, unhappily, that this is not an issue of major concern to scholars in the field of international studies.

Looking beyond technical literatures, we see in the social sciences, an appreciation of the history of struggle and ongoing collective efforts on the part of workers to bring on board new health and safety activists in diverse workplaces. Success in this field could not exist were it not for the specialized knowledge and research skills inherent in occupational psychology and biomedical approaches combined with the political activism of labour movements pushing employers and the state for decent working conditions. This is no small feat. Despite generations of labour struggle, the International Labour Organisation reports that '(e)very 15 seconds, 153 workers have a work-related accident. Every day, 6,300 people die as a result of occupational accidents or work-related diseases – more than 2.3 million deaths per year' (Organization, 2016). How much richer this literature would be if students of world order would consider the gendered social processes that injure and kill workers who have borne the brunt of global economic restructuring, and think of them as worthy subjects as they attend to the disembodied, transnational flows of capital, finance, goods and services in the world economy, or to the conflicts challenging state boundaries in a competitive inter-state system.

References

Amponsah-Tawiah, K. & Mensah, J., 2016. Occupational health and safety and organizational commitment: Evidence from the Ghanaian mining industry. *Safety and Health at Work*, 7, 225–230.

Arcury, T. A., Cartwright, M. S., Chen, H., Rosenbaum, D. A., Walker, F. O., Mora, D. C. & Quandt, S. A., 2014. Musculoskeletal and neurological injuries associated with work organization among immigrant latino women manual workers in North Carolina. *American Journal of Industrial Medicine*, 57, 468–475.

Badami, S., 2014. Suicide as a counter-narrative in Wayanad, Southern India: The invisible death. *South Asia Research*, 34, 91–112.

Baines, D., 2006. Staying with people who slap us around: Gender, juggling responsibilities and violence in paid (and unpaid) care work. *Gender, Work and Organization*, 13, 129–51.

Baylis, J., Smith, S. & Owens, P., 2014. *The Globalization of World Politics: An Introduction to International Relations*, Oxford: Oxford University Press.

Beck-Krala, E. & Klimkiewicz, K., 2016. Occupational safety and health as an element of a complex compensation system evaluation within an organization. *International Journal of Occupational Safety and Ergonomics*, 22, 523–531.

Benach, J., Vives, A., Amable, M., Vanroelen, C., Tarafa, G. & Muntaner, C., 2014. Precarious employment: Understanding an emerging social determinant of health. *Annual Review of Public Health*, 35, 229–253.

Benach, J., Vives, A., Tarafa, G., Delclos, C. & Muntaner, C., 2016. What should we know about precarious employment and health in 2025? Framing the agenda for the next decade of research. *International Journal of Epidemiology*, 45, 232–238.

Bitton, A., Green, C. & Colbert, J., 2011. Improving the delivery of global tobacco control. *Mount Sinai Journal of Medicine: A Journal of Translational and Personalized Medicine*, 78, 382–393.

Bourgois, P. & Hart, L. K., 2011. Commentary on Genberg et al. (2011): The structural vulnerability imposed by hypersegregated US inner city neighborhoods – a theoretical and practical challenge for substance abuse research. *Addiction*, 106, 1975–1977.

Brabcová, I., Vacková, J. & Dvořáčková, O., 2014. Working environment and its impact on the health of immigrants. *Kontakt*, E1–e8. Available: http://dx.doi.org/10.1016/j.kontakt.2014.09.003.

Breslin, F. C., Ibrahim, S., Smith, P., Mustard, C., Amick, B. & Shankardass, K., 2013. The demographic and contextual correlates of work-related repetitive strain injuries among canadian men and women. *American Journal of Industrial Medicine*, 56, 1180–1189.

Carter, B., Danford, A., Howcroft, D., Richardson, H., Smith, A. & Taylor, P., 2013. 'Stressed out of my box': Employee experience of lean working and occupational ill-health in clerical work in the UK public sector. *Work, Employment & Society*, 27, 747–767.

Charlesworth, S. & Baines, D., 2015. Understanding the negotiation of paid and unpaid care work in community services in cross-national perspective: The contribution of a rapid ethnographic approach. *Journal of Family Studies*, 21, 7–21.

Choiniere, J. A., MacDonnell, J. A., Campbell, A. L. & Smele, S., 2014. Conceptualizing structural violence in the context of mental health nursing. *Nursing Inquiry*, 21, 39–50.

Clarke, M., Lewchuk, W., de Wolff, A. & King, A., 2007. 'This just isn't sustainable': Precarious employment, stress and workers' health. *International Journal of Law and Psychiatry*, 30, 311–326.

Confederation, I. T. U. 2016. *One Worker Dies Every 15 Seconds Due to Employer Negligence* [Online]. Brussels. Available: www.ituc-csi.org/one-worker-dies-every-15-seconds [Accessed 09 January 2017].

Connell, R. W. & Messerschmidt, J., 2005. Hegemonic masculinity. *Gender & Society*, 19, 829–859.

Cottini, E., 2012. Is your job bad for your health? Explaining differences in health at work across gender. *International Journal of Manpower*, 33, 301–321.

Cresswell, J. W. 2013. *Qualitative Inquiry and Research Design: Choosing Among Five Approaches*, Los Angeles: Sage.

Daly, T. & Armstrong, P., 2016. Liminal and invisible long-term care labour: Precarity in the face of austerity. *Journal of Industrial Relations*, 58, 473–490.

Ekstedt, E., 1999. Form of employment in a project-intensive economy. *American Journal of Industrial Medicine*, 36, 11–14.

Farmer, P., Nizeye, B., Stulac, S. & Keshavjee, S. 2006. Structural violence and clinical medicine. *PLoS Med*, 3(10), 1686–1691. e449.

Fierke, K. M. 2007. *Critical Approaches to International Security*, Cambridge: Polity.

Flynn, M. A., Eggerth, D. E. & Jacobson, C. J., 2015. Undocumented status as a social determinant of occupational safety and health: The workers' perspective. *American Journal of Industrial Medicine*, 58, 1127–1137.

Forssén, G. & Carlstedt, A., 2001. Work, health and ill health: New research makes women's experiences visible. *Scandinavian Journal of Primary Health Care*, 19, 154–157.

Galtung, J., 1969. Violence, peace, and peace research. *Journal of Peace Research*, 6(3), 167–191.

Galtung, J., 1975 *Peace: Research, Education, Action.* Copenhagen: Christian Ejlers.

Gamlin, J. & Hawkes, S., 2015. Pregnancy and birth in an indigenous Huichol community: From structural violence to structural policy responses. *Culture, Health & Sexuality*, 17, 78–91.

Guldenmund, F., Bryan, C. & Mearns, K., 2013. An exploratory study of migrant workers and safety in three European countries. 92–99.

Harvey, D., 2004. The 'new' imperialism: Accumulation by disposession. *Socialist Register 2004: The New Imperial Challenge*, 40, 63–87.

Harvey, D. 2005. *A Brief History of Neoliberalism*, New York: Oxford University Press.

Howard, J., 2017. Nonstandard work arrangements and worker health and safety. *American Journal of Industrial Medicine*, 60, 1–10.

Jamieson, S., 2005. The neoliberal state and the gendered prosecution of work injury. *Health Sociology Review*, 14, 69–76.

Kadetz, P., 2016. Problematizing the 'global' in global health: An assessment of the global discourse of safety. *Fudan Journal of the Humanities and Social Sciences*, 9, 25–40.

Kensbock, S., Bailey, J., Jennings, G. & Patiar, A., 2015. Sexual harassment of women working as room attendants within 5 star hotels. *Gender, Work & Organization*, 22, 36–50.

Landsbergis, P. A., Grzywacz, J. G. & LaMontagne, A. D., 2014. Work organization, job insecurity, and occupational health disparities. *American Journal of Industrial Medicine*, 57, 495–515.

Lipscomb, H. J., Dement, J. M., Epling, C. A., Gaynes, B. N., McDonald, M. A. & Schoenfisch, A. L., 2007. Depressive symptoms among working women in rural North Carolina: A comparison of women in poultry processing and other low-wage jobs. *International Journal of Law and Psychiatry*, 30, 284–298.

McBride, S., Mahon, R. & Boychuk, G. W. 2015. *After '08: Social Policy and the Global Financial Crisis*. Vancouver and Toronto: University of British Columbia.

Menendez, M., Benach, J., Muntaner, C., Amable, M. & O'Campo, P., 2007. Is precarious employment more damaging to women's health than men's? *Social Science & Medicine*, 64, 776–781.

Messing, K., 1998. *One-Eyed Science: Occupational Health and Women Workers*. Philadelphia, PA: Temple University Press.

Milanovic, B. 2016. *Global Inequality: A New Approach for the Age of Globalization*, Cambridge, MA and London, England: Belknap Press of the Harvard University Press.

Mora, D. C., Arcury, T. A. & Quandt, S. A., 2016. Good job, bad job: Occupational perceptions among Latino poultry workers. *American Journal of Industrial Medicine*, 59, 877–886.

O'Daniel, A. A., 2008. Pushing poverty to the periphery: HIV-positive African American women's health needs, the Ryan White Care Act, and a political economy of service provision. *Transforming Anthropology*, 16, 112–127.

Organization, I. L. 2016. *Safety and Health at Work* [Online]. Geneva. Available: www.ilo. org/global/topics/safety-and-health-at-work/lang--en/index.htm [Accessed 09 January 2017].

Premji, S., Duguay, P., Messing, K. & Lippel, K., 2010. Are immigrants, ethnic and linguistic minorities over-represented in jobs with a high level of compensated risk? Results from a montréal, Canada study using census and workers' compensation data. *American Journal of Industrial Medicine*, 53, 875–885.

Premji, S. & Lewchuk, W., 2014. Racialized and gendered disparities in occupational exposures among Chinese and white workers in Toronto. *Ethnicity & Health*, 19, 512–528.

Quesada, J., Hart, L. K. & Bourgois, P., 2011. Structural vulnerability and health: Latino migrant laborers in the United States. *Medical Anthropology*, 30, 339–362.

Rodriguez, G., Trejo, G., Schiemann, E., Quandt, S., Daniel, S., Sandberg, J. & Arcury, T., 2016. Latina workers in North Carolina: Work organization, domestic responsibilities, health, and family life. *Journal of Immigrant and Minority Health*, 18, 687–696.

Rupert, M. E., 1990. Producing hegemony: State/society relations and the politics of productivity in the United States. *International Studies Quarterly*, 34, 427–456.

Safety, C. C. f. O. H. a. 2016. *Hazards* [Online]. Ottawa: Government of Canada. Available: www.ccohs.ca/topics/hazards/ [Accessed 30 October 2016].

Saussy, H., ed. 2010. *Partner to the Poor: A Paul Farmer Reader*. Berkeley, CA: University of California Press.

Scott-Samuel, Alex, Stanistreet, Debbi & Crawshaw, Paul, 2009. Hegemonic masculinity, structural violence and health inequalities. *Critical Public Health*, 19(3–4), 287–292.

Smith, P. M. & Mustard, C. A., 2009. Comparing the risk of work-related injuries between immigrants to Canada and Canadian-born labour market participants. *Occupational and Environmental Medicine*, 66, 361–367.

Smith, R. J. D., 2012. Immigrant workers and workers' compensation: The need for reform. *American Journal of Industrial Medicine*, 55, 537–544.

Thurston, W. E. & Vissandjée, B., 2005. An ecological model for understanding culture as a determinant of women's health. *Critical Public Health*, 15, 229–242.

Thurston, W. E., Roy, A., Clow, B., Este, D., Gordey, T., Haworth-Brockman, M., McCoy, L., Beck, R. R., Saulnier, C. & Carruthers, L., 2013. Pathways into and out of homelessness: Domestic violence and housing security for immigrant women. *Journal of Immigrant & Refugee Studies*, 11, 278–298.

Vosko, L. F., 2015. Introduction. In: *Comparative Perspectives Database on Precarious Employment*. Available at: www.genderwork.ca/cpd/?page_id¼2 (Accessed 9 March 2015).

Walker, R. B. J., 1990. Security, sovereignty, and the challenge of world politics. *Alternatives: Global, Local, Political*, 15, 3–27.

Walter, N., Bourgois, P. & Margarita Loinaz, H., 2004. Masculinity and undocumented labor migration: Injured latino day laborers in San Francisco. *Social Science and Medicine*, 59, 1159–1168.

Wasilkiewicz, K., Albrechtsen, E. & Antonsen, S., 2016. Occupational safety in a globalized construction industry: A study on Polish workers in Norway. *Policy and Practice in Health and Safety*, 14, 128–143.

11 Public health in the Anthropocene

Exploring population fears and climate threats

Jade S. Sasser

Introduction

Since 2000, earth scientists have argued that we are inhabiting a moment of unprecedented human disruption of natural environments and habitats, in which ecology and planetary systems at all scales have been shaped by human presence and activity. Known as the Anthropocene, this concept holds that human population growth and resource extraction and use have made human beings the primary force behind geological and ecological change on the planet (Crutzen & Stoermer 2000). However, this is not an undisputed fact. Far from a biological given, the 'Anthropocene idea' (Moore 2015) also operates as a political concept resting on anthropogenesis – an assumption that humans stand apart from nature and the environment and act on it in easily discernible ways (Sayre 2012). This idea of the Anthropocene drives much of the discourse around global climate change and its impacts on human bodies, lives, and communities. For example, the Intergovernmental Panel on Climate Change (IPCC) Fourth Assessment Report stated emphatically that global warming is unequivocal and that at least half of this warming is the result of human activity (Pachauri & Reisinger 2007; Liverman 2007). The National Aeronautics and Space Administration (NASA) is more forceful in its language: 'the main cause of the current global warming trend is human expansion of the "greenhouse effect"' (NASA 2016). The range of changes in earth systems impacted by climate change – extreme heat, drought, decreased fresh water availability, geographic shifts in habitats for disease vectors, increased extreme weather events, among others – have both direct and indirect impacts on human health. As a result, public health agencies and researchers are increasingly becoming involved in climate change.

For example, in 2016, the World Health Organization's (WHO) analysis of climate impacts squarely centres human lives:

> the ultimate impact of climate change is on our most precious resource – human lives and health ... [and] the responsibility for protecting lives ultimately falls on the health sector. Investing in health resilience to climate risks can save lives both now, and in the future.
>
> (WHO 2016)

In a widely cited 2009 report, public health researchers described climate change as the biggest threat to human health in the twenty-first century, one that places the lives and wellbeing of billions of people across the globe at risk (Costello *et al.* 2009). Several years later, the Lancet Commission on Health and Climate Change formed in, 2015 to 'map out the impacts of climate change, and the necessary policy responses, in order to ensure the highest attainable standards of health for populations worldwide' (Watts *et al.* 2015: 1861). The international group of academic researchers, policy experts, and public health professionals set their task to conduct a broad, multi-year assessment of the literature on the public health impacts of climate change, and to make a series of policy recommendations, which they organized around their conclusion that 'tackling climate change could be the greatest global health opportunity of the 21st century' (Watts *et al.* 2015: 1861).

However, the impacts of climate change on human health are not the same across all populations or communities. Rather, they impact communities and bodies differently, along the lines of gender, class, and race (Godfrey & Torres 2016). While researchers, policymakers, and government officials concerned with global public health are increasingly drawing attention to the wide range of current and potential future health impacts of climate change, some of these actors have called for greater attention to the links between population growth and climate change. They argue that reproductive health and family planning interventions offer solutions to both mitigate and help communities adapt to climate change. How are these perspectives linked? Do they simply represent diverse approaches to the connections between climate change, human health, and the body? Or do their efforts highlight the ways climate change exacerbates embodied structural and social inequalities?

The remainder of this chapter is organized in three sections. In the first, I argue that climate change exacerbates embodied structural and social inequalities, thus entrenching existing health disparities, particularly along the lines of gender, race, and poverty. Next, I explore how a narrow focus on population and family planning reflects longstanding, interlinked narratives of ecological threat and fear, which threatens to exacerbate embodied inequalities, rather than remedy them. The chapter concludes with a discussion of alternative framings that resist these forms of structural and discursive violence.

Climate change and embodied structural violence

Structural violence was first defined by Johan Galtung (1969) as violence in which there is no particular subject, or person, who acts to inflict violence on others. Rather, violence is 'built into the structure and shows up as unequal power and consequently as unequal life chances' (Galtung 1969: 171). It is characterized by unequal distribution of resources and decision-making over resource distribution. Rather than direct action taken between individuals and groups, structural violence manifests indirectly, through the impacts of highly inequitable or violent social structures, particularly in the context of bodies: '[i]nequality then shows up in differential morbidity and mortality rates, between individuals in a district, between districts in a nation, and between nations in the international system – in a chain of interlocking feudal relationships' (Galtung 1969: 177). Following on Galtung, Farmer (2004) defines structural violence as violence exerted systematically by all interests within a given social order. This kind of violence cannot be understood through assertions of individual blame and responsibility; rather it stems from structures, systems, and the 'social machinery of oppression' (Farmer 2004: 307). Farmer's ethnographic studies among the poor in Haiti demonstrate this point well; connecting joblessness and poverty with migration, transactional sex economies, and inability to adhere to treatment regimens, his analyses point to the fact that not individuals, but systems and structures of entrenched inequality give rise to the conditions in which disease manifests and becomes entrenched among the poor (Farmer 1992).

As noted above, climate change impacts the availability and quality of air, water, and crops, as well as increasing the frequency of extreme heat and weather events such as floods and storms, and expanding the range of habitats for disease vectors like mosquitoes. Changes to the climate have direct and indirect impacts on planetary systems, ecosystems, and social systems, all of which shape the conditions that protect or threaten human health. It is important to note the role of scientific uncertainty that makes it difficult to draw definitive conclusions regarding the impacts of climate change on human health; these uncertainties impact what researchers estimate to be the future health impacts (McMichael *et al.* 2002). In addition, most of the epidemiological studies of the health impacts of climate change have been conducted in industrialized nations. Additional research is needed to understand how climate change, which already exacerbates embodied structural violence among the poor and marginalized, impacts public health among local communities in the global South.

At the same time, we know that climate change does not impact all human populations equally. For example, gendered roles dictate that women are more likely to be responsible for food gathering and production, energy and water collection, and the gathering of medicinal plants. These gender-specific tasks are heavily dependent on natural environments and resources, and are particularly vulnerable to ecological disruption. Degraded environments play an important role in shifting power relationships in society, particularly gendered power relationships. As women lose access to and control over environmental resources, they become more marginalized and less able to meet their own, and their families' health and survival needs (Dankelman 2010). Women, particularly those over 65, are more likely to die during heat waves and extreme weather events, such as major storms, particularly among those who have pre-existing cardiovascular or respiratory diseases (Nagel 2016; McMichael *et al.* 2002).

Weather-related disasters, of which floods are the most common, have strong impacts on public health through accidents and drownings. These events take a particularly gendered toll. For example, of the 140,000 people killed in Cyclone Marian in Bangladesh in 1991, approximately 90 percent were women and children (Schmuck 2002). Sociocultural roles and expectations around childrearing and family caretaking, attitudes toward unaccompanied women in public, and women's lack of knowledge of how to swim all contributed to this dramatic gendered death toll. In addition, women are more likely to suffer poor health outcomes and gender-based violence in the wake of disasters. In the wake of disasters, women have particular health needs that require gender-sensitive planning. Specifically, sexually transmitted infection (STI) prevention and treatment, supplies for contraception and menstrual hygiene, prenatal care, and protection from sexual violence (Enarson & Chakrabarti 2009). Women are disadvantaged at all levels of disaster processes, including 'exposure to risk, risk perception, preparedness, response, physical impact, psychological impact, recovery and reconstruction' (WHO 2005), which is exacerbated by gendered household and community roles and responsibilities, as well as gender based access to resources and decision making.

Gender roles also disproportionately make women vulnerable to the drivers of climate change. For example, everyday household meal preparation, a responsibility predominantly held by women all over the world, frequently exposes women and children to household air pollution based on use of traditional stoves and biomass fuels (including wood, charcoal, animal dung, or crop residues). According to the WHO, 4.3 million people each year die prematurely from illnesses attributable to biomass and other solid fuels (WHO 2012; WHO 2007). Traditional household cooking practices are also linked to climate change. The smoke they produce contains black carbon, which climate researchers have identified as the second most significant contributor to global warming, after carbon dioxide (Bond *et al.* 2013). Often the firewood that fuels them is unsustainably harvested over many hours by women and girls in conditions of extreme scarcity, raising concerns about deforestation and the entrenchment of unequal gender roles and dynamics.

The health disparities of climate change are acknowledged by political leaders as both domestic and global problems requiring policy responses. In 2016, the White House issued a 'Climate and Health Assessment' report documenting the human health impacts of climate change. The report argues that climate change is 'a significant threat to the health of the American people', and that 'every American is vulnerable to the public health impacts associated with climate change' (USGCRP 2016). At the same time, it highlights the fact that certain groups are particularly vulnerable, including those who are 'low income, some communities of color, immigrant groups (including those with limited English proficiency), Indigenous peoples, children and pregnant women, older adults, vulnerable occupational groups, persons with disabilities, and persons with preexisting or chronic medical conditions' (USGCRP 2016). The report calls for prioritizing the needs of vulnerable populations in policy responses to climate change, in order to safeguard their health and wellbeing. Poor and racial and ethnic minority populations are also particularly vulnerable climate related health problems in global context. Climate change exacerbates existing health disparities which disproportionately impact the poor, the world over: '[c]limate change will have its greatest effect on those who have the least access to the world's resources and who have contributed least to its cause' (Costello *et al.* 2009: 1694).

Pointing to the impacts of climate disruptions on water, food security, and extreme weather events, as well as numerous indirect results of climate change, public health leaders are increasingly calling for a coordinated international management response including representatives from government, civil society, and academia. One strategy would be the development of a 'public health movement that frames the threat of climate change for humankind as a health issue' focusing on the unique potential role health professionals can bring to the issue, specifically that of attracting political attention (Costello *et al.* 2009: 1696). With this political attention, public health researchers and practitioners can advocate for recommendations focused on reducing the health impacts of climate change through reducing new greenhouse gas emissions, managing events directly associated with disease, and developing and supporting effective health management systems. However, health inequality is not the only framing used to analyze the relationships between human bodies and climate change. Some researchers and international development actors have chosen to focus on climate change through the lens of population trends, specifically population growth and migration. This focus, often cast through the lens of ecological and health security, casts poor, racialized populations in the global South as global threats – and population interventions targeting women's bodies as the solution. As previously demonstrated, climate change exacerbates existing health and other security threats to vulnerable populations. Characterizing the growth of these populations as a key driver of climate change, thus a driver of climate threats, operates as a form of discursive violence. The next section explores these linked discourses they intersect with discourses emphasizing militarization, and raises questions about how this focus entrenches discursive structural violence.

Producing a climate of fear

Even as women and the poor, particularly in the global South, are more vulnerable to the health and bodily effects of climate change, their fertility, resource use, and migration patterns are frequently subsumed into powerful narratives of environmental threat shaped by fear. Particular fears, such as environmental and biological fears, play a 'particularly powerful role in obscuring and naturalizing social, economic, and political processes and attendant policy choices' (Hartmann *et al.* 2005: 3). For example, looking at population growth as a key driver of climate change distracts from an analysis of the economic and political systems generating climate outcomes. Narratives and images invoking fear and anxiety about the future of the planet and the continued sustainability of life proliferate in environmental discourse. These discourses have been embedded in environmentalist discourse for a very long time, and when they focus on threats to 'our way of life' (Hartmann *et al.* 2005: 1), they play a powerful role in identifying threats to security – individual, national, and global.

Security itself is closely linked to the production of fear. Environmental and biological fears, which are produced through image, narrative, and performance, are translated into security discourses for various purposes – often to influence policy. The Commission on Human Security's, 2003 report, *Human Security Now,* describes human security as 'concerned with safeguarding and expanding people's vital freedoms. It requires both shielding people from acute threats and empowering people to take charge of their own lives', and it requires an international policy response prioritizing 'people's survival, livelihood and dignity, during downturns as well as in prosperity' (Commission on Human Security 2003: iv). The term human security, from which health security derives, does not have a singular or clear definition. It is described with respect to both states and individuals, the security of the nation, the freedoms of individuals, protection from threats and harms, physical security and psychological well-being. Human security is intentionally vague, 'powerful precisely because it lacks precision . . . the term, in short, appears to be slippery by design. Cultivated ambiguity renders human security an effective campaign slogan, but it also diminishes the concept's usefulness as a guide for academic research or policymaking' (Paris 2001: 88). The 1994 UN Human Development Report is the most 'widely cited and authoritative' definition of human security (Paris 2001; Aldis 2008). The broadness and vagueness of definitions pose a challenge for policymakers to narrow down specific problems and solutions/interventions, or for lawmakers to allocate resources (Paris 2001). Struggles over the conceptual apparatus of human security centre on debates over whether to prioritize bodily safety and freedom from harm, or the securing of political rights and economic resources, or military concepts of security focused on protecting and strengthening national borders through surveillance and weaponization. Although much of the work to define and describe human security has moved beyond a focus on military- and state-centred models, it still often centres questions of threats, whether to individuals, groups, communities, and societies. What does this have to do with health?

In the arena of health security, while the literatures and perspectives are diverse, there are common themes: protection from threats; development of novel approaches to respond to new political and economic contexts; involvement of new public health actors, including militaries; and relationship between public health and foreign policy. 'Taken together, the introduction of a threat protection mentality, foreign policy agendas, military interests and bioterrorism concerns into global public health, under the concept of global public health security, have subtly altered our understanding of global public health' (Aldis 2008: 373).

There is no policy or scholarly based consensus on the definition or scope of health security or human security, nor the intent of policy and programmes designed to implement it (Aldis 2008: 373). One of the strategies that has been proposed to address climate change and its impacts on human security is through slowing global population growth. For example, a growing body of research focused on projecting future population trends alongside greenhouse gas emissions (GGEs) suggests that slowing population growth will lead to fewer GGEs overall, and have direct health benefits (O'Neill *et al.* 2012; O'Neill *et al.* 2010; Gaffin & O'Neill 1997). These studies analyze the roles of urbanization, household size and resource consumption, and population aging, concluding that long-term global population reductions would lead to concurrent reductions in GGEs, slowing the pace of climate change. However, this research is not without its challenges. The studies are based on projections of possible futures, modelled on large scale, aggregate trends within and between countries and regions. In other words, they model what could possibly happen many decades into the future, based on trends occurring now.

However, not all projection models point to the same conclusions. An older study points to another issue concerning population projections and climate change. The, 1992 World Bank paper, based on econometric estimates, concludes that 'there is little basis for the view that the South could contribute to major reductions in global warning by taking new and stronger steps to reduce its population' (Birdsall 1992: n.p.). However, the paper also argues that slowing population growth in global South countries through contraceptive provision is 'cost-effective compared with other options to reduce emissions', a strategy that would benefit developed nations:

> The global negative externality represented by rapid population growth in developing countries provides a strong, new rationale for developed countries, in their own interests, to finance programmes that would reduce population growth in developing countries. This is true even though feasible reductions in population growth would represent only a modest contribution to reducing greenhouse gas emissions.

The author ultimately concludes that both educating women and providing universal access to contraceptives are more efficient cost saving measures to reduce GGEs when compared with other strategies such as a carbon tax.

This approach – putting forth population interventions as cost-effective climate change strategies – has continued to gain ground in recent years. The international charity Population Matters (formerly known as Optimum Population Trust) sponsors a website known as PopOffsets, in which financial contributions to reproductive health and family planning programmes are purported to help avert new GGEs through keeping birth rates low in high fertility countries. On its website, the project touts its work as the 'only project in the world that allows for the offsetting of carbon emissions by helping to improve family planning provision' (PopOffsets n.d.). In this model, people, bodies, and greenhouse gases are reduced to dollars and cents, economic models and cost–benefit ratios that collapse all sense of social complexity and completely obscure political and economic conditions. Ironically, it also allows its supporters to feel good about their own resource consumption practices by positing their donations as offsetting the carbon impacts of their, and others' resource consumption behaviours (Sasser 2016).

What these models do not account for is the roles of structural inequality and structural violence. The resource extraction, development, and concurrent GGEs initiated through large-scale institutions such as militaries, are unaccounted for in these models. This is a significant oversight for several reasons. First, military activities contribute significantly to the production of greenhouse gas emissions. The U.S. Air Force, for example, is the world's single largest consumer of petroleum. A study conducted in, 2010 demonstrated that the U.S. military emitted hundreds of millions of megatons of carbon each year during the Iraq War in its bid to protect U.S. access to oil in the region (Liska & Perrin 2010). Second, military institutions' research on climate change is often focused on the arena of security, expressed in militarized terms. This emphasis places resource scarcity and conflict into the arena of threat – and justifies the possibility of military action to address the effects of climate change. For example, the International Institute for Strategic Studies (IISS), a military think tank, puts forth a statement on climate change and security on its website that

> [t]he IISS believes climate change could have a serious effect on regional and global stability, and researches how global warming may affect disputes over territory, water and other resources, or could otherwise threaten peace. It also studies the mechanisms for averting 'climate wars'.
>
> (IISS 2016)

Such "war talk" is a dangerous way of linking back to human security – it positions people in resource-poor or conflict-prone settings as a potential threat to others. For example, Hartmann (2014: 17) demonstrates how military attention to the potential for increased 'resource scarcity, environmental degradation, and climate change' in Africa has been used to argue for increased military engagement on the continent. In addition, in, 2007 UN Secretary General Ban Ki-moon claimed that the violence in Darfur, Sudan, was driven by climate change and resource scarcity, and exacerbated by demographic issues – an argument which he used to justify further military intervention in the region (Ki-moon 2007). These arguments are often buttressed by racialized narratives depicting young men in the Middle East and Africa as poor, mobile, and dangerous- narratives that invoke national security concerns in demographic terms through strategic demography (Hartmann & Hendrixson 2005).

These narratives are linked directly to discourses that circulate and amplify environmental and biological fears, and that identify potential sources of harm: 'environmental and biological fears are implicated in the identification and construction of threats to individual, national, and global security. Fear begets threat, and threat begets fear' (Hartmann *et al.* 2005: 1). What these fears accomplish is the escalation of a public rhetoric centred on threat, as well as scapegoating particular populations as dangerous "others". When populations are characterized through the lenses of difference and fear, the structural inequalities they face can become naturalized as the focus on fear and threat plays a role in obscuring political and economic processes and policy decisions. Fears are materially grounded at the same time that they are constructed and historically contingent. They also can and inform the ways researchers, policymakers, and other influential actors conceptualize global and local problems and allocate resources. What can be done to resist these forms of structural and discursive violence? Below I explore some alternative framings of linkages between climate change, health, and bodies, focusing on strategies that prioritize vulnerable populations.

Reframing the narrative

In 2009 the WHO published a paper advocating contraceptive access as a resource that can help poor nations adapt to the ravages of climate change. Ensuring universal contraceptive access, they argued, would respond to stated needs and desires of less developed countries and communities. For example, a literature review revealed that a significant number of least developed countries submitting strategies to the Global Environmental Facility identified rapid population growth as an element that might impact their ability to adapt to climate change. In addition, 'it is perhaps more conducive to a rights-based approach to implement family planning programmes in response to the welfare needs of people and communities rather than in response to international concern for global overpopulation' (Bryant *et al.* 2009).

While approaches that meet the stated needs of impacted communities are a step in the right direction, focusing primarily on contraceptive access is an inadequate approach. First, it does nothing to undo the problematic narratives connecting the fertility and reproduction of the poor to climate change. Second, it does not account for the myriad other embodied health problems that result, both directly and indirectly, from changes in the climate – and if health-related funding and resources for adaptation are primarily focused on contraceptive access, this would leave significant other health issues out of the picture, which could potentially exacerbate existing health conditions, rather than remedy them. If population interventions threaten to replicate structural violence, what are the alternatives? How can we have approaches to climate change and its impacts on human health that reject structural violence and instead support individual and community resilience?

One example would be to prioritize particularly vulnerable communities in early warning systems, adaptation plans, and other disaster management policies and programs. This would include integrating a gender perspective into planning for the impacts of natural disasters, as well as adaptation programmes in general. One study of communities impacted by drought separately analyzed women's and men's adaptation strategies within the same household (Eriksen *et al.* 2005), and found that specializing in a non-agricultural livelihood strategy helped individuals remain resilient to climate stresses. However, women were far less likely to have alternative livelihood strategies due to gendered norms governing reproductive labour in households, cultural and gendered expectations about men's and women's work outside of the home, and lack of access to financial capital. Financial independence through income generation can increase women's ability to remain resilient during times of climate-driven vulnerability, with positive impacts on food security and other resource access.

Another example concerns women's gendered roles with respect to energy use and food provision in households. As noted, biomass fuels are the primary cooking fuel sources for billions of people around the world, primarily women, and the household air pollution they produce has significant and long-term consequences for women's and children's health, illness, and death. Improved cookstove programmes that burn clean fuels or reduce the amount of fuel and smoke involved in cooking can have a significant impact on this trend. The Global Alliance for Clean Cookstoves (GACC) advocates the universal adoption of clean cookstoves and fuels. A GACC strategy effort in 2010 aims at getting clean stoves into 100 million households by the year 2020, primarily by addressing barriers to the production, availability, and use of clean stoves and fuels. At the same time, the strategy aims to improve gender conditions by reducing the amount of time women and girls spend searching for and collecting fuel and cooking. Significant challenges have arisen in cookstove programmes, including affordability, users' lack of familiarity with stoves, stove failures, and lack of women's participation in stove design (Gunther 2015), prompting some to speculate whether these projects should be abandoned. However, stove projects are designed to address environmental, health, and social problems – and while imperfect, they may have some marginal positive impact. For example, programmes that train women to produce, market, and sell stoves help women attain some level of financial independence, which can provide some measure of resilience against climate-driven vulnerability. In addition, these programmes and their advocates should push for the availability and provision of truly clean stoves – those that operate on clean fuels like gas, electricity, and sunlight – in order to move toward social equity in addition to improving health.

Much more research is needed on the relationships between climate change, public health, and vulnerability, particularly with a gender lens. While feminist researchers have increasingly studied the role of gender, race, poverty and climate change, very little is still known about the specifically gendered health effects of climate change. How are women's bodies and livelihoods impacted differently by climate change, both directly and indirectly? What strategies are women and communities using to adapt to these unequal outcomes? How can women's voices, priorities, and needs be foregrounded in public health arenas so that their unique needs can be met? As these questions are addressed, widening the field of knowledge and centring the research priorities on the needs of the most vulnerable, structural and discursive forms of violence and their impacts will weaken in explanatory power and recede from the centre of the discussion.

At the same time, the challenges of militarization and the characterization of racialized threats must be addressed. The Paris Agreement, which the U.S. withdrew from in June 2017, was a groundbreaking agreement for multiple reasons, among them the fact that U.S. military contributions to GGEs would no longer be concealed. Requiring militaries to report GGE activities would provide a more accurate accounting of annual responsibility for emissions, as well as bolstering activist efforts to secure global climate justice. Activist efforts are also key to challenging and rejecting the racialized discourses that pin the blame for climate change on the poor. Building and sustaining alternative narratives linking climate change firmly to its structural and institutional drivers is a key component of linking diverse grassroots social movements for health, reproductive justice, and climate justice.

176   *Jade S. Sasser*

References

Aldis, W. (2008) 'Health security as a public health concept: a critical analysis', *Health Policy and Planning*, vol. 23, pp. 369–375.

Birdsall, N. (1992) 'Another look at population and global warming', The World Bank Country Economics Department, Policy Research Working Papers, Washington, D.C. Online. Available: http://documents.worldbank.org/curated/en/985961468766195689/pdf/multi-page.pdf (accessed 6 October 2016).

Bond, T.C., Doherty, S.J., Fahey, D.W., Forster, P.M., Berntsen, T., DeAngelo, B.J., Flanner, M.G., Ghan, S., Karcher, B., Koch, D., Kinne, S., Kondo, Y., Quinn, P.K., Sarofim, M.C., Schultz, M.G., Schulz, M., Venkataraman, C., Zhang, H., Zhang, S., Bellouin, N., Guttikunda, S.K., Hoke, P.K., Jacobson, M.Z., Kaiser, J.W., Klimont, Z., Lohmann, U., Schwarz, J.P., Shindell, D., Storelvmo, T., Warren, S.G., and Zender, C.S. (2013) 'Bounding the role of black carbon in the climate system: a scientific assessment', *Journal of Geographical Research*, vol. 118, no.11, pp. 5380–5552.

Bryant, L., Carver, L., Butler, C.D., and Anage, A. (2009) 'Climate change and family planning: least-developed countries define the agenda', *Bulletin of the World Health Organization*, vol. 87, pp. 852–857. Online. Available: www.who.int/bulletin/volumes/87/11/08-062562/en/ (accessed 23 April 2016).

Commission on Human Security. (2003) *Human Security Now: Protecting and Empowering People*, United Nations, New York, NY.

Costello, A., Abbas, M., Allen, A., Ball, S., Bell, S., Bellamy, R., Friel, S., Grace, N., Johnson, A., Kett, M., Lee, M., Levy, C., Maslin, M., McCoy, M., McGuire, B., Montgomery, H., Napier, D., Pagel, C., Patel, J., Oliverira, J.A.P, Redclift, N., Rees, H., Rogger, D., Scott, J., Stephenson, J., Twigg, J., Wolff, J., and Patterson, C. (2009) 'Managing the health effects of climate change', *The Lancet*, vol. 373, pp. 1693–1733.

Crutzen, P.J. and Stoermer, E.F. (2000) 'The "anthropocene"', *Global Change Newsletter*, no. 41, pp. 17–18.

Dankelman, I. (ed.) (2010) *Gender and Climate Change: An Introduction*, Earthscan, London, England, and Washington, D.C.

Enarson, E. and Chakrabarti, P.G.D. (eds) (2009) *Women, Gender and Disaster: Global Issues and Initiatives*, Sage Publications, Thousand Oaks, CA.

Eriksen, S.H., Brown, K., and Kelly, P.M. (2005) 'The dynamics of vulnerability: locating coping strategies in Kenya and Tanzania', *Geographical Journal*, vol. 171, no. 4, pp. 287–305.

Farmer, P. (1992) *AIDS and Accusation: Haiti and the Geography of Blame*, University of California Press, Berkeley and Los Angeles, CA.

Farmer, P. (2004) 'An anthropology of structural violence', *Current Anthropology*, vol. 45, no. 3, pp. 305–325.

Gaffin, S.R. and O'Neill, B.C. (1997) 'Population and global warming with and without CO2 targets', *Population & Environment*, vol. 18, pp. 389–413.

Galtung, J. (1969) 'Violence, peace and peace research', *Journal of Peace Research*, vol. 6, no. 3, pp. 167–191.

Godfrey, P. and Torres, D. (eds) (2016) *Systemic Crises of Global Climate Change: Intersections of Race, Class, and Gender*, Routledge, London, England and New York, NY.

Gunther, M. (2015) 'These cheap, clean stoves were supposed to save millions of lives. What happened?' *Washington Post*, October 29, 2015. Online. Available: www.washingtonpost.com/opinions/these-cheap-clean-stoves-were-supposed-to-save-

millions-of-lives-what-happened/2015/10/29/c0b98f38-77fa-11e5-a958-d889faf
561dc_story.html?utm_term=.6de1c8e09a3a (accessed 1 August 2016).

Hartmann, B. (2014) 'Converging on disaster: climate security and the Malthusian anticipatory regime for Africa', *Geopolitics*, vol., 19, no. 4, pp. 757–783.

Hartmann, B. and Hendrixson, A. (2005) 'Pernicious peasants and angry young men: the strategic demography of threats', in Hartmann, B., Subramaniam, B., and Zerner, C. (eds), 2005, *Making Threats: Biofears and Environmental Anxieties*, Rowman & Littlefield, Lanham, MD.

Hartmann, B., Subramaniam, B., and Zerner, C. (eds) (2005) *Making Threats: Biofears and Environmental Anxieties*, Rowman & Littlefield, Lanham, MD.

International Institute for Strategic Studies (IISS). (2016) 'Climate change and security' Online. Available HTTP: www.iiss.org/en/research/climate-s-change-s-and-s-security (accessed 1 August 2016).

Ki-moon, B. (2007) 'A climate culprit in Darfur', *Washington Post*, 16 June 2007. Online. Available: www.washingtonpost.com/wpdyn/content/article/2007/06/15/AR200706 1501857.html (accessed 1 August 2016).

Liska, A.J. and Perrin, R.K. (2010) 'Securing foreign oil: a case for including military operations in the climate change impact of fuels', *Environment: Science and Policy for Sustainable Development*. Online. Available: www.environmentmagazine.org/ Archives/Back%20Issues/July-August%202010/securing-foreign-oil-full.html (accessed 1 August 2016).

Liverman, D. (2007) 'From uncertain to unequivocal', *Environment: Science and Policy for Sustainable Development*, vol. 49, no. 8, pp. 28–32.

McMichael, A.J., Woodruff, R.E., and Hales, S. (2002) 'Climate change and human health: present and future risks', *Lancet*, vol. 367, pp. 859–869.

Moore, A. (2015) 'Anthropocene anthropology: reconceptualizing contemporary global change', *Journal of the Royal Anthropological Institute*, vol. 22, pp. 27–46.

Nagel, J. (2016) *Gender and Climate Change: Impacts, Science, Policy*, Routledge, New York, NY, and London, England.

NASA. (2016) 'Global climate change: vital signs of the planet'. Online. Available: http:// climate.nasa.gov/causes/ (accessed 20 July 2016).

O'Neill, B.C., Dalton, M., Fuchs, R., Jiang, L., Pachauri, S., and Zigova, K. (2010) 'Global demographic trends and future carbon emissions', *Proceedings of the National Academy of Sciences*, vol. 107, no. 41, pp. 17,521–17,526.

O'Neill, B.C., Liddle, B., Jiang, L., Smith, K.R., Pachauri, S., Dalton, M., and Fuchs, R. (2012) 'Demographic change and carbon dioxide emissions', *The Lancet*, vol. 380, no. 9837, pp. 157–164.

Pachauri, R.K. and Reisinger, A. (eds) (2007) 'Climate change, 2007: synthesis report', *IPCC*, Geneva, Switzerland. Online. Available: www.ipcc.ch/publications_and_data/ publications_ipcc_fourth_assessment_report_synthesis_report.htm (accessed 19 May 2016).

Paris, R. (2001) 'Human security: paradigm shift or hot air?' *International Security*, vol. 26, no. 2, pp. 87–102.

PopOffsets. n.d. Online. Available: www.populationmatters.org/popoffsets/ (accessed 10 May 2016).

Sasser, J.S. (2016) 'Population, climate change, and the embodiment of environmental crisis', Ch. 9 in Godfrey, P. and Torres, D. (eds), *Systemic Crises of Global Climate Change: Intersections of Race, Class, and Gender*, Routledge, London, England and New York, NY.

Sayre, N.F. (2012) 'The politics of the anthropogenic', *Annual Review of Anthropology*, vol. 41, pp. 57–70.

Schmuck, H. (2002) 'Empowering women in Bangladesh', *International Federation of Red Cross and Red Crescent Societies*. Online. Available: www.ifrc.org/en/news-and-media/news-stories/asia-pacific/bangladesh/empowering-women-in-bangladesh/ (accessed 1 August 2016).

USGCRP. (2016) '*The Impacts of Climate Change on Human Health in the United States: A Scientific Assessment.*' In Crimmins, A., Balbus, J., Gamble, J.L., Beard, C.B., Bell, J.E., Dodgen, D., Eisen, R.J., Fann, N., Hawkins, M.D., Herring, S.C., Jantarasami, L., Mills, D.M., Saha, S., Sarofim, M.C., Trtanj, J., and Ziska, L. (eds). U.S. Global Change Research Program, Washington, DC, 312 pp. Available: https://health2016.globalchange. gov (accessed 7 January 2016).

Watts, N., Adger, W.N., Agnolucci, P., Blackstock, J., Byass, P., Cai, W., Chaytor, S., Colbourn, T., Collins, M., Cooper, A., Cox, P.M., Depledge, J., Drummond, P., Ekins, P., Galaz, V., Grace, D., Graham, H., Grubb, M., Haines, A., Hamilton, I., Hunter, A., Jiang, X., Li, M., Kelman, I., Liang, L., Lott, M., Lowe, R., Luo, Y., Mace, G., Maslin, M., Nilsson, M., Oreszczyn, T., Pye, S., Quinn, T., Svensdotter, M., Venevsky, S., Warner, K., Xu, B., Yang, J., Yin, Y., Yu, C., Zhang, Q., Gong, P., Montgomery, H., and Costello, A. (2015) 'Health and climate change: policy responses to protect public health', *The Lancet*, vol. 386, no. 10006, pp. 1861–1914.

World Health Organization. (2005) 'Gender and health in natural disasters', WHO Department of Gender, Women, and Health, Geneva, Switzerland. Online. Available: http://apps.who.int/gender/gwhgendernd2.pdf?ua=1 (accessed 20 July 2016).

World Health Organization. (2007) 'Indoor air pollution: national burden of disease estimates', WHO Press: Geneva, Switzerland. Online. Available: www.who.int/indoorair/ publications/indoor_air_national_burden_estimate_revised.pdf (accessed 2 April 2016).

World Health Organization. (2012) 'Global health observatory data: mortality from household air pollution'. Geneva, Switzerland. Online. Available: www.who.int/gho/ phe/indoor_air_pollution/burden/en/ (accessed 2 April 2016).

World Health Organization. (2016) 'Protecting health from climate change', WHO Global Programme on Climate Change & Health, Geneva, Switzerland. Online. Available HTTP: www.who.int/globalchange/mediacentre/news/WHO-Climate-change-Programme-Summary-2016-2017.pdf?ua=1 (accessed 20 July 2016).

12 Bewitched or deranged

Access to health care for transgender persons

Chloe Schwenke

Introduction

It was a very big step for me, but my therapist had convinced me that the time had come. I really hadn't needed much persuasion; she had taken me through an exhaustive diagnostic process and the outcome was not in question. I was now secure; I had an authoritative expert's opinion of what I already intuitively knew was true; that I am a transgender woman. It was therefore time to begin my journey to health, my gender transition, and one key role player in that process would be the endocrinologist who would manage and monitor my hormone therapy.

We were all still using fax machines in 2008, and my therapist had sent a fax to my selected endocrinologist (whom I shall simply call 'Dr C') describing her diagnosis and offering him her considered judgment in support of my hormone therapy. When I arrived at Dr C's office at the prestigious George Washington University Hospital on the afternoon of June 13, I was met with a warm and very welcoming smile by the doctor. This wasn't going to be so bad . . .

I inquired if he'd read the fax from my therapist. He hadn't, but he promptly found it and began reading. Within less than a minute, he left his office without a word or any eye contact, his eyes still on that fax. I waited a very long time, but when he did return the smiles were gone. Instead, he addressed me in a manner that was both rude and patronizing, and he could barely bring himself to answer my questions or look me in the eyes. In the deprecating way in which he addressed me, it was painfully clear that Dr C resented my presence in his office, and had no interest in providing the support that I sought. I left, feeling truly disrespected and thoroughly humiliated.

For a very vulnerable and insecure transgender woman (still then presenting as male) just beginning her long and complicated gender transition, being so poorly received by a medical practitioner in the presumed safety of a relatively liberal East Coast city in the United States was my first unsettling experience engaging as a transgender person with the medical establishment. Other incidences were to follow, including during the next year when I was living my life full time as Chloe. I visited a dermatologist for a routine annual examination, and I disclosed my transgender status at the outset. She was so flustered by this disclosure that all she could do was ask me to leave before the examination ever began. Somehow, she found sufficient composure to request that I never come back.

These two personal experiences need to be seen in context. I'm very non-threatening, healthy, extremely well-educated, and articulate – in short, I am a privileged and relatively secure white American of the middle class. With but a few exceptions, I have faced only relatively mild forms of the harsh daily realities so common to most of my transgender sisters and brothers around the world: persistent unemployment, lack of familial support, violence, stigma, and comprehensive patterns of discrimination that often qualify as structural violence. Other realties common to my demographic I had missed entirely: dependence on drug and alcohol abuse, reliance on sex work for economic survival, abuse and discrimination from rule-of-law institutions and unjustified incarceration in gender-inappropriate settings, and homelessness. Yet one commonality I did share: along with an alarmingly large percentage of transgender persons I had given very serious consideration to suicide.[1]

These two personal health care anecdotes (unfortunately, I also have several others) are at best indicative of the state of knowledge about transgender issues among the medical establishment in Washington, D.C. eight years ago, and the structural violence imposed then (and to a considerable extent even still) by health insurance companies that routinely excluded any transgender-related medical procedures from coverage. In time, I was able to find very competent medical services from doctors who hadn't the slightest problem with my 'gender history,' although the costs for these services were totally mine to bear. I share these two unhappy accounts, however, only because they represent a much more comprehensive and challenging issue facing transgender persons around the world – the widespread and often institutionalized exclusion of trans people from health care, the multiple (and often intersecting) societal and environmental challenges to the health of transgender persons and particularly transgender women, and the resulting pervasive sense of insecurity that ensues from such treatment – particularly when it is endemic within a society. And while I had approached Dr C for very transgender-specific care, there wasn't anything uniquely transgender about my annual dermatological exam. Yet for health care that is either routine or transgender-specific, access for transgender persons to such services is fraught with insecurities.

In many countries, anecdotal evidence consistently demonstrates that transgender and gender nonconforming persons must run the gauntlet whenever they seek health care, and those on the feminine end of the gender continuum often confront health care standards that already discriminate against women and girls. Some policy efforts are underway to mitigate this reality, but their impact has yet to be felt widely.[2] For now, it is appropriate to recognize that we each claim multiple intersecting identities, and transgender women will frequently face discrimination on many counts (gender nonconforming, being female, race and ethnicity, age, and so on). Assume that you are a transgender person with a probable strep throat, and you know that this condition needs medical attention. You are also well aware that you can be turned away by the clinic immediately upon arrival if your appearance is deemed to be incongruous in some manner with 'normal' expectations. You can also be rejected upon arrival at the clinic when you attempt to register, and your identity documents describe someone with a name and gender marker that is not aligned with the authentic gender identity that you now claim. In most countries that is unavoidable, since in nearly two thirds of the world's countries there exists no realistic prospect of ever obtaining new legal identity documents that recognize a transgender change in status.[3] You also realize that you can feel rejected by the behavior of clerical and office staff, who have had no training about how to interact with transgender patients and who are likely to assault your dignity with accusations that you are somehow unnatural, immoral, sinful, or who cannot imagine why anyone classified as male would 'wish' to become female. You're also sensitive to the possibility that you'll be accused of being a homosexual (this category still being deemed repugnant by many people), regardless of the fact that the sexual orientation of transgender persons is not linked to their sense of authentic identity. Many transgender persons do not identify as homosexual.

Staff at the clinic may also decide that you are mentally incompetent or deranged, or they may patronize you as being simply an 'amusing' spectacle. And if these many institutional challenges were not daunting enough, you also stand a very good chance of being rejected by the evident homophobic, transphobic, and occasionally misogynistic attitudes and behaviors of the other patients waiting for treatment, who may (and frequently do) take great offense at your presence. These entrenched social norms and the resulting patterns of exclusion, and the often severe personal consequences that ensue for the transgender persons so affected, fit the description of structure violence (Galtung, 1969).

All of this is likely to happen before you've even seen a trained medical practitioner. Assuming that you have the fortitude to withstand those initial slights, challenges, and insecurities, there remains a very real prospect that the trained medical staff will find your presence in their clinic to be unacceptable or disruptive. Most will have had no training in the transgender phenomenon, even though a strep throat is ungendered. Still, some training in the health needs and realities routinely endured by transgender people – and in the most effective and respectful ways to communicate with transgender people – would go a great distance in making transgender persons feel respected, safe, and welcome when they come seeking health care.

Conditions vary widely between highly developed countries (HDCs) and less developed countries (LDCs). Should you, as a transgender person in an LDC, have the temerity to approach the medical establishment to seek specific health care associated with your transgender status or your desire to pursue hormonal, surgical, or other medical procedures to assist you in your transition to your authentic gender, your reception may be far worse than your plight with that strep throat. Whether in search of routine or specialized health care, transgender people around the world confront enormous obstacles and plausible threats to their safety, yet we only know this from anecdotal evidence such as the two personal incidences that I described above, and from the narratives shared by trans people globally.[4] With the important exception of research that is directly associated with the HIV pandemic, there's almost no empirical data recorded or routinely acquired regarding the quality, effectiveness, or safety of health care for transgender persons, and few donors seem to be in any hurry to fund or implement such research.[5] Even in the relatively well-funded field of HIV/AIDS research, the focus until as little as three years ago has been almost exclusively on gay men, and on a category of men who do not self-identify as gay or bisexual but who do acknowledge at least some sexual contact with other men (and are hence classified as 'men who have sex with men', or MSM). Only relatively recently was it (finally) discovered that transgender women have the highest HIV prevalence rates of all, and while that information (if inexcusably belated) is very valuable, it addresses only a small part of the overall health and security spectrum of transgender persons.[6]

Anecdotal narratives from around the world are compelling both in their number and their common characteristics, which should suffice in making the case that urgent steps are needed to remedy this widespread denial of a very basic human right: the right to safe and secure access to health care. And while it is beyond the scope of this chapter to provide a comprehensive global overview of denial of safe access to health care, I offer below brief examples and commentary on these challenges as they affected a small sample of transgender persons in four countries: Jamaica, Kenya, Russia, and the United States. This does not represent a robust survey, and is at best formative research based on key informant interviews with persons many of whom – for reasons of maintaining their personal safety – must remain anonymous. In time, hopefully, funding will be found for rigorous research employing the most effective methods of safely accessing what are classified in the research community as 'hidden populations,' but for now these observations must remain anecdotal and linked to personal contacts by the author. As a researcher, I wish that it were otherwise and that appropriately robust qualitative and quantitative research was underway around the world. It isn't. Still, while each example that I describe below has unique attributes, together they share many disturbing common parameters.

Jamaica[7]

Jamaica is not alone among Caribbean countries in navigating the divisive boundaries and the phenomenon of gendered, sexualized, and racialized bodies that together form complex inter-relationship between respecting the rule of law (mostly inherited from Victorian British social norms) and adherence to societal attitudes and behaviors that concentrate on class respectability and male privilege. In this context, feminist activism in Jamaica is deeply immersed in confronting that culture where violence against women and girls (including but not limited to domestic violence and intimate partner violence) remains widespread, and where strong traditional religious and cultural values still exert a compelling influence in defining the socially acceptable roles of women and girls. There have been some cross-overs into the larger spectrum of lesbian, gay, bisexual, transgender, queer, and intersex (LGBTQI) concerns, such as some forceful advocacy against the 'corrective rape' of lesbians. Also of note was the precedent-setting Caribbean Conference on Domestic Violence and Gender Equality. This was held in Jamaica in March 2014 and was a gathering that explicitly targeted gender-based violence within the LGBTQI community from a human rights framework, and showed no reticence in calling attention to the necessity of getting men and boys committed to the struggle against gender-based violence.[8]

Still, the issues around transgender Jamaicans have yet to be unpacked in any adequate way,[9] or focused on in their own context. Transgender persons experience intense levels of discrimination, exclusion, and violence in Jamaica, where transgender status is generally (but wrongly) almost entirely conflated with being homosexual. A tragic illustration of this was the brutal death of a 16-year-old transgender woman in July 2013, who came out of the closet and attended a party dressed as the woman she knew herself to be. Her debut was met with gunshots and stab wounds, and while her death was widely reported in the Jamaican and international press, and by organizations such as Human Rights Watch, she was almost always referred to as a 'cross-dressing man' and not as a transgender woman. She had suffered violence at the hands of her father for many years, and had been forced to leave school at 14 due to intense bullying. Ironically, only her male name 'Dwayne Jones' and male pronouns were ever cited in the media, and she went to her death denied any respect for her authentic gender identity.

Jamaican law criminalizes (male) homosexual conduct, and prevailing cultural and religious attitudes stigmatize and often lead to violence against homosexual Jamaicans of all genders. In 2011, the Jamaican government amended its Constitution, adding a new Charter of Fundamental Rights and Freedoms (Charter). Clause 2 of that Charter articulates a right to freedom from discrimination 'on the grounds of being male or female.' but makes no provisions for protection of Jamaicans on the basis of gender identity or sexual orientation. Under Jamaican law, there also exists no provision to enable a transgender person to achieve legal recognition in their authentic gender identity, effectively making them legally and economically non-persons.[10] Left with only their pre-transition documentation which doesn't align with what they claim as their authentic gender, they are unable to get a job, sign a lease, travel internationally, drive a vehicle, vote, and so on. Jamaican transgender persons also complain of the existence of many arbitrary laws that police use to justify their arrest and detention, for example on charges of 'gross indecency' (Jamaica Forum for Lesbians, All-Sexuals & Gays, Shadow Report, 2011).

Most Jamaican transgender people have long experience with exclusion, and therefore most suffer from lower levels of education, widespread unemployment, poverty, and an inability to afford basic services – including health care. Few Jamaicans openly identify as transgender men,[11] although recent indications are that this may now be starting to change. Relative to the general population, transgender Jamaicans are disproportionately affected by HIV and are very vulnerable to a range of sexually transmitted infections, often associated with the economic survival need to pursue high risk sex work.

In the context of accessing health care, the health sector (health care providers, insurance companies, public health officials, policy-makers, and health-focused legislators) is generally poorly informed about and generally insensitive to the characteristics and needs of their transgender community. Doctors, nurses, and other medical staff and clinicians are not trained in the care of transgender persons, and the Jamaican transgender community frequently finds that their authentic gender identities are not respected by such providers who often misgender them or refuse to use their preferred pronouns and names. Some of this treatment may be ascribed to ignorance or lack of training, but based on some reports the transgender community in Jamaica frequently finds such encounters very unsettling and even offensive, which is hardly conducive to ensuring regular access to safe and secure health care.

Given the high prevalence rates among transgender persons for HIV and sexually transmitted diseases,[12] and the overall low level of understanding of such diseases among the general population in Jamaica, transgender Jamaicans with HIV or who are at high-risk of contracting HIV suffer additional discrimination when seeking health-related services.[13]

Other concerns about health care providers expressed by Jamaican transgender persons include the tendency of such providers to view all health needs of transgender Jamaicans exclusively in terms of gender affirming surgeries or other health needs associated with gender transitioning. More prosaic and routine health needs are often ignored by the more sensationalized focus on those factors that make transgender people 'different.'

There have been some efforts made to redress this situation. In 2014, the U.S. Agency for International Development (USAID) funded the Health Policy Project, which included the roll out of a training pilot program and facilitators' manual (Health Policy Project, 2013) to help health care providers in Jamaica to better and more safely serve the transgender community. About 20 physicians, psychologists, psychiatrists, and nurses attended, together with transgender individuals and representatives from Jamaica's National Family Planning Board. Also, as of 2016 under a pilot project being carried out by ITECH (International Training and Education Center for Health), clinicians are being trained on appropriate and respectful ways to work with LGBTQI clients/patients.[14]

In other initiatives, the National Family Planning Board (NFPB) has also been hosting workshops from the middle of 2015 to the present for government employees to foster awareness of transgender realities and associated health concerns, making the distinction clearly between sexual orientation and gender identity. Jamaica Aids Support for Life, under funding by the Elton John Foundation, has also been reaching out to the transgender community, offering counseling and access to medical services (although such services do not include hormone therapy or access to an endocrinologist). UWIHARP, PRIDE in Action, and NFPB are also embarking on a project to introduce transgender and general LGBTQI health services on the campus of the University of the West Indies and its extended campus on the north coast.[15]

Kenya[16]

As in any country where homophobia and transphobia are widespread and entrenched within social norms, and the patriarchy firmly in place, Kenyan transgender people are not easy to find. Still, some transgender Kenyans are making themselves known through civil society organizations and through the media. As with transgender people everywhere, they remain few in number, but their voices are beginning to share their perspectives in ways that were simply unavailable before. Many of these public narratives describe a highly patriarchal and inflexible medical establishment and health sector that places less emphasis on the health needs of women and girls compared with men and boys,[17] and that excludes, demeans, humiliates, and rejects transgender Kenyans.

Among the most publicly vocal and best-known of Kenya's transgender community is Audrey Mbugua, who prefers to identify herself as a 'transsexual' (a term generally understood to mean a transgender person who lives exclusively and consistently in their authentic gender identity). Her own words convey a harrowing sense of the insecurities that she and other Kenyan transgender persons face:

> Hostility from members of the public against transsexual Kenyans continues to be the hallmark of transsexual people's lives. These can take the form of name-calling, physical assaults, rape and the destruction of one's property. The excuse Kenyans give to justify such hostility is that transsexualism is un-African and un-Christian and so must be discouraged within Kenyan society . . . Religious and cultural fundamentalism plays a big role in promoting and condoning these dehumanizing acts.
>
> Transsexual Kenyans face entrenched prejudice in Kenya's medical sector. Despite incessant requests for medical services such as hormone therapy and sex-reassignment therapy, government officials and public hospitals continue to play the dirty games of tossing transsexual people from one government official to another. Discrimination in the medical sector is both overt and covert. For example, there was an incident of a chief executive officer of a hospital cancelling gender-reassignment therapy for a 25-year-old transsexual woman and asking her to have her parents send him a 'no objection' letter. This individual then revealed in the company of his friends that he will never allow his hospital to change what God had created . . .
>
> (Mbugua, 2009)

Despite the outspoken comments of activists such as Audrey Mbugua,[18] transgender people also experience a continuing invisibility in Kenya. As is so common in much of the world, transgender Kenyans are conflated with lesbians, gay men, and bisexuals. Even the U.S. State Department's recent human rights report fails to make any specific references to the plight of transgender Kenyans, focusing instead exclusively on issues associated with Kenyans who are homosexual (U.S. State Department, 2016).

The plight of Kenya's transgender women is particularly vexing, linked as it is with the traditional values that constrain women and girls to specific roles, but which also provide a widely understood and culturally attenuated level of meaning through such roles. Kenyan feminists struggle to reconcile their allegiance with traditions that on the one hand provide them with such valued identity, but on the other hand diminish their full human dignity and agency. Despite some modest recent legal reforms, Kenyan women remain largely subordinate to men and often are still perceived as the property of husbands or fathers. Many face arranged marriages at very young ages, are subject to widespread gender based violence, and through customary practices face vast inequalities in asset control and in access to quality health care, inheritance rights, entitlement to land ownership and use, employment, education, and personal opportunities for improving their well-being. Female genital cutting, while technically illegal in Kenya, remains at very high levels in many parts of the country, and women's participation in Kenya's democratic decision-making is still highly constrained. Among younger and better educated Kenyans of all genders in urban centers like Nairobi there are positive signs of improvements in gender equality awareness, but for the vast majority of Kenyans the old values and practices persist without revision, and with minimal evidence of any sustained effort by Kenyan men to embrace and act upon principles of gender equality.[19] Given this context, expecting traditional Kenyan society to embrace and respect the equal human dignity of Kenya's transgender women may be nothing short of folly for the foreseeable future.

This absence of a clear and obvious trajectory for transgender inclusion in Kenya doesn't mean that a vacuum exists in advocacy by Kenyan feminists for transgender Kenyans. In a 2013 posting on the Kenyan blogsite *Feministloft*, blogger Neo Musangi considers Audrey Mbugua's public narrative and calls Kenyans to account for their rejection of transgender realities:

> . . . we refuse to engage with our own sex/sexual/sexuality inconsistencies. We refuse to think of sexuality as a continuum . . . That's how hetero-patriarchal normativity works . . . Men have to be men and women must remain women . . . Audrey is . . . putting masculinities on the spot. How dare she?[20]

The data doesn't yet exist to provide a comprehensive view into the systemic constraints faced by Kenya's transgender community in accessing routine health care. To date, the emphasis has been the media's sensationalism-driven focus only on requests for health services by Kenyans seeking to transition genders. Transgender persons are more than their gender confirming surgeries and hormone therapies, but a holistic assessment of their dignity experience in the context of secure and safe health care is yet to be told.

Russia[21]

The plight of transgender Russians is shrouded in obscurity, misinformation, bureaucratic obfuscation, insecurity, and confusion. As is generally the case globally, based on numerous first-hand anecdotal reports most Russians appear to conflate the transgender phenomenon with sexual orientation, although in recent years the Russian media has also frequently been witnessed to link transgenderism to pedophilia and to forms of sexual conduct associated with gay men.[22]

Under Russian law, transgender persons are entitled to undergo gender affirming medical and surgical treatments, and to have their authentic gender (gender marker and gender-appropriate name) recognized in official documents, including a revised birth certificate. In reality, however, the procedures to obtain legal recognition after a gender transition are so burdensome, time-consuming, expensive, and lengthy that they are nearly impossible to achieve. One example of these constraints is the requirement that those seeking legal recognition of their authentic names and gender submit a 'certificate of gender change' – the template of which doesn't exist in any approved format. Russian state registry offices then frequently refuse to issue an amended birth certificate due to the lack of a submission using the proper form.[23]

It has also become common within Russia to associate LGBTQI status with an agenda to corrupt the morals of minors, and laws have been put into effect to prevent 'LGBTQI propaganda' as a measure to 'protect' Russian youth from accessing relevant information. An additional and very unfortunate consequence of this legislative tactic is that transgender Russian youth, who are often aware of (if not well informed about) their transgender status from a very early age, are unable to access counseling and therapeutic help in the early and highly insecure stages of their gender identity struggles. In other countries, anecdotal evidence suggests that a similar lack of access to such information and to competent psychological support may be linked to high rates of suicidal ideation, but in such countries as in Russia there is no data collected on this phenomenon. The Russian medical establishment and public health officials have made negligible efforts, formally or informally, to address either the health needs of transgender Russians or the insecurity and discrimination that they face in seeking health care. Both the Fundamentals of Legislation of the Russian Federation on Health Care and the 2010 Draft Federal Law on the Fundamentals of the Care for Health of the Citizens in the Russian Federation articulate anti-discrimination standards (Article 17, and Article 5 respectively), yet the lists of discrimination parameters cited by both documents fail to include gender identity or sexual orientation.

Pragmatically, most Russian medical professionals and specialists (particularly in rural areas) have inadequate or no training in health issues pertaining to transgender persons. For example, while some medical practitioners are amenable to prescribing hormone replacement therapy, their lack of knowledge of the correct endocrine profile that should be achieved exposes many of their transgender patients to considerable health risks. This widespread lack of competence among Russian physicians regarding medical support for gender transitions is now well-known within the Russian transgender community, and many transgender Russians also have had experiences of physicians who have been transphobic or otherwise hostile to them. Not surprisingly, many transgender Russians prefer self-medicating with hormones purchased on the black-market, a practice that is inherently high in health risks.

Overall, the daily realities faced by transgender Russians are grim. In written comments dated 10 June 2015 submitted to the European Court of Human Rights in the Case of Bogdanova vs. Russia, it was noted that:

> Transgender people are more likely to be homeless than the general population . . . Many transgender people report feeling lonely or isolated, and some but not all experience mental health issues. Research undertaken in different European countries consistently shows higher suicide rates and self-harming behavior among transgender people. Transgender people surveyed typically cite a number of trans-related reasons for such behavior, including gender dysphoria, not having their gender recognized, social stigma, frustrations with treatment delays, lack of access to treatment, worry that they would never 'fully' or 'successfully' transition, having their identity misunderstood by health professionals and not feeling supported by gender identity specialists . . . Transgender people face systemic discrimination trying to access general health care services, which includes being treated with contempt or refused care. . . . Health care professionals may be ignorant of the specific health needs of transgender people, lack the professional training to meet their health needs, or refuse to provide treatment due to transphobic prejudice.
>
> (TGEU, 2015)

One distinctive feature of the transgender phenomenon in Russia is that based on the social norms held by the majority of the Russian public, it would appear that the majority of Russians generally hold their transgender population in contempt. This will need to be validated through robust research, as will the many anecdotal reports that Russian attitudes toward female-to-male transgender people are more positive than their views of male-to-female transgender persons. Such gender-skewed attitudes may also account for the rough estimates (again, such data is very anecdotal) that transgender men outnumber transgender women in Russia, which may well be indicative of the powerful influence of Russian society's assignment of much higher status to men. If so, this is unlikely to change anytime soon. Currently, feminism in Russia is beleaguered, and certainly Russian feminists are not well positioned to advocate on behalf of Russia's transgender population (Sundstrom, 2010).

Russian President Vladimir Putin has ushered in an age of exaggerated patriarchy in which male values and attributes are widely praised (often in crude locker-room language), in a society that already had deep patriarchal roots despite the superficial assertions of gender equality under Communism. Simultaneously, Putin and the Russian political elite have nurtured an expanding narrative intended to reinforce the traditional domestic dependency role of women and girls, and bolstered this messaging with the passage of repressive legislation that significantly cuts the funding of women's crisis centers, along with stronger regulations restricting access to abortions. The highly gendered power dynamics in Russia have been anything but subtle, as described by Nicola-Ann Hardwick:

Russia's transition period from communism to a new regime was fundamentally linked to gender. In the tumultuous Gorbachev and Yeltsin eras, women faced a myriad of challenges, some of them, once again, rather paradoxical. On the one hand, the policies of glasnost and perestroika led to a belated sexual revolution in Russia . . . male homosexuality was decriminalized in 1993 and a new criminal code in 1997 redefined rape and the age of consent. Yet, the developments in the early 1990s soon also revealed that the narrative on sex and gender roles would remain in the state's control. With the upsurge in rampant consumerism, the post-Soviet market has objectified women 'as trophies and servants to men.' Political discourses reconstructed the role of women as belonging to the domestic sphere, feminism continued to be linked with negative connotations such as ugliness, hatred of men, and lesbianism (as it had been since the Brezhnev period), and women's organizations received little grassroots support.

(Hardwick, 2014)

For now, most Russian transgender people keep a low profile, and while 'LGBTQI' civil society groups do exist in Russia it is very difficult to find any transgender (or intersex) members within them. Instead, the voice of transgender Russia is subdued and repressed by the structural violence of a society that rejects them, and consequently their prospects for achieving higher standards of quality, safety, and inclusiveness in accessing health care is unlikely to improve within the foreseeable future.

United States

As I write this, the United States is immersed in a heated public controversy about whether civil and political rights protections extend to gender identity. Specifically, this debate is about access to public school toilet facilities and locker rooms, whether transgender youth in public schools or any transgender persons seeking to use any public toilet facility that aligns with their authentic gender identity should be allowed to do so (versus being required to use the facilities that align with the gender marker on their original birth certificate), and whether transgender persons should be allowed to serve in the armed forces. This political, media, and cultural firestorm directed at transgender persons (and transgender youth and young adults in particular) is characterized by a rancorous display of misinformation, fear, prejudice, sexism, ignorance, religious extremism, and bombast that undercuts any sense of security for this very vulnerable demographic. In due course the news cycle will have its way; the American media and public will move on and the political and civil rights of transgender Americans will be left to the courts and legislators (federal and state, and in some cases even to municipal and local governments) to decide. What is left unanswered is how and when transgender Americans will find our way to a durable sense of safety and security in accessing public accommodations, and by inference, public services.

There may be some unintended benefits from this current heightened focus on transgender people and our 'issues' arising out of this controversy, bolstered by the recent high-profile attention directed at celebrity transgender women such as Caitlyn Jenner, Janet Mock, Laverne Cox, and numerous transgender models and fashion designers. American consciousness is being raised to the reality and existence of at least a 'glamorous' celebrity stereotype of transgender women (and to a much lesser extent to transgender men). It remains an open question, however, whether this awakening will begin to translate into a transformation of social norms and a softening of attitudes among the American general public, or any better understanding of the many intersectionality issues that have significance in the context of claiming an authentic identity, and consequently to progress in achieving improved quality of life and security for ordinary transgender persons in the United States. In the interim, American transgender women – especially transgender women of color – are facing exceptionally high rates of violence, humiliation, and insecurity.[24]

At least in the United States there is some data – the beginnings of an empirical baseline from which to track changes. It is still only a beginning, but a number of key public health organizations have recognized that critical gaps exist in the identification and application of appropriate health indicators to gather health sector performance data in meeting the specific needs of minority and marginalized populations, including transgender Americans (Stroumsa, 2014). In 2015 the U.S. Trans Survey (USTS) was carried out, as a follow-up to the National Transgender Discrimination Survey. With over 27,000 respondents (age 18 and older) from every state and U.S. territory, the USTS is the largest on-line survey ever carried out to date on the lives and experiences of trans people in any country. That original study was developed and conducted by the National LGBTQ Task Force and the National Center for Transgender Equality in 2008–09, and the results were released in the 2011 report: 'Injustice at Every Turn.' The later study was the product of the National Center for Transgender Equality in Washington, D.C. (which the author has supported both as a member and as a paid consultant), and was released in December of 2016.

In the context of accessing health care, the data from these two surveys is very sobering. Transgender Americans randomly selected to participate in the initial survey were clearly seen to be experiencing high levels of insecurity, due to being discriminated against not only in their access to American health care but in nearly every aspect of American society. More than 25% of the respondents cope with this insecurity and discrimination by turning to drugs or alcohol. The elevated level of insecurity is also registered in the HIV rates reported by transgender respondents, which were over four times the national average, with exceptionally high HIV prevalence rates (15.32%) for transgender women who engaged in sex work. With respect to accessing health care specifically, 19% of the initial survey's sample reported that they were refused health care services due to their transgender or gender nonconforming status, with even higher numbers among people of color in the survey. Nearly a third of respondents (28%) reported that they had been subjected to harassment in a medical setting, and half of respondents related having had to teach their medical providers about transgender care (Grant *et al.*, 2011: 1). In the later survey, respondents encountered high levels of mistreatment when seeking health care, with one-third (33%) of those who saw a health care provider in the year prior to the survey having had at least one negative experience related to their transgender status. Examples cited in the 2015 survey include being verbally harassed or refused treatment because of their gender identity. In addition, almost one-quarter (23%) of the 2015 survey respondents acknowledged that they had not even sought needed health care based on their expectation of a hostile reception (James, 2016).

These grim statistics should not be assumed to speak to patriarchal attitudes alone. Some second-wave American feminists also have been and remain outspoken critics of transgender persons – especially transgender women. Arguably, this polemic began back in 1973 at the West Coast Lesbian Conference, held in Los Angeles. At that event, keynote speaker Robin Morgan offered a thoroughly excoriating rebuke to the inclusion of a transgender folksinger on the conference agenda, saying:

> I will not call a male 'she'; thirty-two years of suffering in this androcentric society, and of surviving, have earned me the title 'woman'; one walk down the street by a male transvestite, five minutes of his being hassled (which he may enjoy), and then he dares, he *dares* to think he understands our pain? No, in our mothers' names and in our own, we must not call him sister.
>
> (Goldberg, 2014)

Thankfully such extreme views are becoming a fringe phenomenon by this stage, and transgender women have also become progressively more effective and secure in pushing back strongly against such views. With the coming of third-wave feminism with its focus on individual identity, its embrace of diversity and intersectionality, the recognition of the degree to which economic advantages and related privileges are distributed on the basis of gender, gender identity, sexual orientation, and other subjugated identities, and its rejection of an American feminism anchored in a universal female identity (as defined by upper middle class white American women), feminists in contemporary America have come to embrace transgender women as sisters and to also find some solidarity with transgender men. Currently feminism in the United States is much more about sensitivity to gender identity, the meaning of gender, the economic and political impacts and realities associated with gender, and the use of gender-inclusive language than it is about defending the purity of the claim to womanhood. American feminists now are sensitized not only to the subjugation and disadvantages faced by American women and girls due to patriarchy, but are increasingly aware of the impact of 'cisgender privilege' (cisgender being a term for all non-transgender people) on their ability to empathize comprehensively with their transgender sisters and brothers. And while patriarchy in the United States is recognized and understood more thoroughly than ever before, the power of that patriarchy remains very strong – as recent political attacks on women's reproductive rights have made clear.

Health care in America still places women at a disadvantage, with complex health insurance arrangements that foster a sense of dependence on health care providers and that limit public access to certain information. With access to affordable and effective health care so tightly linked to formal sector employment, there's a perceived hierarchy of who is most valuable within American society – and that remains white males in formal employment. Mothers who have elected to stay at home rely as dependents on their spouse's employment to achieve security in their access to health care, and since American women typically do not rise to the same higher levels in their employment as American men do, such women face fewer health care benefits associated with higher income positions. In this context, transgender Americans are among the most marginalized and insecure, as transgender Americans experience extremely high rates of unemployment and hence are very exposed to the lack of health care insurance coverage.

Unaffordable or ineffectual health insurance isn't the only challenge for transgender Americans to achieve security in accessing health care. There simply are not enough physicians and medical staff who have the knowledge, competence, or inclination to provide quality health care to transgender patients.

Conclusion

These examples from four countries illustrate how far we have to go to achieve societies where not only women and girls receive equivalent access to health care as do men and boys, but also where marginalized groups and sexual minorities are also included and respected as valuable, dignified, and equal persons. These brief case studies also show the negative impact on transgender access to health care that have their origin in the resilience of traditional cultural values and patriarchal attitudes, in the lack of information and training on transgender realities, and in the conflation between gender identity and sexual orientation. The many negative influences affecting the health of transgender persons frequently become so engrained and institutionalized that they constitute a pernicious form of structural violence, with deeply deleterious impacts on the well-being of transgender persons. And while not all of the anecdotal reports are dire – an alternative but small literature of more positive narratives does exist[25] – the preponderance of such accounts are very troubling.

While we might like to consider the United States to be leading a trend for acceptance of transgender diversity in health care, strong contrary voices remain influential. Robert P. George, who is the McCormick Professor of Jurisprudence at Princeton University and who is widely respected as a prominent academic, lawyer, conservative Roman Catholic thinker, and legal theorist, recently issued his opinion: 'There are few superstitious beliefs as absurd as the idea that a woman can be trapped in a man's body & vice versa . . .'.[26]

Is the transgender phenomenon the product of superstition, or mental delusion? Are transgender persons best thought of as people who are somehow bewitched or deranged? Such opinions from prominent persons are themselves outrageous and irresponsible. The growing inventory of transgender narratives from all over the world – narratives that demonstrate a remarkable degree of consistency in the shared experience of transgender people sensing and claiming our true gender identity – is hard to dismiss so blithely. Transgender people have demonstrated, time and again, our need to put at jeopardy everything we hold dear to claim the security that comes from being authentically oneself. As long as Prof. George and people of his mindset continue to feel emboldened to pass their ill-informed judgment of an entire global demographic who have experienced extreme discomfort, discrimination, abuse, humiliation, violence and even death in order to claim our authenticity, transgender people will remain insecure. When intellectual, political, religious, social, professional, or other leaders and opinion-shapers assault the fundamental dignity of an entire class of persons by accusing us of being irrational or deranged, they strengthen a culture in which the humanity, safety, and security of the people they demean is undercut and diminished. The result is clear: access to health services are withheld or severely compromised for those who dare to be 'different' by being ourselves.

Notes

1   There is very little reliable evidence of incidence rates of suicidal ideation, or attempted suicides, among transgender persons. One exception is the U.S. Transgender Survey 2015, which found that in the United States 40% of its survey respondents have attempted suicide in their lifetime – nearly nine times the attempted suicide rate in the U.S. population (4.6%). See James, S. E., Herman, J. L., Rankin, S., Keisling, M., Mottet, L., & Anafi, M. (2016). *The Report of the 2015 U.S. Transgender Survey*. Washington, DC: National Center for Transgender Equality, at http://www.ustrans survey.org/report.
2   The World Health Organization (WHO) is beginning to address these issues of transgender exclusion to medical care, through: (1) recommended changes to relevant sections of the 11th edition of the *International statistical classification of diseases and related health problems (ICD-11)*; (2) the adoption of a person-centered approach to transgender people's health; and (3) a policy and practice framing of the health of transgender persons based on human rights and equity parameters. See Rebekah Thomas, Frank Pega, Rajat Khosla, Annette Verster, Tommy Hanaa & Lale Sayc: 'Ensuring an inclusive global health agenda for transgender people,' *Bull World Health Organ* 2017;95:154–156 | doi: http://dx.doi.org/10.2471/BLT.16.183913.
3   See http://www.nationalgeographic.com/magazine/2017/01/gender-identity-map-where-you-can-change-your-gender-on-legal-documents/.
4   There is a very small but growing global literature in this context. See, for example, 'The search for international consensus on LGBT health' by Scherdel, Martin, Deivanayagam, Adams, and Shanahan in www.thelancet.com/lancetgh Vol. 2 June 2014; 'Health equity for LGBTQ people through education' by Duvivier and Wiley in www.thelancet.com Vol 387 April 2, 2016; and illustrative of press coverage: 'Transgender patients face challenges at the hospital' by Ellin, in the *New York Times* of February 16, 2016 at http://well.blogs.nytimes.com/2016/02/16/for-transgender-patients-challenges-at-the-hospital.
5   See the entire issue on 'HIV epidemics among transgender populations: on the importance of a trans-inclusive response,' with guest editors Poteat, Keatley, Wilcher and Schwenke in www.jiasociety.org/index.php/jias/issue/view/1480 of July 2016.
6   The CDC has estimated the HIV prevalence among transgender women was 22% in five high-income countries, including the United States, and that 28% of transgender

women had HIV infection while 12% of transgender women self-reported having HIV. This discrepancy suggests many transgender women living with HIV don't know their HIV status. The CDC also report that black/African American transgender women were most likely to test HIV positive, compared with those of other races/ethnicities: 56% of black/African American transgender women had positive HIV test results compared to 17% of white or 16% of Hispanic/Latina transgender women. Among the 3.3 million HIV testing events reported to the CDC in 2013, the highest percentages of newly identified HIV-positive persons were among transgender persons. Although HIV prevalence among transgender men is relatively low (0–3%), a 2011 study suggests that transgender men who have sex with men are at substantial risk for acquiring HIV. See http://www.cdc.gov/hiv/group/gender/transgender/.

7   This section was developed with the advice and review of Jamaican transgender activist Laura Garcia and others in the Jamaican transgender community who shall remain anonymous.

8   See https://feministactivism.com/tag/caribbean-conference-on-domestic-violence-and-gender-equality/.

9   For example, through social norms analysis, or through research specifically on social inclusion.

10   Jamaicans are able to obtain a legal change of name through a deed poll process, but transgender people who have pursued this option report that they are treated with disdain and are subject to intense humiliation and disrespect. It is not possible under current Jamaican law to have one's gender marker changed.

11   The BBC filmed a short documentary in 2015 about two young Jamaican transgender men, now resident in the U.K., who return on a brief visit to Jamaica to seek acceptance from their respective families. See http://transguys.com/videos/trans-men-jamaica.

12   See www.cdc.gov/hiv/group/gender/transgender/.

13   As noted in the Shadow Report of 2011: 'Health workers in Jamaica reportedly routinely mistreat patients with HIV or AIDS by providing inadequate care or by denying treatment altogether. In certain cases, doctors are afraid to touch infected patients, effectively preventing them from conducting adequate examinations . . . Those who have made it to clinics are sometimes turned away and subjected to abusive comments from health care providers, decreasing the chances that they will get treatment. Cases have been documented in which health workers have released confidential medical information about HIV/AIDS patients to the public and other patients by segregating the HIV positive patients from the other patients.'

14   This program is being rolled out not only in Jamaica but also in Trinidad and two other Caribbean countries.

15   Details of these programmatic interventions were made available to the author by the Jamaican transgender activist Laura Garcia.

16   This section was developed with the advice and peer review of Kenyan transgender activist and queer African feminist blogger Barbra Wangare Maruga, and Neo Sinoxolo Musangi, Humanities Research Fellow at the British Institute in Eastern Africa.

17   Kenya still has one of the highest maternal mortality rates in the world, at an estimated 400 deaths per 100,000 births in 2013. See www.google.com/search?q=Kenya%2C+less+emphasis+on+the+health+needs+of+women+and+girls+&ie=utf-8&oe=utf-8#q=Kenya,+gender+gap+in+health,+women&start=10.

18   Audrey Mbugua also shares a short narrative of her life in the video https://www.youtube.com/watch?v=f7ngUWtTtuQ.

19   See 'Gender Inequalities in Kenya', edited by Creighton and Yieke, UNESCO 2006 at www.unesdoc.unesco.org/images/0014/001458/145887e.pdf.

20   See www.feministloft.com/audrey-mbugua-is-in-the-news-again-bebecomingbeing-transgender-in-kenya/#comments.

21   This section was developed with the advice and review of Russian LGBTI activist Oleg Tomilin.

22 See https://mic.com/articles/58649/russia-s-anti-gay-law-spelled-out-in-plain-english#.
    ENDaYoeQK.
23 See www.sutyajnik.ru/documents/4995.pdf.
24 See www.avp.org/storage/documents/ncavp_transhvfactsheet.pdf .
25 Such a positive literature regarding transgender realities (although not specifically
    about health and security) remains small and highly personal, largely accessible only in
    memoirs of transgender persons who have transitioned successfully to lives of greater
    peace and meaning. Illustrative examples would include *Redefining Realness: My Path
    to Womanhood, Identity, Love & So Much More* (2014, Atria Books) by Janet Mock;
    She's Not There: A Life in Two Genders (2013, Broadway Books) by Jennifer Boylan;
    and *Through the Door of Life: A Jewish Journey between Genders* (2012, University of
    Wisconsin Press) by Joy Ladin.
26 This opinion was stated in a Tweet on May 15, 2016. See www.breitbart.com/big-
    government/2016/05/16/princeton-prof-transgenderism-not-scientific-superstitious-
    belief.

References

Center for Disease Control and Prevention (2013). Online. Available: www.cdc.gov/hiv/
    group/gender/transgender/ (accessed June 3, 2016).
Galtung, Johan (1969). 'Violence, peace, and peace research,' *Journal of Peace Research*,
    Vol. 6, No. 3, pp. 167–191. Available: www.gsdrc.org/document-library/violence-peace-
    and-peace-research/ (accessed August 30, 2016).
Goldberg, Michelle (2014). 'What is a woman? The dispute between radical feminism and
    transgenderism.' *The New Yorker*, August 4, 2014.
Grant, Jaime M.; Lisa, A.; Mottet, Justin; Tanis, Jack; Harrison, Jody; Herman, L., and
    Keisling, Mara (2011). *Injustice at Every Turn: A Report of the National Transgender
    Discrimination Survey*. Washington: National Center for Transgender Equality and
    National Gay and Lesbian Task Force.
Hardwick, Nicola-Ann (2014). 'Reviewing the changing situation of women in Russian
    society.' Online. Available: www.e-ir.info/2014/12/20/reviewing-the-changing-situation-
    of-women-in-russian-society (accessed June 6, 2016).
Health Policy Project. (2013). *Understanding and Challenging HIV and Key Population
    Stigma and Discrimination: Caribbean Facilitator's Guide*. Washington, DC: Futures
    Group, Health Policy Project.
Jamaica Forum for Lesbians, All-Sexuals & Gays (2011). *Human Rights Violations of
    Lesbian, Gay, Bisexual, and Transgender (LGBT) People in Jamaica: A Shadow Report*.
    Online: www2.ohchr.org/english/bodies/hrc/docs/ngos/LGBT_Jamaica103.pdf.
James, S. E., Herman, J. L., Rankin, S., Keisling, M., Mottet, L., & Anafi, M. (2016). *The
    Report of the 2015 U.S. Transgender Survey*. Washington, DC: National Center for
    Transgender Equality.
Mbugua, Audrey (2009). Untitled article in Pambazuka News, Online. Available: www.
    pambazuka.org/governance/hardships-faced-transsexual-people-kenya (accessed June
    8, 2016).
Stroumsa, Daphna (2014). 'The state of transgender health care: Policy, law, and medical
    frameworks,' *American Journal of Public Health*; 104(3), pp. e31–e38. Available: www.
    medscape.com/viewarticle/821141_3 (accessed June 8, 2016).
Sundstrom, Lisa McIntosh (2010). 'Russian women's activism: Two steps forward, one
    step back' in *Women's Movements in a Global Era*, ed. Amrita Basu. Boulder: Westview
    Press, 253.

Thomas, R.; Pega, F.; Khosla, R.; Verster, A.; Hanaa T.; and Sayc, L. (2017). 'Ensuring an inclusive global health agenda for transgender people,' *Bulletin of the World Health Organization*; 2017; 95:154–156.

Transgender Europe (TGEU). Coming Out, The European Region of the International Lesbian, Gay, Bisexual, Trans and Intersex Association (ILGA-Europe), The European Professional Association for Transgender Health (EPATH) joint submission (2015). 'Written Comments dated 10 June 2015 in the European Court of Human Rights in the Case of Bogdanova v. Russia' (Application No. 63378/13). Available: www.google.com/search?q=Written+Comments+dated+10+June+2015+in+the+European+Court+of+Human+Rights+in+the+Case+of+Bogdanova+v.+Russia&ie=utf-8&oe=utf-8 (accessed June 8, 2016).

U.S. State Department (2016). 'Country reports on human rights practices for 2015.' Available: www.state.gov/j/drl/rls/hrrpt/humanrightsreport/index.htm#wrapper (accessed June 11, 2016).

13 Development as violence

Corporeal needs, embodied life, and the sustainable development goals

Colleen O'Manique and Pieter Fourie

Introduction

This chapter casts a critical eye on the prospects for securing girls' and women's health through the UN Sustainable Development Goals (SDGs), which were endorsed by member states of the United Nations as the *de facto* global instrument for development from 2016 to 2030. We consider two United Nations (UN) outcome documents, namely 'Transforming Our World: the 2030 Agenda for Sustainable Development' (TOW), which the UN General Assembly ratified on 25 September 2015, and 'The Addis Ababa Action Agenda of the Third International Conference on Financing for Development' (FfD), which the UN General Assembly endorsed on 27 July 2015. Transforming Our World sets out the SDGs '. . . that seek to build on the [Millennium Development Goals] and complete what these did not achieve' (Preamble 2030 Agenda), while FfD is the final outcome document of negotiations on the financial architecture for funding the SDGs.

TOW is the most recent UN grand scheme to end global poverty. Crafted by the UN General Assembly through a three-year process of consultations with a wide range of stakeholders across the globe, the 17 SDGs and the 169 associated targets replace the eight MDGs that were launched in 2000 and expired at the end of 2015. The SDGs take over as the development establishment's global instrument for development and poverty alleviation. Both the MDGs and SDGs contain an explicit as well as an implicit focus on gender equality and the empowerment of women: three of the eight original MDGs had girls and women in sight, and there was a stated understanding that all eight goals applied equally to all people. While only one of the 17 SDGs, Goal 5 ('Achieve gender equality and empowering all women and girls') focuses explicitly on women, women and gender are integrated throughout both TOW and FfD.

With regards to 'women's empowerment', it has been widely recognized, even within the UN, that the MDGs failed to deliver on their promise. But those who have crafted the SDGs maintain that the highly consultative process of civil society engagement leading to the final consensus has created a potentially transformative document that contrasts with the technocratic and top-down nature of the MDGs. While scepticism remains in terms of how impactful the SDGs will be for securing gender justice, there has been a palpable optimism that the SDGs are different.

However, there are visible contradictions between the aspirations contained in TOW and a global financing framework that embraces the model of global geopolitical and financial governance foundational to the current economic and eco-systemic crisis. Both documents reflect the central role of the private sector and multinational corporations (MNCs) in the SDG project in ways that render invisible their current role in the intensification of inequality, environmental destruction, and gender injustice. We argue that the promise of the SDG project will be limited for the same reason that the MDGs have failed women: gender injustice is implicated in the network of social and economic relations that constitute the current structurally violent dynamics of the global economy.

This chapter reflects on the following questions: What constitutes 'gender equality' and 'women's empowerment' in both agendas? And to what extent can they be achieved within the context of the SDGs and its proposed financing framework? We identify the stable meanings contained in both documents that construct a particular view of sustainable development and women's 'empowerment', a view that naturalizes the continued exploitation of gendered, classed, and racialized bodies in the global economy. We examine the relationship between the SDG project, women's wage labour, and social reproduction: the material and ideological spaces where the demands of socially necessary labour, much of it unwaged, have intensified over the past four decades of neoliberalism. We also examine how the SDGs fall short on sexual and reproductive health and rights. We begin with the basic understanding that bodily autonomy and integrity and control over one's sexual and reproductive life, secure livelihoods and incomes that include time for rest and leisure; access to nutritious food, clean water, unpolluted, stable and peaceful environments; and access to public goods such as quality education, health care, and democratic participation are foundational to health security. These fundamental requirements for health mirror many of the requirements for human development that are codified in the Universal Declaration of Human Rights: food, water, shelter, security, a non-threatening physical environment, education, and self-determination. SRHR are indivisible from other rights claims, given that they are foundational to the enjoyment of other rights. The gendered division of reproductive labour has been normalized as the 'natural' extension of biological reproduction, with women's unpaid care labour subsidizing the productive economy still a universal constant. The guarantee of the exercise of SRHR is therefore critical to girls' and women's overall health and well-being, and is foundational to challenging the deeply engrained impulse for male control of girls' and women's bodies that is written into and religious and state laws, and the hierarchy of labouring bodies in local and global economies.

To calibrate our analysis we interviewed 14 key informants – civil society representatives, government officials, and development practitioners – from South Africa and Canada who were either part of or closely observed the process leading up to the publication of the SDGs. As we have stated elsewhere (O'Manique and Fourie, 2016), Canada and South Africa are interesting contexts, as they are both exemplars of middle power states aiming to consolidate their soft power. Both countries wish to be viewed as good global citizens, but they do so within different geopolitical contexts. Both countries have participated in the global neoliberal turn in the last three decades, and both have signed up to the MDGs and the SDGs, and institutionally embrace the framework. The interviews were conducted between November 2015 and May 2016, and in order to enable reflections that are free of institutional and other constraints, we anonymized the respondents' reflections. Our interview schedule consisted of unstructured questions, allowing respondents with as much freedom as possible to reflect and to raise issues and pursue lines of thinking. Our discussions focused on respondents' views on both the TOW and the FfD, and more specifically, on the prospects for gender justice through the 2030 Agenda, and some of their responses appear in italics. We interpreted our interview data in tandem with the most recent analyses of the SDGs to have emerged since September 2015, and some of our respondents' comments appear in indented italics.

We begin with a brief historical context and account of gender justice in the MDGs and their reshaping in the SDGs as the backdrop to this critique. The chapter then provides an account of how gender issues have been framed discursively within both TOW and FfD. We make explicit our reservations about the SDGs' silence around social reproduction and SRHR, thus perpetuating a particularly misogynistic, neoliberal structural violence. We conclude with a reflection on the prospects for women's labour, SRHR, and for gender justice through the 2030 agenda and the long-term viability of the development industry's stated aspiration to be transformative, rather than regressive.

The context

The development industry emerged in earnest after World War II, ostensibly as a corollary of the decolonisation movement of the 1950s and 1960s (and thus steeped in Cold War considerations and geopolitical pragmatics) and since the post-War period has increasingly evolved as a neoliberal project. The Eurocentric notion of 'development' has its antecedents in the

> . . . colonization people's cultures, economies, and political and social systems by marginalizing the indigenous, taking away the control of their land, extracting their labour and other resources, and creating an international division of labour designed to stimulate the industrialization and enrichment of the colonizer and force the decline of native industries.
>
> (Trietler and Boatcă, 2016: 161)

We acknowledge that there have always been and there remain progressive voices both inside and outside the UN galaxy; there is no simple and unified narrative, and people working within UN bodies, bilateral aid programmes, granting institutions and non-governmental, and civil society organizations have different standpoints, perspectives, and intents. But over time, their influence has been subject to the same political and ideological forces that have led to neoliberalism's consolidation: the failure to address intransigent structural and political inequalities between the global North and South forged through colonization, and the deepening professional-ization, de-politicization, and the capture of the development project by private actors (Banks, Hulme, and Edwards, 2014: 709; Adams and Martins, 2015).

Development assistance is still able to vaccinate children and provide HIV drugs, deliver contraceptives and clean cookstoves, and build roads and schools, but most interventions are palliative, and cannot address the increasing corporate concentration of power and the crises that it creates. Development has become a multi-billion dollar enterprise; a set of knowledges, technologies and practices that are understood as relatively autonomous from geopolitical realities and the governance of the global political economy, despite the fact that the neoliberal project within which the development industry is embedded shapes today's obscene levels of inequality and life chances that development ostensibly addresses. Hawkesworth (2016) portrays the politics of twenty-first century development as disembodied to the extent that 'difference' has become naturalized. Centuries of colonial domination and their continuities in both nation-state and global policies have authorized 'a racialized gendering that masks embodied power and raced-gendered systems of privilege and advantage' (p. 18). While population and development policies have been designed to foster economic growth, they have been intricately involved in shaping the life chances of differently classed, and racialized women, their intimate lives and their gendered labour across the globe (Hawkesworth, 2016: 162).

> Operating through national legislation, moral prohibitions, informal mecha-nisms of social control, appeals to the conscience of the world community, sexual and racial divisions of labour . . . international conventions support and maintain regulatory sexual and racial regimes that undermine the autonomy of certain subjects while shoring up the power of others.
>
> (Hawkesworth, 2016: 162)

The common sense understanding is that the market determines the value of various labouring bodies in the global economy, with those at the top of the wealth pyramid, the most entrepreneurial, hard-working and risk-taking, and therefore deserving of their wealth. Those labouring at the bottom need only be 'empowered' through targeted investments in education, health, micro-entrepreneurship, and access to family planning to reap the benefits of development. Amancio Ortega, the owner of Zara, is one of the eight richest men in the world today; his collective wealth is as much as the poorest 3.6 billion people on the planet, the majority who happen to be female. In the factories of Vietnam and Myanmar that make clothes sold at Zara, women work up to 18 hours a day, and sometimes through the night, yet do not earn enough to sustain themselves and their families (Oxfam, 2017: 3). There is a general blindness to the structural violence of the foundations and realities of the most deeply entrenched injustices, because they have been naturalized by ideologies that justify the value attached to different bodies and different lives.

Since its inception in the post-war period, the development industry has evolved into a top-down, technical project to deliver progress to the poor through the recasting of problems from the political realm to the ostensibly more 'neutral' realm of science, technology and economics. The disastrous Structural Adjustment Programmes of the 1980s gave way to the Poverty Reduction Strategy Papers of the 1990s, and then at the turn of the millennium these efforts coalesced into a truly global project: the MDGs, which became the lodestar of the development narrative until 2015. The MDGs were negotiated in the late 1990s, a small group of technocrats under the primary influence of key European countries, the United States and Japan, with sponsorship from the International Monetary Fund (IMF), the World Bank, and the Organization for Economic Co-operation and Development (OECD). In September 2000 all member-states of the UN signed on to the MDGs' 21 measurable targets and 60 indicators that were designed to guide developmental interventions until 2015. Three of the MDGs were directed explicitly at women and girls: MDG 3: 'Promote gender equality and empower women', and the separate but twinned goals, MDG 4: 'Reduce child mortality' and MDG 5: 'Improve maternal health'.

Shaping the framing of women's empowerment' in the MDGs was the backlash against the gains of the transnational women's health movement that had been codified in the declaration emerging from the International Conference on Population and Development (held in Cairo, 1994) and the Plan of Action from the Beijing Women's Conference (held in 1994). A major step forward for women's health rights was a consensus of what constituted SRHR.

The definitions articulated in both documents encompassed access to health's social determinants; comprehensive health care including reproductive health care; the right to a satisfying sex life and the freedom to decide if and when to reproduce; freedom from coerced sexual relations and violence, sterilization/forced contraception and involuntary maternity; and rights to family planning (Petchesky, 2003; Hawkesworth, 2006; Nowicka, 2011). Both the Cairo and Beijing conferences had placed on the map the understanding that SRHR were indivisible from basic human rights to bodily autonomy and integrity, were foundational to girls' and women's exercise of other fundamental rights, and could only be achieved in the context of economic, gender and racial justice and poverty alleviation. The progress that was won for SRHR was the product of a global struggle by feminist health rights activists supported by the International Women's Health Coalition (see Germain, this volume, Chapter 6).

But in the processes that culminated in the MDGs, the 'conspicuous absence' (Kabeer, 2015: 382) of feminist voices allowed pressure from the Vatican, Islamic States, and the conservative Christian lobby to ensure that women were reduced to mothers, that non-normative sexual identities were invisible, and that what constituted women's health was maternal health narrowly conceived (Vanwesenbeeck, 2008; Sen and Mukherjee, 2013; Kabeer, 2015). In short, the voices of civil society and women's human rights advocates were shut out. Feminist/civil society scholars and activists pointed to the uncontroversial conception of women's equality and empowerment contained in the MDGs as a diversion from critical issues central to gender justice and SRHR, and raised concerns that the MDGs' economistic framework was unable to capture complex dimensions of women's poverty and exclusion. MDGs 4 and 5 were purged of the human rights framing of reproductive health, and exclusively focused on the reduction of maternal mortality. A recent statement on the promotion, protection and fulfilment of SRHR made by the Science & Technology Advisory Group and the Gender rights Advisory Panel describes the global situation with regard to SRHR as marked by

> ... [a] sustained lack of sufficient funding; stigmatisation of both users and providers of sexual and reproductive health services; continued support for harmful practices such as child marriage and female genital mutilation; paring down of legislation that protects women's rights; tolerance of violence against women and girls; increasing restrictions on access to, and provision of, scientifically accurate sexual and reproductive health information, including comprehensive sexuality education; unnecessary restrictions on the availability of contraceptive methods; and the imposition of legal barriers, such as third party consent requirements, to sexual and reproductive health services.
>
> (UNDP/UNFPA/UNICEF/WHO/WB 2017)

MDG 3, the separate goal of 'Women's empowerment' was understood as equity with males within specific domains of the public sphere. The aggregated metrics for measuring girls' and women's empowerment were gender parity in primary and secondary school enrolment, and ratios of women to men in non-agricultural wage employment, and formal parliamentary positions (O'Manique and Fourie, 2016). The goalposts could be measured and quantified: as Kabeer (2015: 348) noted, more elusive goals, such as the advancement of democracy and the exercise of women's human rights were 'too difficult to measure'. The MDGs left intact the situation of many racialized poor, rural women who faced systematic cultural/ ethnic, spatial, political, and economic forms of discrimination, with national statistics hiding deeply entrenched inequalities (Kabeer, 2011). With regards to gender justice, it has been widely recognized, even within the UN, that the MDGs failed to deliver even on their limited promises. The report of the UN Secretary General on the 'Challenges and Achievements of the Implementation of the SDGs for Women and Girls' reported limited progress, citing the need for a broader rights-based approach to health in general and SRHR:

> This approach should address the risk factors contributing to maternal mortality, including the inadequate provision of care or lack of sexual and reproductive health-care services; inaccessibility of care owing to other reasons, such as social barriers including women's limited autonomy and freedom of movement, distance and cost; early marriage; and women's constrained reproductive and sexual choices, such as if and when and how many children to have. Conflict also undermines maternal health. The average maternal mortality ratio is 50 per cent greater in conflict-affected contexts, compared with the global average.
>
> (UN Commission on the Status of Women, 2014: 9)

Gender in the SDGs

The preamble to the SDGs states:

> ... seek to build on the Millennium Development Goals and complete what they did not achieve. They seek to realize the human rights of all, and to achieve gender equality and the empowerment of all women and girls.

In September 2015 nearly 200 members of the UN General Assembly ratified the MDGs' successor: 'Transforming our World: The 2030 Agenda for Sustainable Development (TOW)'. Crafted by the UN General Assembly through a three-year process of consultations with a wide range of stakeholders across the globe, the 17 SDGs and the 169 associated targets replaced the eight MDGs with their 2015 expiry, taking over as the development establishment's global instrument for development and poverty alleviation. The process was led by UN member states but in 2012 the process was extended to broader stakeholder groups that were invited to participate though UN organized consultations, civil society networks, public meetings and online forums. Some participants in the SDG process view the outcome for gender justice as an improvement over the MDGs, pointing to the hard work of the Women's Major Group, whose members pressed for the recognition and inclusion of rights-based perspectives on social reproduction and SRHR. The successes that were celebrated were the inclusion of monitoring and follow-up of the SDGs through the use of 'high-quality, timely and reliable data disaggregated by sex, age, geography, income, race, ethnicity, migratory status, disability, and other characteristics relevant in national contexts' (UN, 2015b: para. 126), a welcome change from the absence of disaggregated data in the monitoring of the MDGs. FfD also goes to some length to mainstream gender into the financing framework, and also states close to the outset, '[w]e reiterate the need for gender mainstreaming, including targeted actions and investments in the formulation and implementation of all financial, economic, environmental, and social policies' (UN, 2015b: para. 6). UN (2015a) claims '[t]he goals and targets are the result of over two years of public consultation and engagement with civil society and other stakeholders around the world, which paid particular attention to the voices of the poorest and most vulnerable'.

Other observers of the process counter the view expressed in the preamble of TOW that the voices of the poorest and most vulnerable were central to the outcome document. Lou Pingeot exposed the central role of large MNCs in the consultations, documenting their privileged access of these particular 'stakeholders' in the central processes through which the final agenda culminated. His in-depth account concluded that corporations and business associations lobbied hard to centre their own interests, closing off civil society voices by radically constructing sustainable development in voluntary, multi-stakeholder terms (Pingeot, 2014: 29). The language of stakeholders masks the power and privilege of certain interests over others, and shuts out the voices of those most impacted, while creating the assumption or illusion that all groups are on equal footing. Our interviews told a similar story, with one UN respondent describing the process:

> To my knowledge there was very little consultation with civil society on these [gender] issues. The South African Government sees this as a high level issue to be managed by high level people, so there is no consultation with civil society. The Office for the Status of Women does not really consult with members of civil society in the consultations with people going to discuss this in New York. There has been no consultation with women, poor women, on what should go into the SDGs. Donor agencies give input. There is no fieldwork or work on the ground, to go and ask the women about what they would like to see done about their lives. Most of the negotiations and fighting about what must go into the SDGs took place in hotels far away from women.

The following comment sums up the consensus of about the consultation process in Canada:

> There was the exact opposite of what meaningful consultation should be. It happened after the bulk of the agenda had been finalized.
> In Addis, [FfD] civil society was ignored. The understanding was that TOW is the soft, well-meaning folks while Addis are the real-world economists. You can't have poverty reduction without reigning in inequality. Innovative financing is just pocket change.

While only one of the 17 SDGs, Goal 5, 'Achieve gender equality and empowering all women and girls' focuses explicitly on women, women and gender are mentioned 31 times in the 29-page TOW document, with attempts at mainstreaming into nine other goals. Goal 5 with its associated targets is as follows:

Target 5.1 End all forms of discrimination against all women and girls everywhere.
Target 5.2 Eliminate all forms of violence against all women and girls in the public and private spheres, including trafficking and sexual and other types of exploitation.
Target 5.3 Eliminate all harmful practices, such as child, early and forced marriage and female genital mutilation.
Target 5.4 Recognize and value unpaid care and domestic work through the provision of public services, infrastructure and social protection policies and the promotion of shared responsibility within the household and the family as nationally appropriate.
Target 5.a Undertake reforms to give women equal rights to economic resources, as well as access to ownership and control over land and other forms of property, financial services, inheritance and natural resources, in accordance with national laws.
Target 5.b Enhance the use of enabling technology, in particular information and communications technology, to promote the empowerment of women.

Target 5.c Adopt and strengthen sound policies and enforceable legislation for the promotion of gender equality and the empowerment of all women and girls at all levels.

(UN 2016)

Paragraph 41 of FfD states:

> We are committed to women's and girls' equal rights and opportunities in political and economic decision-making and resource allocation and to removing any barriers that prevent women from being full participants in the economy. We resolve to undertake legislation and administrative reforms to give women equal rights with men to economic resources, including access to ownership and control over land and other forms of property, credit, inheritance, natural resources and appropriate new technology. We further encourage the private sector to contribute to advancing gender equality through striving to ensure women's full and productive employment and decent work, equal pay for equal work or work of equal value, and equal opportunities, as well as protecting them against discrimination and abuse in the workplace. We support the Women's Empowerment Principles established by UN-Women and the Global Compact and encourage increased investments in female-owned companies or businesses.

(UN 2015b: para. 41)

Both documents are expressed in broad and aspirational language, as one would expect, with the entire development project constructed as an enterprise of change. Paragraphs 14–17 of TOW admit to billions living in poverty, rising inequalities within and between countries, and enormous disparities in opportunities, wealth, and power. They list trends that threaten to reverse any progress to date: national disasters, conflict, extremism, terrorism, humanitarian crises and forced displacements, national resource depletion, and climate change (UN, 2015a: paras 14–17). But while the documents acknowledge the on-going crises, they retreat into technical expertise as the solution: the Basel III process, mentioned in paragraph 106 of FfD is seemingly the only structural adjustment required to address the continued financial crisis.

Both documents are on the same page about what they refer to as the dimensions of sustainable development, namely that it results from the nexus of three dimensions: economic, social, and environmental, which are left largely unspecified. Both documents declare a number of agents and vectors of sustainable development. Economic growth is framed as the *key* requirement for sustainable development, and current global financial and trade policies remain largely untouched. The main policy recommendations proposed are an intensified and even more central role of the private sector and market-based instruments to stimulate growth, and of business as the new enabler of development and empowerment. Any possibility of market failure is ignored. Where economic growth is not immediately indicated or apparent, technological advances, expressed as a focus on science, technology, and innovation, are framed in almost messianic terms. FtD more explicitly affirms the status quo through a strong affirmation of 'private business activity, investment and innovation [as] main drivers of productivity, inclusive economic growth, and job creation' (UN, 2015b: para. 35). International trade is described as '. . . an engine for inclusive economic growth and poverty reduction, and contributes to the promotion of sustainable development', while the WTO is '. . . a universal, rules-based, open, transparent, predictable, inclusive, non-discriminatory and equitable multilateral trading system' (UN 2015b: para. 79). Given the right conditions (infrastructure, and an educated work force and 'supportive policies') it can '. . . help to promote productive employment and decent work, women's empowerment and food security, as well as a reduction in inequality, and contribute to achieving the sustainable development goals' (UN, 2015b: para. 79). The 'rapid growth' of philanthropy is celebrated as providing significant contributions to achieving 'common goals' (UN, 2015b: para. 42), while foreign direct invest-ment, when aligned with national development strategies, can also contribute to sustainable development.

Given that the responsibility for the achievement of the SDGs is nested in nation-states, 'modernized, progressive tax systems, improved tax policies, and more efficient tax collection at national levels' (UN, 2015b: para. 22), becomes the main source of development finance, with the role of the IMF, WB and UN to 'assist in combating illicit financial flows' and developing 'regulatory frameworks' to align with 'nationally owned sustainable development strategies' (UN, 2015b: para. 5). Where domestic public resources are lacking, 'multistakeholder partnerships' and 'blended finance' are named as the financial mechanisms for 'humanitarian finance' to address specific needs of the poorest. The 'sustainable' in development refers 'incentivising changes in financing as well as consumption and production patterns . . . harnessing the potential of science, technology and innovation' and '. . . following existing agreements and conventions in international law on climate and biodiversity' (UN, 2015b: para. 3). The impacts and gravity of the current ecosystemic crisis is not addressed in any meaningful way.

Gender justice?

Both documents view women's empowerment as instrumental to their incorporation into wage labour. The acknowledgement of the existence of women's unpaid labour, to the extent that it needs to be measured, is seen as a strategic victory for some. In the words of an 'insider-outsider' working in the UN sector:

> It's very easy to be cynical; the agenda itself so broad, far too imprecise . . .
> but there has been a recognition that generations of policy have been based on
> crappy evidence. The desire to transform gender stats, to push toward better
> gender data which has not existed, is really good. There is a need to revise stat
> instruments to capture things that are missing, such as national time use
> surveys. The 5.4 target: recognize unpaid care work and domestic work as
> nationally appropriate: if you take a long-term feminist perspective and create

an internationally agreed upon target, this is revolutionary. Better data is not just a technocratic exercise. Behind all this, my pragmatic, cynical self is agnostic . . . you can probably achieve the targets without changing much.

The recognition that women's unwaged and domestic labour needs to be alleviated through 'provision of public services, infrastructure and social protection' contradicts the reality that specific policies of austerity, privatization, and sub-subsistence wages are attached to the intensification of women's unpaid labour. The foundation and the breadth of crises of social reproduction that continue to intensify are trivialized. The justification for freeing women from their unpaid care labour is that it can free up time for their participation in the wage economy. As FfD states, '[e]vidence shows that gender equality, women's empowerment and women's full and equal participation and leadership in the economy are vital to achieve sustainable development and significantly enhance economic growth and productivity' (UN, 2015b: para. 21).

There is nothing feminist about integrating women into labour markets that are themselves precarious and insecure, characterized by poor pay, and segregated along the lines of gender and race (see Healy, this volume, Chapter 10). Indeed, the (female) labour of social reproduction that keeps families and communities alive, is excluded from economic calculation. Giving it the label of 'empowerment' can operate as form of violence.

> *The primary justification of women's empowerment in UN documents is that it makes economic sense. Nothing about what is moral or ethical. The economic is devoid of any morality. States are in the process perpetuating and creating new sets of violence.*
>
> *There is no deep understanding about what this [empowerment] means, especially, for local women, for small-scale farmers, food security. Economic empowerment and microcredit is the way they want to go, but that's it. A lot of the gender activism is trapped in a liberal feminist rhetoric, a numbers game. There's not a really deep look at reproductive rights, race, historical analysis . . . we haven't unpacked that.*

There have been no shortage of feminist analyses of the global political economy that challenge the idea that gender justice can be realized within this current climate of neoliberal globalization (Bergeron, 2011; Gill and Roberts, 2011; Marchand and Runyan, 2011; Chant, 2012; Peterson, 2012). While the neoliberal project privileges capital and the 'productive' economy, household and informal spaces of social reproduction are rendered invisible. This is despite the fact that it is in these latter spaces where a growing range of activities that sustain human life are carried out, essentially absorbing the costs of reproducing labouring bodies for capital. This work is largely (although not exclusively) the invisible work of women and girls. This invisibility is made possible only through the increasingly accepted understanding that the main role of the state is to secure 'an enabling environment' for investment and increased growth (Gill and Roberts, 2011). Post-2008 austerity has further intensified the 1980s policies of structural adjustment, absolving the state of responsibility for maintaining even the most basic conditions of social reproduction.

Feminist political economists have traced the dialectical relationship between the production of capital and social reproduction under neoliberal globalization. In aggregate, the world has witnessed the steady erosion of the conditions required to ensure the daily and generational reproduction of human life and labour. Globally, we see a number of broad trends that have manifested differently in different locations, resulting from the dramatic reshaping of classed, gendered and racialized divisions of labour oriented toward sustaining profitability. States that formerly supported social reproduction through welfare state policies have been subject to austerity resulting in a re-privatization of the social wage, the public expenditure provided to the social sectors to improve the living and working conditions for households. In others, where a welfare state never existed, the commodification of the means of sustaining life (water, food, fuel, shelter, education, and so on) has intensified. Local and subsistence economies have been undermined and sub-subsistence wages in the absence of basic social protections have become the norm. The women who have been absorbed into the 'productive' economy at the tail end of global commodity chains in such sectors as electronics, health and elder care, cleaning, sex work, and seasonal agriculture are the new members of the growing labour precarity.

> *There's still an invisibility of the care economy in the SDG document . . . in this country we have a massive home-based care economy that is parasitic on women . . . this goes unaddressed . . . in this country voluntary work is their fulltime profession. There is a celebration of the virtue of home based care, but no serious discussion about how this is paid for. It's not virtuous, it's violent. It keeps women outside the formal economy. Women are exploited, they don't have healthcare. The UN makes me quite cross. They just don't think.*
>
> *The SDGs are not truly transformative. At a policy level, things have shifted here and there, but . . . it's very difficult to interpret them and make them have any bearing on how normal women live . . . they do not touch the lives of women in rural villages.*

Despite the discourse of 'national ownership' and the 'universality' of the agenda (all countries, not just ones in the Global South, have signed on to the SDGs and have the obligation to report on their implementation) states exist in a global context in which they have been evacuated of much of the economic and financial policy space required to fulfil the SDGs. Rules governing global trade and finance have locked in certain rights of capital that have evacuated the state of much of the power and the autonomy to 'develop' as its population see fit, despite the rhetoric of 'country ownership'. The binding rights of capital trump human rights, including laws to protect local economies, control over resources, and the natural environment. This universal frame is stated in such general terms that it does not give the SDGs any sense of implementable traction.

That being said, again and again both documents are at pains to clarify that the values, principles and norms that they purport to espouse need to be 'domesticated', or that their implications need to be 'nationally appropriate'. Yet the rights of states consistently trump citizen's human rights when it comes to certain women's human rights, and the human rights of LGBTQ people. Sceptics of Agenda 2030 point out that, in the words of one respondent, this '*dilutes the promise of the development project as a truly transformative global compact – a "new social contract"'* – between governments and citizens.

It was a hard battle to get sexual and reproductive health into the agenda . . . never mind rights. The rights perspective is still not there. Governments can look at a whole range of issues and just cherry-pick.

If governments are provided with such a get-out-of-jail-free card, the implications are dire for notions of states' human rights obligations towards their citizenry, or of government obligations to implement challenging but truly transformative legislation.

States are often the most egregious violators of their citizens' human rights. Although there is a dedicated goal to 'Achieve gender equality and empower women and girls', the goal remains significantly free of any meaningful reference to human or women's rights. States can simply ignore this broad aspiration, in the name of what is deemed 'nationally appropriate'. The current economic and geopolitical climate doesn't bode well for gender justice and women's empowerment with the rise of nativist populist movements and religious fundamentalisms. Gender identities have always been constituted in relation to militarized and religious nationalism, and militarism itself is a central feature of the contemporary global political economy. The new president of the United States openly campaigned on a misogynist platform and on his first day in office signed an executive order to defund all organizations in the US and globally that fund information on, or access to abortion. The rise of nativist populism in the EU and religious fundamentalisms around the world are predictable responses to deepening and multiple crises, as is the xenophobic 'othering' of immigrants and refugees. The rise of highly masculinized authoritarian states originate in deepening inequalities and related insecurities, as do resource wars and low-intensity violence. None of these forces bode well for the bodily autonomy and integrity of racialized, gendered and non-normative sexualised bodies living in places of insecurity.

The SDG project is also silent on the millions of people live their lives outside of national borders and stateless. According to the UNHCR, in 2015 there were 65.3 million forcibly displaced people (UNHCR, 2015) and 2014 estimates 10 million as stateless (UNHCR, 2014). As Pugh (this volume, Chapter 5) asserts, 'states are responding to migration pressures with an increasingly control-oriented and securitised approach, tightening or attempting to close borders, criminalising irregular and often low-skilled migrants, and framing migrants broadly in the language of social, political and economic threat' (p. 65). Whilst the SDGs have nothing to say about refugees, both documents 'recognize[s] the positive contribution of migrants for inclusive growth and sustainable development' and that migration requires 'coherent and comprehensive responses' (UN, 2015a: para. 35; UN, 2015b: para. 40), which amounts to the vague promise of protection of labour rights and humane treatment. Female migrants sending home remittances are constructed as the heroes of their nations, with states, NGOs and IFIs actively promoting migratory remittances as a source of development finance and social reproduction (Kuntz, 2010: 920). The only concrete goal in TOW concerning migration amounts to a pledge to provide adequate and affordable financial services to migrant families, both abroad and at home, by reducing the cost of remittances by 2030 to less than 3 per cent of the amount transferred, and by promoting 'cheaper, faster and safer' transfer of remittances (UN, 2015a: 20).

Migration for work, regionally and internationally, has risen exponentially as a family survival strategy. In countries of the Global North, some middle-class families have been able to resolve their own crises of social reproduction by relying on domestic labour from abroad, the marketization of the care economy intensifying inequalities as the rich are able to purchase domestic services cheaply (Kuntz, 2010: 913). The burden of family and household care is left to other girls and women, and some tasks simply go unfulfilled, as evidence suggests that male family members tend not to fill-out the domestic labour void (Pareñnas, 2000; Elias, 2010; Kuntz, 2010). Yet both TOW and FfD are silent on the human and psychological costs to migrants and to family members left behind, the children, and the elderly. And while migrants get named amongst the most vulnerable, it is *forced* migrants only who are singled out. TOW pledges to 'eradicate forced labour, end modern slavery and human trafficking and . . . child labour in all its forms' (UN, 2015a: Goal 8.7). Feminist scholars have challenged this forced versus voluntary' dichotomy, illuminating that one's decision to migrate is often not a real choice, but a necessity for personal or family survival. At all stages of migration, various gendered insecurities can arise and are shaped by intersecting power relations and geopolitical contexts. Vulnerability and exploitation can extend to many 'voluntary' migrants who make dangerous journeys, are subject to sexual violence, and end up in exploitative or isolated workplaces without full citizenship rights (Outshoorn, 2005; Freedman, 2012).

Conclusion

While many feminist civil society advocates view the SDGs as an improvement from the MDGs with regard to the language on women's empowerment, we have suggested that there are visible contradictions between the aspirational language and goals for gender justice, and the means of implementation encoded in FfD that is unquestioning of the model of global financial governance that is responsible for the ongoing economic and eco-systemic crisis. Both TOW and FfD reiterate the central role of the private sector and corporate capital in the SDG project in ways that render invisible their current role in the intensification of inequality, environmental crises, and gender injustice. A range of civil society critics (DAWN, WWG, 2015; Women's Major Group, 2015) have questioned whether gender equality and 'women's empowerment' (an over-used linguistic icon of the development industry) are achievable in a context that ignores such contradictions.

Both the TOW and FfD align with the broader global corporate agenda that has financialized growing sectors of the economy, intensified the commodification of life's necessities rendering their price subject to volatile market forces, while destroying nature and consolidating wealth in a tiny elite. Both documents construct a particular Eurocentric and economistic view of sustainable development and women's empowerment, a view that maintains the existing hierarchical distribution of power and resources, and a political economy that requires, for continued capital accumulation, an intensification of both unpaid care labour, and low paid and precarious gendered and racialized wage labour at the bottom of the social hierarchy. Furthermore, we suggest that the reversal of many of the hard-won gains of women's SRHR need to be understood as an effect of the blunt misogyny and racism that characterize the populist responses around the world to deepening global inequality and insecurity. We may well see isolated gains in women's SRHR, particularly around the less politically charged issues from various targeted interventions around specific measurable goals. A number of our respondents expressed that in some ways, the SDGs are a strategic advance despite their consistency with the market model of development. One South African government representative was refreshingly forthright:

> *The SDGs are not an accountability mechanism for civil society to hold governments to account. The SDGs will never be a stick; we governments will find an argument out of it. The SDGs are good for the big picture, the big frame.*

The promise of the SDG project will be limited for the same reason that the MDGs have failed women: gender injustice – and particularly the intensification and exploitation of women's labour – both waged and unwaged – and the denial of SRHR are implicated in the network of social and economic relations that constitute the current structurally violent dynamics of the global economy. In the SDGs, 'rights' become conflated with 'unleashing one's potential', which simply means becoming a productive worker and consumer within local, national, and global economies. By not questioning the systemic, structural impediments of women's and girls' human rights, Goal 5 is not only un-feminist, but anti-feminist; it is not only apolitical, but part of what James Ferguson (1994) calls the 'anti-politics machine' that is development. Issues such as gender-based violence, SRHR, and social reproduction are exposed in the documents with no meaningful redress through obligated and accountable national governments; nor are the global actors at the forefront of the implementation the SDG project accountable to anyone. The link between the personal and the political is missing in the SDGs, as it was missing in the MDGs. The overarching norms of neoliberal economism and (deeply circumscribed) state sovereignty constitute the essence of the SDGs and the contemporary development industry as a whole. One interviewee said:

> *True transformation is not part of the formal discourse. What I see is business as usual. There s no great challenge to how the global economy is run. We are not questioning basic growth models and we sanction environmental degradation.*

Some members of civil society do see *Transforming our World* as a document, despite its deep flaws, that can hold governments to account. The challenge, then, is perhaps not only to critique, but to find the room to manoeuvre within the project.

> *The good thing about the SDGs is that they shine a spotlight on the domestic work [in Canada] we need to do. . . . The issue is, if you are an international development organization, how do you situate yourself? What are we saying about our own accountability? OUR mining companies are over there, doing the damage . . . we need to look at things in a tactical way. Where is real change going to happen?*

So, where does this leave us? The reality is that the TOW is deeply flawed in terms of its contents, but it is also powerful in terms of how it has been institutionalized and legitimized at the level of global governance. We may not like it, and determined radicals may want us to throw it out and start afresh, but the reality is that this document will significantly shape the development agenda for the next 15 years. To address these issues, to get them back on the global development agenda, will require 'new struggles for interpretation over the scope of concepts, responsibilities, policies and achievements, and new terrains for contestation' (Esquivel, 2016: 18). Without this, the development frame on the one hand and the human (and women's) rights frame on the other will remain separate, and sterile. To repoliticize the development project globally will require creativity and subversion:

> Creatively, this can happen by braiding together the policies that can be gleaned from the resolution itself and the body of human rights texts, various UN declarations and the [International Labour Organization] labour conventions. Subversively, this would show the urgent need to give full attention to both gender equality and climate justice, to ensure the survival and well-being of humanity. This would ultimately shake up the entire rationale for 'development'.
>
> (Koehler, 2016: 65)

New allies need to be identified and new alliances forged, across the Global North and South. Interestingly, our most radically feminist interlocutors were also the ones who expressed the most optimism, for the long term:

> *There's always agency. It depends on your ability to keep looking and not to get discouraged. Nothing stays the same. We have to watch for those shifts. The 'ideal state' won't be permanent either. It's about being able to read where power is and where the opportunities may be; it'll take a while to identify where you can influence.*

Acknowledgement

This research was supported by the Social Sciences & Humanities Research Council (SSHRC), Canada [Grant number 55-51431].

References

Adams, Barbara and Jen Martins. 2015. *Fit for Whose Purpose? Private Funding and Corporate Influence in the U.N.* New York: Global Policy Forum.
Banks, Nicola; David Hulme and Michael Edwards. 2014. 'NGOs, States, and Donors Revisited: Still too Close for Comfort?', *World Development* 66: 707–718. Available at www.sciencedirect.com/science/article/pii/S0305750X14002939, accessed 19 April 2017.
Bergeron, Suzanne. 2011. 'Economics, Performativity and Social Reproduction in Global Development', *Global Development* 3(2): 151–61.
Chant, Sylvia. 2012. 'The Disappearing of 'Smart Economics?' The World Development Report 2012 on Gender Equality: Some Concerns about the Preparatory Process and the Prospects for Paradigm Shift', *Global Social Policy* 12(2): 198–218.
DAWN/Women's Working Group on Financing for Development. 2015. 'Intervention by Nicole Bidegain Ponte, DAWN and WWGon FFD', CSO Opening Plenary CSO Financing for Development (FfD) Forum 11 July 2015. Available at www.dawnnet.org/feminist/resources/sites/default/files/articles/20150711_nicole-opening_cso_session.pdf, accessed 12 February 2016.
Elias, Juanita. 2010. 'Making Migrant Domestic Work Visible: The Rights Based Approach to Migration and the Challenges of Social Reproduction', *Review of International Political Economy* 17(5): 848–59.
Esquivel, Valeria. 2016. 'Power and the Sustainable Development Goals: A Feminist Analysis', *Gender & Development* 24(1): 9–23.
Ferguson, James. 1994. *The Anti-Politics Machine: 'Development', Depoliticization and Bureaucratic Power in Lesotho.* Minneapolis, MN: University of Minnesota Press.
Freedman, Jane. 2012. 'Analyzing the Gendered Insecurities of Migration: A Case-Study of Female Sub-Saharan Migrants in Morocco', *International Feminist Journal of Politics* 14(1): 36–55.
Gill, Stephen and Adrienne Roberts. 2011. 'Macroeconomic Governance, Gendered Inequality, and Global Crises', in Brigitte Young, Isabella Bakker and Diane Elson (eds) *Questioning Financial Governance from a Feminist Perspective*, London and New York: Routledge: 152–172.
Hawkesworth, Mary. 2006. *Globalization and Feminist Activism.* Oxford: Rowman and Littlefield.
Hawkesworth, Mary. 2016. *Embodied Power: Demystifying Disembodied Politics.* New York: Routledge.
Kabeer, Naila. 2011. 'MDGs, Social Justice and the Challenge of Intersecting Inequalities', Centre for Development Policy and Research. Available at www.soas.ac.uk/cdpr/publications/pb/file66938.pdf, accessed 12 February 2016.
Kabeer, Naila. 2015. 'Tracking the Gender Politics of the MDGs: Struggles for Interpretive Power in the International Development Agenda', *Third World Quarterly* 36(2): 377–95.
Koehler, Gabrielle. 2016. 'Tapping the Sustainable Development Goals for Progressive Gender Equity and Equality Policy?' *Gender & Development* 24(1): 53–68.

Kuntz, Rahel. 2010. 'The Crisis of Social Reproduction in Rural Mexico: Challenging the "Reprivatization of Social Reproduction" Thesis', *Review of International Political Economy* 17(5): 913–45.

Marchand, Marianne H. and Anne Sisson Runyan. 2011. *Gender and Global Restructuring.* London: Taylor and Francis.

Nowicka, Wanda. 2011. 'Sexual and Reproductive Rights and the Human Rights Agenda: Controversial and Contested', *Reproductive Health Matters* 19(38): 119–28.

O'Manique, Colleen and Pieter Fourie. 2016. 'Gender Justice and the MDGs: South Africa and Canada Considered', *Politikon* 43(1): 97–116.

Outshoorn, Joyce. 2005. 'The Political Debates on Prostitution and Trafficking of Women', *Social Politics: International Studies on Gender, State and Society* 12(1): 141–55.

Oxfam 2017. 'An Economy that Works for Women', Briefing Paper, March, 2017. Available at www.oxfam.org/sites/www.oxfam.org/files/file_attachments/bp-an-economy-that-works-for-women-020317-en-summ.pdf, accessed 13 April 2017.

Pareññas, Rachel Salazar. 2000. 'Migrant Filipina Domestic Workers and the International Division of Domestic Labor', *Gender and Society* 14(4): 560–78.

Petchesky, Rosalind. 2003. *Global Prescriptions: Gendering Health and Human Rights.* London: Zed Books.

Peterson, V. Spike. 2012. 'Inequalities, Informalization and Feminist Quandaries', *International Feminist Journal of Politics* 14(1): 5–35.

Pingeot, Lou. 2014. 'Corporate Influence in the Post-2015 Process', Global Policy Forum Working Paper. Available at www.globalpolicy.org/component/content/article/252-the-millenium-development-goals/52572-new-working-paper-corporate-influence-in-the-post-2015-process.html, accessed 17 March 2016.

Sen, Gita and Avanti Mukherjee. 2013. 'No Empowerment without Rights, No Rights without Politics: Gender-Equality, MDGs and the Post 2015 Development Agenda', Working Paper. Available at https://cdn2.sph.harvard.edu/wpcontent/uploads/sites/5/2013/09/SenMukherjee_PowerOfNumbers_HSPHDRAFT_2013_jg_revisions.pdf, accessed 17 March 2016.

Trietler, Vilna and Manuela Boatca. 2016. 'Dynamics of Inequalities in Global Perspective', *Current Sociology* 64(2). Available at http://journals.sagepub.com/doi/abs/10.1177/0011392115614752 (accessed 14 April 2017).

UN. 2015a. 'Transforming our World: The 2030 Agenda for Sustainable Development', Available at https://sustainabledevelopment.un.org/content/documents/21252030%20Agenda%20for%20Sustainable%20Development%20web.pdf, accessed March 2016.

UN. 2015b. 'Addis Ababa Action Agenda of the Third International Conference on Financing for Development', New York: United Nations. Available at www.un.org/esa/ffd/wp-content/uploads/2015/08/AAAA_Outcome.pdf, accessed 17 March 2016.

UN. 2016. Metadata, Goal 5 Achieve Gender Equality and Empower all women and Girls (Updated 31 March 2016). Available at https://unstats.un.org/sdgs/files/metadata-compilation/Metadata-Goal-5.pdf (accessed 21 April 2017).

UNDP/UNFPA/UNICEF/WHO/WB. 2017. 'Statement on the Promotion, Protection and Fulfilment of SRHR of the Science & Technology Advisory Group and the Gender Rights Advisory Panel', Available at www.who.int/reproductivehealth/STAG-STATEMENT.pdf?ua=1 (accessed 14 April 2017).

UN Commission for the Status of Women. 2014. 58th Session Challenges and Achievements in the Implementation of the MDGs for Girls and Women, Report of the Secretary-General. Available at www.un.org/ga/search/view_doc.asp?symbol=E/CN.6/2014/3 (accessed 21 April).

UNHCR. 2014. *Global Action Plan to End Statelessness*, 4 November 2014. Available at http://www.refworld.org/docid/545b47d64.html (accessed 22 April 2017).

UNHCR. 2015. 'Figures at a Glance: Global Trends 2015', Available at www.unhcr.org/en-us/figures-at-a-glance.html (accessed 21 April 2017).

Vanwesenbeeck, Ine. 2008. 'Sexual Violence and the MDGs', *International Journal of Sexual Health* 20(1–2): 25–49.

Women's Major Group. 2015. 'Women's Major Group Disappointed with Action Agenda on Financing for Development', Available at www.awid.org/news-and-analysis/womens-major-group-disappointed-action-agenda-financing-development (accessed 17 March 2016).

Index

Page numbers in **bold** refer to figures, page numbers in *italic* refer to tables.

Milton Keynes UK
Ingram Content Group UK Ltd.
UKHW040103071024
449327UK00019B/771